6th EDITION

Mosby's WORKBOOK for NURSING ASSISTANTS

RELDA T. KELLY, RN, MSN
Professor Emeritus
Kankakee Community College
Kankakee, Illinois
Parish Nurse, Wesley United Methodist Church
Bradley, Illinois

Procedure Checklists by
HELEN CH[illegible] RS, MSN, CRRN, CNS
Professor
[illegible]munity College
[illegible]ankakee, Illinois
Parish Nurse, St. Teresa [illegible] Catholic Church
Kankakee, Illinois

Mosby

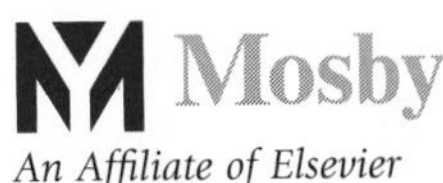

An Affiliate of Elsevier

11830 Westline Industrial Drive
St. Louis, Missouri 63146

MOSBY'S WORKBOOK FOR NURSING ASSISTANTS ISBN 0-323-02581-1

International Standard Book Number 0-323-02581-1

Executive Editor: Susan R. Epstein
Senior Developmental Editor: Maria Broeker
Publishing Services Manager: Gayle May
Project Manager: Joseph Selby
Designer: Dana Peick, GraphCom Corporation
Cover Art: Kathi Gosche
Design Manager: Kathi Gosche

Printed in the United States of America

Last digit is the print number: 9 8 7 6 5 4 3 2 1

This workbook is dedicated to my husband Earl,
who provided endless support and encouragement during this production

and

to my grandchildren—Samuel, Michela, and Ian,
who are my investment in the future.

REVIEWERS

Ann Bennett, RN, MSN
Allied Health Tech Prep Instructor
Scioto County Joint Vocational School
Lucasville, Ohio

Jeanne Heki, RN
Nursing Assistant Instructor
Ventura County Superintendent of Schools
Camarillo, California

Debra McMenamin, RN,C
Laboratory/Clinical Instructor
Howard Community College
Columbia, Maryland

ILLUSTRATION CREDITS

p. 97: Unnumbered figure. Courtesy J.T. Posey Co., Arcata, Calif.

p. 177: Unnumbered figure. Courtesy U.S. Department of Agriculture, Washington, D.C.

p. 178: Unnumbered figure. Courtesy OSF St. Joseph Medical Center, Bloomington, Ill.

p. 230: Unnumbered figure Courtesy OSF St. Joseph Medical Center, Bloomington, Ill.

PREFACE

Mosby's Workbook for Nursing Assistants is written to be used with *Mosby's Textbook for Nursing Assistants*, 6th edition. The student will not need other resources to complete the exercises presented in this *Workbook*. It is designed to help the student apply what has been learned from his or her study of the material presented in each chapter of the textbook.

Four sections are found in every chapter in this *Workbook*: (1) Key Terms, (2) Circle the BEST Answer, (3) Optional Learning Exercises, and (4) Independent Learning Activities. The "Key Terms" listing provides a review of all of the terms listed in the textbook. The "Circle the BEST Answer" section provides a thorough review of the textbook chapter using multiple-choice questions. This section will also give the student practice to take the NAACEP test. "Optional Learning Exercises" section provides alternative exercises that will give the student more practice in the studying the materials. "Independent Learning Activities" section provides practical application exercises for the student to carry out alone or with classmates.

Other exercises are provided in some chapters to help review content using a variety of learning methods. These include fill-in-the-blank statements, multiple-choice exercises, crossword puzzles, and labeling exercises. Questions related to *Mosby's Nursing Assistant Skills Videos* are included in appropriate chapters, which will help the student focus on the videos as they watch them.

In addition, "Procedure Checklists" that correspond with the procedures of the textbook are provided. These checklists are designed to help the student practice the skills to become competent at performing procedures that will affect quality of care.

The answer key for the *Workbook* is found in the *Instructor's Guide.* This key allows the instructor to use the content in the *Workbook* in a variety of study or testing situations. The instructor can give answers to the students as needed.

Assistive personnel are important members of the health team. Completing the exercises in this *Workbook* will increase the student's knowledge and skills. The goal is to prepare the student to provide the best possible care and to encourage pride in a job well done.

Relda T. Kelly

CONTENTS

1 Introduction to Health Care Agencies

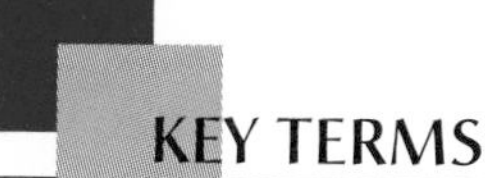

KEY TERMS

Acute illness
Assisted living facility
Case management
Chronic illness
Functional nursing
Health team
Hospice
Licensed practical nurse (LPN)
Licensed vocational nurse (LVN)
Nursing assistant
Nursing team
Patient-focused care
Primary nursing
Registered nurse (RN)
Team nursing
Terminal illness

Fill in the Blanks: Key Terms

1. ______________________________ is a nursing care pattern in which the RN is responsible for the person's total care.
2. A person who gives basic nursing care under the supervision of an RN or LPN/LVN is a ______________________________.
3. When an illness is ongoing, is slow or gradual in onset, and has no known cure, it is a ______________________________ illness.
4. A nurse who has completed a 1-year nursing program and has passed a licensing test is a ______________________________.
5. The ______________________________ are individuals who provide nursing care—RNs, LPNs/LVNs, and nursing assistants.
6. A sudden illness from which the person is expected to recover is an ____________________.
7. When a nursing care pattern focuses on tasks and jobs and each nursing team member has certain tasks and jobs to do, it is called ______________________________.
8. An ______________________________ provides housing, personal and support services, health care, and social activities in a homelike setting.

9. An illness or injury for which there is no reasonable expectation of recovery is a

_______________________ illness.

10. _______________________ is a health care agency or program for persons who are dying.

11. In some states, LPNs are called

_______________________.

12. _______________________ is a nursing care pattern in which a case manager (for example, an RN) coordinates a person's care from admission through discharge and into the home setting.

13. A _______________________ is a nurse who has completed a 2-, 3-, or 4-year nursing program and has passed a licensing test.

14. Staff members who work together to provide health care are called the

_______________________.

15. _______________________ is a nursing care pattern in which an RN who decides the amount and kind of care each person needs leads a team of nursing staff.

16. When services are moved from departments to the bedside, this nursing care pattern is called a

_______________________.

Circle the BEST Answer

17. All health care agencies work to
    A. Cure illness
    B. Give daily personal care
    C. Meet the person's needs
    D. Provide care after surgery or injury

18. Health promotion includes
    A. Immunizations against infectious diseases
    B. Respiratory, physical, and occupational therapies
    C. Learning skills needed to live, work, and enjoy life
    D. Receiving counseling about healthy living

19. Diagnostic tests, physical examinations, surgery, emergency care, and drugs are used in
    A. Health promotion
    B. Detection and treatment of disease
    C. Rehabilitation and restorative care
    D. Disease prevention

20. The goal of rehabilitation and restorative care is
    A. To teach the person about healthy living
    B. To return persons to their highest possible level of physical and psychological functioning
    C. To return the person completely to normal functioning
    D. To treat the illness with diet, exercise, and medications

21. A person with an acute illness will probably be treated in
    A. A hospital
    B. A long-term care center
    C. An assisted living facility
    D. A rehabilitation agency

22. An example of a care need that may be given in a subacute care agency is
    A. Minor surgery
    B. Wound management of a chronic wound
    C. Help with personal care and drugs
    D. Care for the person who is dying

23. A person may have an apartment and receive help with personal care when living in
    A. A long-term care center
    B. An assisted living facility
    C. A rehabilitation care agency
    D. A skilled nursing facility

24. Persons in a long-term care center
    A. Need hospital care
    B. Are acutely ill
    C. Are usually older and have chronic diseases
    D. Are never able to return home

25. Skilled nursing facilities
    A. Provide needed nursing care until death
    B. Are for persons with health problems that do not require hospital care
    C. Provide care in the person's home
    D. Provide outpatient care

26. Persons who have problems dealing with life events may be treated in a
    A. Mental health center
    B. Skilled care facility
    C. Long-term care center
    D. Hospice

27. Home care agencies provide
    A. Health teaching and supervision
    B. Bedside nursing care
    C. Physical therapy and rehabilitation and food services
    D. All of the above

28. Hospices
    A. Provide short-term care until the person recovers
    B. Give care only in the home
    C. Allow the person and family to have control over the person's quality of life
    D. Only provide care to meet the person's physical needs

29. Health care systems are
    A. Agencies that join together as one provider of care
    B. Members of the health team that give bedside care
    C. Members of the health team that work in a hospital
    D. The hospitals in a community

30. All of the following are members of the health team *except* the
    A. Occupational therapist
    B. Housekeeper
    C. Social worker
    D. Cleric

31. The person responsible for nursing service is
    A. A medical doctor
    B. An RN with a bachelor's or master's degree
    C. A person with many years experience in giving nursing care
    D. The board of trustees

32. Nursing education staff may teach all of these *except*
    A. Basic nursing skills needed to begin employment
    B. Instruction on the use of new equipment
    C. New employee orientation programs
    D. Providing the nursing team with new and changing information

33. An RN who completes a college or university program will be in school for
    A. 2 years
    B. 1 year
    C. 3 years
    D. 4 years

34. An RN
    A. Assesses, plans, implements, and evaluates nursing care and makes nursing diagnoses
    B. Is supervised by licensed doctors and licensed dentists
    C. Only gives care when the person's condition is stable and care is simple
    D. Is always able to diagnose diseases or illnesses

35. An LPN/LVN
    A. Must pass a licensing test to work
    B. Assists RNs in caring for acutely ill person and with complex procedures
    C. May supervise nursing assistants
    D. All of the above

36. When a team leader delegates the care of certain persons to other nurses, the nursing care pattern is called
    A. Patient-focused care
    B. Team nursing
    C. Functional nursing
    D. Primary nursing

37. An example of functional nursing is
    A. An RN coordinates a person's care from admission through discharge.
    B. Nursing tasks and procedures are delegated to nursing assistants.
    C. One nurse gives all treatments.
    D. Services are moved from departments to the bedside.

38. When the number of people caring for each person is reduced, this nursing care pattern is
    A. Functional nursing
    B. Case management
    C. Patient-focused care
    D. Team nursing

39. Medicare
    A. Is bought by individuals and families from an insurance company
    B. Helps pay medical costs for low-income families
    C. May be provided by an employer
    D. Is a federal health insurance program for person 65 years and older

40. A system that limits the amounts paid by insurers, Medicare, and Medicaid by determining the amount paid before care is called
    A. Prospective payment
    B. Medicaid
    C. Managed care
    D. Group insurance

41. In a preferred provider organization (PPO)
    A. The patient may choose any doctor in the community.
    B. The focus is on preventing disease and maintaining health.
    C. A group of doctors and hospitals provide health care at reduced rates.
    D. All of the above are true.

42. When a health care agency is accredited
    A. It is voluntary and signals quality and excellence.
    B. The agency is licensed by the state to operate and provide care.
    C. It allows the agency to receive Medicare and Medicaid funds.
    D. The agency meets standards set by the federal and state governments.

43. If a deficiency is found during a survey of a health care agency, the agency
    A. Is usually given 60 days to correct it
    B. Will be closed immediately
    C. Can decide whether or not to correct the deficiency
    D. Can sue the survey team

Matching

Match the type of health care agency with the service provided

44. ________ Serves people who are dying.
45. ________ Provides complex care while the person recovers from illness or surgery before returning home.
46. ________ Provides services to persons who do not need hospital care but who cannot care for themselves at home.
47. ________ Serves people of all ages for acute, chronic, or terminal illnesses.
48. ________ Treats people who may have difficulty dealing with events in life.
49. ________ Provides housing, personal care, and other services in a homelike setting.
50. ________ Serves people with stable conditions but who need complex care and equipment.
51. ________ Provides care to persons at home.

A. Hospital
B. Rehabilitation agency
C. Long-term care
D. Mental health care
E. Home care agency
F. Hospice
G. Skilled nursing facility
H. Assisted living

Fill in the Blanks

Write the name of the health team member described.

52. ______________________ supervises LPNs/LVNs and assistive personnel.

53. ______________________ diagnoses and treats diseases and injuries.

54. ______________________ collects samples and performs laboratory tests on blood, urine, and other body fluids and secretions.

55. ______________________ takes x-rays and processes film for viewing.

56 ______________________ gives respiratory treatments and therapies.

57. ______________________ assesses and plans for nutritional needs.

58. ______________________ assists persons with musculoskeletal problems.

59. ______________________ helps persons learn or retain skills needed to perform activities of daily living (ADL).

60. ______________________ treats persons with speech, voice, hearing, communication, and swallowing disorders.

61. ______________________ assists persons with their spiritual needs.

62. ______________________ helps patients and families with social, emotional, and environmental issues affecting illness and recovery.

63. ______________________ tests hearing and prescribes hearing aids.

Labeling

64. Fill in members of nursing service on the organizational chart.

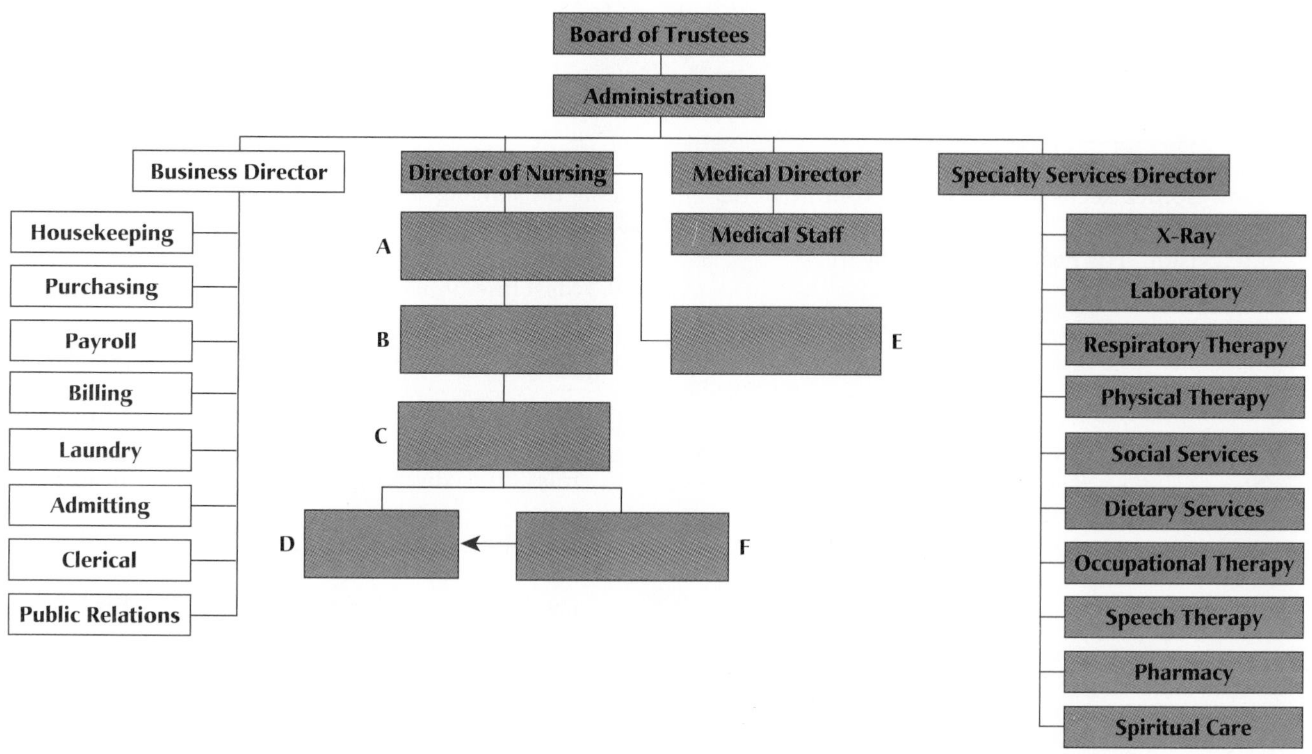

65. The nursing assistant reports to two groups of nursing service. They are

 A. ______________________________

 B. ______________________________

Optional Learning Exercises

Name the member of the health team who provides the service described.

66. Mr. Williams needs assistance to regain skills to dress, shave, and feed himself (for example, ADL). He is assisted by the ______________________________.

67. The nurse has a concern about a drug action, so he calls the ______________________________.

68. Mrs. Young needs the corns on her feet treated. The nurse notifies the ______________________________.

69. Ms. Stewart has the responsibility of performing physical examinations and health assessments and for providing health education for the center where she works. She is a ______________________________.

70. Mr. Gomez keeps turning up the volume of his television. His hearing is tested by the ______________________________.

71. The ______________________________ meets with a new resident and his family to discuss his nutritional needs.

72. Mr. Fox has had a stroke and has weakness on his left side. The ______________________________ assists him by developing a plan that focuses on restoring function and preventing disability from his illness.

73. The doctor orders x-rays after Mr. Jackson falls. The x-rays are provided by the ______________________________.

74. Mr. Ling has chronic lung disease and needs respiratory treatments. These are given by the ______________________________.

75. Ms. Walker plans the recreational needs of a nursing center. She is an ______________________________.

76. After a stroke, Mr. Stubbs has difficulty swallowing. He is evaluated by the ______________________________.

77. When the doctor orders blood tests, the samples are collected by the ______________________________.

Name the nursing care pattern described in the following examples.

78. Ms. Hines works with Dr. Hogan. When his patient, Harry Forbes, is admitted to the hospital, Ms. Hines coordinates the patient's care from admission to discharge. She also communicates with the insurance company and community agencies involved in Mr. Forbes' care. This is an example of ______________________________.

79. When Mr. Holcomb reports for work as a nursing assistant, he is assigned to make all the beds on the unit. The RN gives all the drugs, and the LPN gives all the treatments. This nursing care pattern is ______________________________.

80. Ms. Conroy works on the same nursing unit each day. She has a group of patients and provides total care to each of them. She teaches and counsels the person and family and plans for home or long-term care when needed. This is an example of ______________________________.

81. Ms. Ryan is a nursing assistant. She provides care that is delegated by an RN. The RN leads a team of nursing staff members and decides the amount and kind of care each person needs. This is an example of ______________________________.

82. Mrs. Young receives her care and physical therapy on the nursing unit. She does not have to go to different departments to receive treatments and care. This care is provided by the nursing team rather than by other health team members. This is an example of

______________________________.

Independent Learning Activities

Gather the following information about health care agencies in your area.

- How many hospitals are located in your area? Select one hospital, and answer the following questions.
  - What services are provided by this hospital?
  - How many beds are available for patients?
  - How many staff members work there?
  - How many staff members are RNs? LPNs? Nursing assistants?
  - What care is provided by nursing assistants?
  - Does the hospital have a skilled nursing facility? What types of patients are admitted to this unit?
  - Does the hospital have a rehabilitation or subacute unit? What care is provided in this unit?
  - What services are provided for the person who needs care at home after discharge?

- How many long-term nursing centers are located in your area? Select one center, and answer the following questions.
  - What types of residents are accepted in the center? (For example, does the center consider the level of care needed, resident's disease, or method of payment?)
  - What rehabilitation services are given?
  - How many residents live in the center?
  - How many staff members work there?
  - How many staff members are RNs? LPNs? Nursing assistants?
  - What care is provided by nursing assistants?

- How many nursing centers in your area provide skilled nursing care? Select one center, and answer these questions.
  - How many residents live in the center?
  - How many staff members work there?
  - How many staff members are RNs? LPNs? Nursing assistants?
  - What care is provided by nursing assistants?

- How many assisted living facilities are located in your area? Select one center, and answer the following questions.
  - Is the facility independent or part of a long-term care center?
  - How many residents live in the facility?
  - What kind of living quarters do the residents have? (For example, does each resident have an apartment or studio? Do they share kitchen facilities, or does each person have a kitchen?)
  - How many staff members work there?
  - How many staff members are RNs? LPNs? Nursing assistants?
  - What care is provided by nursing assistants?

- What agency provides care for persons with mental illnesses? What type of care is provided?

- Does your area have a hospice program? If so, answer the following questions about the program?
  - Is this program located within a center, or does it provide care in the person's facility?
  - What type of care is provided?
  - What special training is given to the staff?
  - What duties can be performed by a nursing assistant?

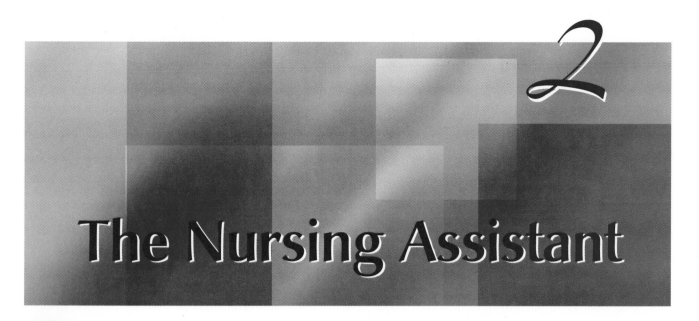

KEY TERMS

Abuse
Accountable
Assault
Battery
Civil law
Crime
Criminal law
Defamation
Delegate
Ethics
False imprisonment
Fraud
Invasion of privacy
Job description
Law
Libel
Malpractice
Negligence
Responsibility
Slander
Standard of care
Task
Tort
Will

Fill in the Blanks: Key Terms

1. A ______________________________ is a function, procedure, activity, or work that does not require an RN's professional knowledge or judgment.
2. ______________________________ is negligence by a professional person.
3. Saying or doing something to trick, fool, or deceive another person is ______________________________.
4. ______________________________ is concerned with offenses against the public and society in general.
5. A ______________________________ is a legal statement of how a person wishes to have property distributed after death.
6. Being responsible for one's actions and the actions of others who perform delegated tasks is called being ______________________________.

7. A rule of conduct made by a government body is a ____________________.

8. ____________________ is the unauthorized touching of a person's body without the person's consent.

9. The intentional mistreatment or harm of another person is ____________________.

10. ____________________ is defamation through oral statements.

11. Injuring a person's name and reputation by making false statements to a third person is ____________________.

12. ____________________ is a knowledge of what is right and wrong conduct.

13. Intentionally attempting or threatening to touch a person's body without the person's consent is ____________________.

14. A ____________________ is a wrong committed against a person or a person's property.

15. ____________________ is concerned with relationships between people.

16. A ____________________ is a listing of responsibilities and functions the agency expects you to perform.

17. The duty or obligation to perform some act or function is called ____________________.

18. Violating a person's right not to have his or her name, photograph, or private affairs exposed or made public without giving consent is ____________________.

19. ____________________ is the skills, care, and judgment required by the health team member under similar circumstances.

20. To ____________________ means authorizing another person to perform a task.

21. An act that violates a criminal law is a ____________________.

22. ____________________ is the unlawful restraint or restriction of a person's movement.

23. Defamation through written statements is ____________________.

24. ____________________ is an unintentional wrong in which a person fails to act in a reasonable and careful manner and causes harm to a person or to a person's property.

Circle the BEST Answer

25. Until the 1980s, nursing assistants
    A. Attended nursing assistant classes approved by the state
    B. Were not used to provide basic nursing care
    C. Received on-the-job training from nurses
    D. Only worked in hospitals

26. Efforts to reduce health care costs include
    A. Nursing shortages
    B. Changes made by Omnibus Budget Reconciliation Act (OBRA) of 1987
    C. Hospital closings and mergers
    D. Changes in nurse practice acts

27. When staff members are given training to perform basic skills that are provided by other health team members, it is called
    A. Staffing mixing
    B. Cross training
    C. Managed care
    D. Scope of practice

28. Laws about the roles and functions of a nursing assistant are based on
    A. Joint Commission of Hospital Accreditation
    B. The nurse practice act
    C. The state medical society
    D. Insurance companies

29. If you perform a task beyond the legal limits of your role, you could be
    A. Protected by the nurse practice act
    B. Practicing nursing without a license
    C. Protected by the nurse who supervises your work
    D. Accused of a criminal act

30. OBRA requires that the nursing assistant training and competency evaluation program have at least __________ hours of instruction.
    A. 16
    B. 75
    C. 120
    D. 200

31. Which of these areas of study is *not* included in a training program for nursing assistants?
    A. Communication
    B. Elimination procedures
    C. Resident rights
    D. Phlebotomy (drawing blood)

32. The competency evaluation for nursing assistants has two parts. They are a
    A. Written test and a skills test
    B. Multiple-choice test and a true-false test
    C. Skills test and a complete bed bath demonstration
    D. Written test and an oral question-and-answer test

33. If you fail the competency evaluation the first time it is taken, you
    A. Can retest a second time
    B. Must repeat your training program
    C. Can retest two more times for a total of three times
    D. Can retest as often as necessary, free of charge

34. All of the following information is contained in the nursing assistant registry information, *except*
    A. Information about findings of abuse or neglect and of dishonest use of property
    B. Date of birth
    C. Number of dependents
    D. Date the competency examination was passed

35. OBRA requires that retraining and a new competency evaluation test must be taken if you have not worked as a certified nursing assistant for
    A. 2 consecutive years
    B. 5 years
    C. 1 year
    D. 6 months

36. Your work as a nursing assistant is supervised by
    A. An RN or LPN/LVN
    B. The doctor
    C. The director of nursing
    D. A nursing assistant with more experience

37. You are alone in the nurses' station and you answer the phone. Dr. Smith begins to give verbal orders to you. You should
    A. Hang up the phone.
    B. Politely give him your name and title, and ask him to wait while you get the nurse.
    C. Quickly write down the orders, and give them to the nurse.
    D. Politely give him your name and title, and ask him to call back later when the nurse is there.

38. As a nursing assistant, you never give medications unless
    A. The nurse is busy and asks you to give them.
    B. The person is in the shower, and the nurse leaves the medications at the bedside.
    C. You have completed a state-required medication and training program about giving medications.
    D. You are feeding the person, and the nurse asks you to mix the medications with the food.

39. The nurse asks you to carry out a task that you do not know how to do. You should
    A. Ignore the order because it is something you cannot do.
    B. Perform the task as well as you can.
    C. Ask another nursing assistant to show you how to carry out the task.
    D. Promptly explain to the nurse why you cannot carry out the task.

40. The nurse asks you to assist him as he changes sterile dressings. You should
    A. Assist him as needed.
    B. Tell him you cannot assist to perform any sterile procedures.
    C. Tell him that this is something you cannot do.
    D. Report his request to the supervisor.

41. Who can tell the person or the family a diagnosis or prescribe treatments?
    A. Director of nursing
    B. RN
    C. Doctor
    D. Experienced nursing assistant

42. When you read a job description, you should not take a job if it requires you to
    A. Carry out duties you do not like to do
    B. Maintain required certification
    C. Attend in-service training
    D. Function beyond your training limits

43. Which of the following is *not* acceptable?
    A. An RN delegates a task to an LPN/LVN.
    B. An LPN/LVN delegates a task to a nursing assistant.
    C. An RN delegates a task to a nursing assistant.
    D. A nursing assistant delegates a task to another nursing assistant.

44. When a nurse considers delegating tasks, the decision
    A. Must result in the best care for the person, based on the person's needs at the time
    B. Depends on whether the nurse likes the nursing assistant
    C. Depends on how busy the nurse is that day
    D. Depends on how well the nurse likes the person

45. You have been caring for Mr. Watson for several weeks. The nurse tells you that she will give his care today. Her delegation decision is primarily based on
    A. How well you performed his care yesterday
    B. Changes in Mr. Watson's condition at this time
    C. Whether the nurse knows you
    D. How much supervision you need

46. Which of the following is *not* a right of delegation?
    A. The right task
    B. The right person
    C. The right time
    D. The right supervision

47. You agree to perform a task the nurse delegates to you. Which of these statements tells you it is the right circumstance for you to do this?
    A. You understand the person's physical, mental, emotional, and spiritual needs at this time.
    B. You are comfortable performing the task.
    C. You have reviewed the task with the nurse.
    D. You were trained to do the task.

48. You may refuse to carry out a task for all of the following reasons *except*
    A. The task is not in your job description.
    B. You do not know how to use the supplies or equipment.
    C. You are too busy.
    D. The person could be harmed if you carry out the task.

49. It is unethical if you
    A. Carry out a task you have not been trained to do
    B. Give care to a person whose values or standards differ from yours
    C. Perform a task that is against your religious or moral beliefs
    D. Carry out a task beyond the legal limits of your role

50. Which of the following is *not* good conduct for a nursing assistant?
    A. Carry out every task assigned even when you are unfamiliar with the task.
    B. Take only drugs that have been prescribed by your doctor.
    C. Know the limits of your role and knowledge.
    D. Consider the person's needs to be more important than your own needs.

51. A nurse failed to do what a reasonable and careful nurse would have done. Legally, this is called
    A. A crime
    B. A tort
    C. Negligence
    D. Malpractice

52. If you fail to identify a person properly and perform a treatment on him intended for another, you are
    A. Committing a crime
    B. Legally responsible for your actions
    C. Not responsible legally but are unethical
    D. Guilty of an intentional tort

53. A nursing assistant writes a note to a friend that injures the name and reputation of a person by making false statements. This is called
   A. Libel
   B. Slander
   C. Malpractice
   D. Negligence

54. A nursing assistant tells a person she is a nurse. She has committed
   A. Fraud
   B. Libel
   C. Slander
   D. Negligence

55. When a person is confined to his room by a caregiver, he is a victim of
   A. Physical abuse
   B. False imprisonment
   C. Invasion of privacy
   D. Battery

56. If a person tells you that he does not want you to dress him and you go ahead and touch him, you may be accused of
   A. Fraud
   B. Battery
   C. Assault
   D. False imprisonment

57. If you are asked to obtain a person's signature on an informed consent, you should
   A. Make sure the person is mentally competent.
   B. Refuse. You are never responsible for obtaining a written consent.
   C. Make sure the person understands what he is signing.
   D. Ask a family member to witness the signed consent.

58. If a person is confused or unconscious, informed consent
   A. Is not necessary
   B. Cannot be obtained, and so no treatments can be given
   C. Can be given by a husband, wife, son, daughter, or legal representative
   D. Can be given by the director of nursing

59. You can refuse to sign a will if
   A. You are named in the will.
   B. You do not believe the person is of sound mind.
   C. Your nursing center has policies that do not allow employees to witness wills.
   D. All of the above are true.

60. Which of the following is *not* an element of abuse?
   A. Willfully causing injury
   B. Intimidation
   C. Expecting a person to feed and dress himself within his abilities
   D. Depriving a person of food as punishment

61. What kind of abuse occurs when an older person is left to sit in urine or feces?
   A. Physical
   B. Involuntary seclusion
   C. Mental
   D. Sexual

62. An example of verbal abuse can be
   A. Failing to answer a signal light
   B. Locking a person in a room
   C. Oral or written statements that speak badly of a person
   D. Making threats of being punished

63. Depriving a person of needs such as food, clothing, or a place to sleep is
   A. Verbal abuse
   B. Involuntary seclusion
   C. Physical or mental abuse
   D. Sexual abuse

64. Which of the following may be a sign of elder abuse?
   A. The person answers questions openly.
   B. The family makes sure the hearing aides have new batteries.
   C. A caregiver is present during all conversations.
   D. All medications are taken as scheduled.

65. A sign of sexual abuse can be
   A. Small circle-like burns on the body
   B. Bleeding or bruising in the genital area
   C. Weight loss with signs of poor nutrition
   D. Lack of personal hygiene

66. If you suspect a person is being abused, you should
   A. Call the police.
   B. Discuss the matter and your observations with the nurse.
   C. Discuss the situation with the family.
   D. Notify community agencies that investigate elder abuse.

67. OBRA requires that if a nursing assistant is found guilty of abuse, neglect, or mistreatment of a person, the incident is
    A. Reported to the abused person's family, and the nursing assistant must apologize
    B. Reported to the state nursing assistant registry
    C. Reported to the state board of nursing
    D. Recorded on the nursing assistant's record in the facility

68. Which of these persons could be a child abuser?
    A. Person with little education
    B. Person with a high income
    C. Person who was abused as a child
    D. All of the above

69. Children who are deprived of food, clothing, shelter, and medical care are victims of
    A. Physical neglect
    B. Emotional neglect
    C. Physical abuse
    D. Sexual abuse

70. Children who are kissed, touched, or fondled in sexual areas are victims of
    A. Physical neglect
    B. Emotional neglect
    C. Incest
    D. Molestation

71. If you suspect a child is being abused, you should
    A. Share your concerns with the RN.
    B. Talk with the child.
    C. Inform the doctor.
    D. Call a child protection agency.

72. A husband does not allow his wife to use the car, leave the home, or visit with family and friends. This form of domestic violence is called
    A. Verbal abuse
    B. Social abuse
    C. Physical abuse
    D. Economic abuse

Matching

Match the examples with the correct tort.

73. ________ While cleaning a person's dentures, the nursing assistant drops and breaks them.

74. ________ A nursing assistant opens a person's mail and reads it without permission.

75. ________ Instead of allowing the person a choice, the nursing assistant tells him that he will get a shower whether he wants one or not.

76. ________ An individual touches a person's body without the person's consent.

77. ________ An individual tricks or fools another person.

78. ________ An individual restrains or restricts a person's freedom of movement without a doctor's order.

79. ________ A nurse gives a treatment to the wrong person.

80. ________ A nursing assistant injures the name and reputation of a resident by making false statements to a third person.

81. ________ A nursing assistant falsely writes notes that accuses another nursing assistant of stealing her purse.

A. Negligence
B. Malpractice
C. Libel
D. Slander
E. False imprisonment
F. Assault
G. Battery
H. Fraud
I. Invasion of privacy

Crossword Puzzle

Fill in the crossword puzzle by answering the clues with words from this list.

abuse	delegate	malpractice
accountable	ethics	negligence
assault	fraud	slander
battery	libel	task
defamation		

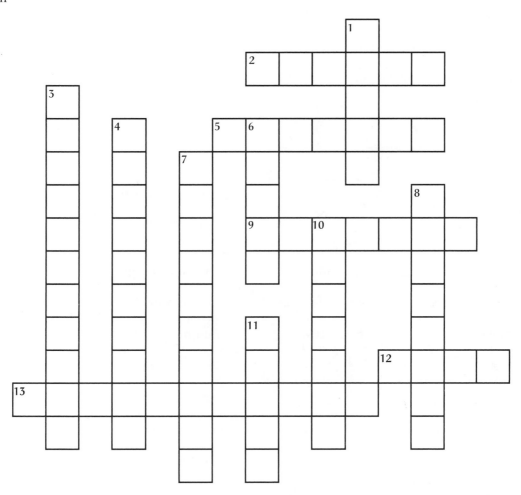

1 2 3 4 5 6 7 8 9 10 11 12 13

Across

2. Knowledge of what is right and wrong conduct
5. Touching a person's body without his or her consent
9. Making false statements orally
12. Functions, procedure, activity, or work that does not require an RN's professional knowledge or judgment
13. Being responsible for one's actions and the actions of others who perform delegated tasks

Down

1. Making false statements in print, writing, or through pictures or drawings
3. Negligence by a professional person
4. Injuring a person's name and reputation by making false statements to a third person
6. Intentional mistreatment or harm of another person
7. Unintentional wrong in which a person fails to act in a reasonable and careful manner
8. To authorize another person to perform a task
10. Intentionally attempting or threatening to touch a person's body without the person's consent
11. Saying or doing something to trick, fool, or deceive a person

Nursing Assistant Skills Video Exercise

View the **Basis Principles** *video to answer these questions.*

82. Federal and state laws and ____________________ policies define the roles and responsibilities of the nursing team.

83. The nursing team is responsible for meeting four needs of the patient or residents and family members. These needs are

    ______________________________,

    ______________________________,

    ______________________________,

    and ______________________________.

84. An ______________________________ identifies nursing care problems, develops and implements nursing care plans, and evaluates the effectiveness of care.

85. An ______________________________ can give simple care to a person whose condition is stable.

86. A ______________________________ helps the nurse with bedside care.

87. What four things do you need to know before you perform a procedure?

    A. ______________________________

    B. ______________________________

    C. ______________________________

    D. ______________________________

88. An RN ______________________________ tasks, activity, or work that does not require an RN's professional judgment.

89. What are the five rights of delegation?

    A. ______________________________

    B. ______________________________

    C. ______________________________

    D. ______________________________

    E. ______________________________

Optional Learning Exercises

OBRA requirements that affect the Nursing Assistant

90. If a home care agency receives Medicare funds, home health care assistants or home health aides must meet ______________________________.

91. OBRA requires ____________________ hours of instruction. ____________________ hours must be supervised practical training. Where can the practical training take place?

    ______________________________ or

    ____

92. OBRA requires 15 areas of study. Write the area of study during which you learn the skill in each example.

    A. You make a bed.

    ____

    B. You close Mr. Smith's door to give him privacy.

    ____

C. You tell Mrs. Forbes the time of day and the day of week frequently during the day.

____

D. You apply lotion to a resident's dry skin.

____

E. You assist a person to put on his shirt.

____

F. When assigned to a new unit, you check to find the location of the fire alarm.

____

G. Practice hand hygiene procedure before and after giving care.

____

H. You get help to move a person from his bed to the chair.

____

I. When speaking to Mr. Jackson, you maintain good eye contact.

____

J. The nurse tells you to exercise a person's extremities (limbs).

____

K. You shave Mr. Stewart.

____

L. You position a urinal for a resident in bed.

____

M. You assist Mrs. Young to walk in the hall.

____

N. You notice Mrs. Peck has an elevated temperature and her skin is warm.

____

O. You cut up the meat on Mr. Johnson's plate before helping him to eat.

____

The National Nurse Aide Assessment Program (NNAAP) (see Appendix A)

93. The NNAAP written test has ________ questions. List the percent of questions in each area.

A. ________ ADL

B. ________ Basic nursing skills

C. ________ Restorative skills

D. ________ Emotional and mental health needs

E. ________ Spiritual and cultural needs

F. ________ Communications

G. ________ Client rights

H. ________ Legal and ethical behavior

I. ________ Member of the health care team

94. List the skills that are tested on the NNAAP.

A. ______________________________

B. ______________________________

C. ______________________________

D. ______________________________

E. ______________________________

F. ______________________________

G. ______________________________

H. ______________________________

I. ______________________________

J. ______________________________

K. ______________________________

L. ______________________________

M. ______________________________

N. ______________________________

O. ______________________________

P. ______________________________

Q. ______________________________

R. ______________________________

S. ______________________________

T. ______________________________

U. ______________________________

V. ______________________________

W. ______________________________

X. ______________________________

Y. ______________________________

Job Description

95. The nursing assistant assists with assessing when he recognizes abnormal ______________ and reports them ______________.

96. When the nursing assistant consistently strives to use time effectively, he or she is assisting with ______________________________.

97. When a nursing assistant reviews basic care provided to patients and reports when changes are needed, this assists with ______________________________.

98. A nursing assistant assists with teaching and learning information when he or she serves as a resource person for ______________________________.

99. When a nursing assistant practices hand hygiene before and after each patient contact, this meets the job description criterion that maintains ______________________________.

100. Nursing assistants are expected to attend and participate actively in unit meetings ______________________________ of the time.

Independent Learning Activities

- Make a list of tasks that would conflict with your moral or religious beliefs.
  - How would you feel about performing these tasks in your job?
  - What would you say to your employer or co-workers?
- Role-play a situation in which you are asked to perform one of the tasks you identified in the previous activity. Have one student play the person asking you to perform the task. Have a second student observe and answer these questions.
  - What was your reaction when asked to perform a task that is in conflict with your moral or religious beliefs?
  - In what way did you communicate your discomfort?
  - What suggestions did you offer to make sure the task was done?
- Identify agencies in your community that help victims (elder, child, domestic) of abuse. Visit one of the agencies and ask these questions.
  - How do you find out about the victim?
  - What services do you offer?
  - What happens to the victim after you identify a problem?
  - Do you have a place where they can be protected?

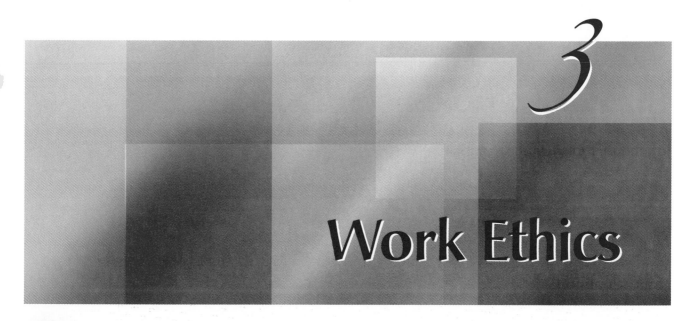

3 Work Ethics

KEY TERMS

Confidentiality
Courtesy
Gossip
Harassment
Preceptor
Stress
Stressor
Work ethics

Fill in the Blanks: Key Terms

1. A staff member who guides is a ______________________________.
2. A ______________________________ is the event of factor that causes stress.
3. Trusting others with personal and private information is ______________________________.
4. ______________________________ is behavior in the workplace.
5. ______________________________ is to spread rumors or talk about the private matters of others.
6. The response or change in the body caused by any emotional, physical, social, or economic factor is ______________________________.
7. ______________________________ is a polite, considerate, or helpful comment or act.
8. ______________________________ means to trouble, torment, offend, or worry a person by one's behavior or comments.

Circle the BEST Answer

9. Work ethics involve
   A. How well you do your skills
   B. What religion you practice
   C. How you treat others and work with others
   D. Cultural beliefs and attitudes

10. Your diet will maintain your weight if you
    A. Avoid salty and sweet foods.
    B. Take in fewer calories than your energy needs require.
    C. Include foods with fats and oils.
    D. Balance the number of calories taken in with your energy needs.

11. Adults need about _______________ hours of sleep daily.
    A. 7
    B. 10
    C. 4
    D. 12

12. Exercise is needed for
    A. Rest and sleep
    B. Muscle tone and circulation
    C. Good body mechanics
    D. Good nutrition

13. Smoking odors
    A. Disappear quickly when the person finishes smoking
    B. Can be covered up by chewing gum
    C. Are only noticed by the smoker
    D. Stay on the person's breath, hands, clothing, and hair

14. The most important reason a person should not work under the influence of alcohol or drugs is either
    A. Can affect the safety of residents and patients
    B. Can cause the person to be disorganized
    C. Can make co-workers angry
    D. Is not allowed by your nursing center

15. Which of these is not part of good personal hygiene for work?
    A. Bathe daily and use a deodorant.
    B. Practice good hand hygiene technique.
    C. Cut toenails straight across.
    D. Keep fingernails long and polished.

16. Tattoos should be covered when working because they
    A. May offend persons you care for, their families, and co-workers
    B. Can become infected
    C. May confuse persons
    D. Increase the risk of skin injuries

17. When working, the nursing assistant may wear
    A. Jewelry in pierced eyebrow, nose, lips, or tongue
    B. Wedding and engagement rings
    C. Multiple earrings in each ear
    D. Nail polish

18. When working, the nursing assistant should *not* wear
    A. A beard or mustache that is clean and trimmed
    B. Hair that is off the collar and away from the face
    C. Perfume, cologne, or aftershave lotion
    D. A wristwatch with a second hand

19. Displaying good work ethics at your clinical experience site may help you find a job because
    A. You will pass the course.
    B. It will show you care.
    C. You will get better grades.
    D. The staff always looks at students as future employees.

20. You should be well-groomed when looking for a job because it
    A. Shows you are cooperative
    B. Makes a good first impression
    C. Shows you are respectful
    D. Shows you have values and attitudes that fit with the center

21. How does an employer know you can perform required job skills?
    A. They will request proof of training and will check your record in the state nursing assistant registry.
    B. They will have you give a demonstration of your skills.
    C. You will be asked many questions about performing certain skills.
    D. You will be required to take a written test.

22. Which of these is *not* an OBRA requirement to work in long-term care?
    A. You must complete a state-approved training and competency evaluation program.
    B. You must have three references from former employers.
    C. The employer checks your record in the state nursing assistant registry.
    D. The nursing center cannot hire persons who were convicted of abusing, neglecting, or mistreating a person.

23. You can get a job application from
    A. Personnel or the human resources office
    B. A friend who works at the center
    C. The director of nursing
    D. The receptionist in the lobby of the center

24. You should take a dry run to a job interview to
    A. Show you follow directions well.
    B. Show you listen well.
    C. Know how long it takes to get from your home to the personnel office.
    D. Look over the center to see whether you want to work there.

25. When you are interviewing, it is correct to
    A. Have a glass of wine before going.
    B. Look directly at the interviewer.
    C. Wear a sweat suit and athletic shoes.
    D. Shake hands very gently.

26. What is a good way to share your list of skills with the interviewer?
    A. Verbally tell the person what you can do.
    B. Ask for a list of skills, and check the ones you know.
    C. Bring a list of your skills, and give it to the interviewer.
    D. Tell the interviewer you will send a list as soon as possible.

27. It is important for you to ask questions at the end of the interview because it
    A. Shows the interviewer you are interested in the job
    B. Helps you to decide whether the job is right for you
    C. Shows you have good communication skills
    D. Shows you are dependable

28. After an interview, it is advised that you
    A. Send a thank-you note within 24 hours of the interview.
    B. Call the interviewer every day to see whether you are being hired.
    C. Wait for the employer to contact you.
    D. Call 1 week after the interview to thank the person for the interview.

29. When a preceptor is assigned to a nursing assistant, the preceptor may be
    A. An RN
    B. Another nursing assistant
    C. An LPN/LVN
    D. Any of the above

30. When you have a job, it is most important to plan good childcare and transportation in advance because it will
    A. Prevent absences and tardiness
    B. Show you are a responsible person
    C. Prevent stress
    D. Show you are a good parent

31. What is a common reason for losing a job?
    A. Not knowing how to perform a task
    B. Frequent absences or excessive tardiness
    C. Being disorganized
    D. Lacking self-confidence

32. When you are scheduled to begin work at 3:00 PM, you should
    A. Plan to arrive by 2:30 PM.
    B. Arrive at exactly 3:00 PM.
    C. Plan to arrive at few minutes early and be ready to work at 3:00 PM.
    D. Arrive within a few minutes before or after 3:00 PM.

33. Which of these statements would signal you have a good attitude?
    A. "I will do that right away."
    B. "It's not my turn. I did that yesterday."
    C. "That's not my patient."
    D. "It's not my fault."

34. You can avoid being part of gossip by
    A. Remaining quiet when you are in a group where gossip is occurring
    B. Only talking about persons and family members to co-workers
    C. Only repeating comments in writing
    D. Removing yourself from a group or situation where gossip is occurring

35. The person's information can be shared
    A. With the person's family
    B. Only among health team members involved in his or her care
    C. With your family
    D. With friends who know the person

36. When you are working, you should *not* wear
    A. A wristwatch with a second hand
    B. Colored undergarments
    C. A shirt with the top button open
    D. White socks

37. Slang or swearing should not be used at work because
    A. Words used with family and friends may offend persons and family members.
    B. The person may not understand you.
    C. The person may have difficulty hearing.
    D. Co-workers may overhear it.

38. You should say "please" and "thank-you" to others because
    A. Courtesies mean so much to people; they can brighten someone's day.
    B. They show respect to the person.
    C. They are required by your job.
    D. They show you like the person.

39. It is acceptable at work if you
    A. Take a pen home to use.
    B. Sell cookies for your child's school project.
    C. Use a pay telephone on your break to call your child.
    D. Make a copy of a letter on the copier in the nurse's station.

40. When you leave and return to the unit for breaks or lunch you should
    A. Tell each person.
    B. Tell any family members present.
    C. Tell the nurse.
    D. All of the above.

41. Safety practices are important to follow because
    A. They help you to be more organized.
    B. Negligent behavior affects the safety of others.
    C. They save the center money.
    D. You will get promoted more quickly.

42. Which of these would *not* be a good safety practice?
    A. Know the contents and policies in personnel and procedure manuals.
    B. Question unclear instructions and things you do understand.
    C. Do not tell anyone when you make a mistake.
    D. Ask for any training that you might need.

43. Care should be planned around
    A. Your break and lunch time
    B. Resident mealtimes, visiting hours, activities, and therapies
    C. Co-workers' schedules
    D. The time scheduled by the nurse

44. Stress occurs
    A. Only when you have unpleasant situations in your life
    B. Because you do not handle your problems well
    C. Because you are in the wrong job
    D. Every minute of every day and in everything you do

45. What physical effects of stress can be life threatening?
    A. High blood pressure, heart attack, strokes, ulcers
    B. Increased heart rate, faster and deeper breathing
    C. Anxiety, fear, anger, depression
    D. Headaches, insomnia, muscle tension

46. Which of these actions is harassment?
    A. Offending others with gestures or remarks
    B. Offending others with jokes or pictures
    C. Making a sexual advance or requesting sexual favors
    D. All of the above

47. If you resign from a job, it is good practice to give
    A. 1 week's notice
    B. 2 weeks' notice
    C. 4 weeks' notice
    D. No notice

Matching

Match the qualities and characteristics of good work ethics with the examples.

48. ________ While working with Mr. Smith, you try to understand and feel what it must be like to be paralyzed on one side.
49. ________ You realize you are very good at giving basic care. You know you need to improve your communication skills.
50. ________ When caring for older residents, you try to do small things to make them happy or to find ways to ease their pain.
51. ________ You thank co-workers when they help you and remember to wish residents happy birthday as appropriate.
52. ________ When Mrs. Gibson is upset and angry, you remember to respect her feelings and to be kind.
53. ________ You accurately report the blood pressure and temperature readings to the nurse.
54. ________ You realize giving care to residents is important and you are excited about your work.
55. ________ Your supervisor tells you she knows she can count on you because you are always on time and perform delegated tasks as assigned.
56. ________ Although Mr. Acevado has different cultural and religious views than yours, you value his feelings and beliefs.
57. ________ Before you left home today, you had an argument with your child. When you get to work, you make every effort to put that aside and be pleasant and happy.
58. ________ The nurse discusses a resident problem with you and states she knows you will keep the information confidential.
59. ________ When you are assigned to give care to a resident, you make sure his or her care is performed thoroughly and exactly as instructed.
60. ________ Your co-worker says she needs help to turn her resident, and you cheerfully offer to help

A. Caring
B. Dependability
C. Consideration
D. Cheerfulness
E. Empathy
F. Trustworthiness
G. Respectfulness
H. Courtesy
I. Conscientiousness
J. Honesty
K. Cooperation
L. Enthusiasm
M. Self-awareness

Fill in the Blanks

61. Work ethics involves

A. ________________________________

B. ________________________________

C. ________________________________

D. ________________________________

E. ________________________________

62. Personal health is important when you are on the job and caring for other persons. Name a part of your health that is described in the examples:

A. You use good hand hygiene techniques and good personal hygiene to prevent odors.

____

B. If you are fatigued, show a lack of energy, and are irritable, it may mean you need more of this.

____

C. You will feel better physically and mentally if you walk, run, swim, or bike regularly.

____

D. Some of these affect thinking, feeling, behavior, and function. This may affect patient and resident safety.

____

E. Avoid foods from the fats, oils, and sweets group. In addition, avoid salty foods and crash diets.

____

F. You may not be able to read instructions and take measurements accurately if you do not have these checked.

____

G. Practice this when you bend or carry heavy objects, as well as lift, move, and turn persons.

____

H. This substance depresses the brain and affects thinking, balance, coordination, and mental alertness.

____

63. List eight places you can find out about jobs.

A. ______________________________

B. ______________________________

C. ______________________________

D. ______________________________

E. ______________________________

F. ______________________________

G. ______________________________

H. ______________________________

64. When an employer requests proof of required training, give the person these items:

A. ______________________________

B. ______________________________

C. ______________________________

65. If a job application asks you to print in black ink, why is it a poor idea to use blue ink?

____

66. Your writing on a job application should be readable so the agency can

______________________________.

67. When a section on a job application does not apply to you, you should

______________________________.

68. When you provide information about employment gaps, it gives the employer a good impression about your ______________________________.

69. When filling out an application, you should be prepared to provide

A. ______________________________

B. ______________________________

C. ______________________________

D. ______________________________

70. If you lie on a job application, it is

______________________________.

If you do this, what can happen?

____

71. You should ask questions at the end of an interview because the agency wants to hire someone who ______________________________.

Crossword Puzzle

Fill in the crossword puzzle by answering the clues with words from this list.

caring	dependability	harassment
confidentiality	empathy	honesty
cooperation	enthusiasm	preceptor
consideration	gossip	stressor
courtesy		

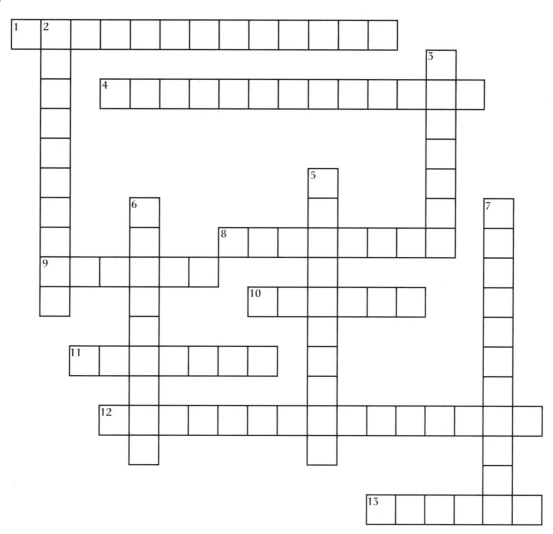

Across

1. Report to work on time when scheduled
4. Respect the person's physical and emotional feelings
8. Polite, considerate, or helpful comment or act
9. Response or change in the body caused by any emotional, physical, social, or economic factor
10. Spreading rumors or talk about the private matters of others
11. Seeing things from the other person's point of view
12. Trusting others with personal and private information
13. Having concerns for the person

Down

2. Being eager, interested, and excited about your work
3. Accurately reporting the care given, your observations, and any errors
5. To trouble, torment, offend, or worry a person by one's behavior or comments
6. A staff member who guides another staff member
7. Willingly helping and working with others

Optional Learning Exercises

Applying for a job in home care

72. When the RN is not at the bedside to help you if problems occur, you are expected to be able to ______________________.

73. When you arrive at homes on time, you are using ______________________.

What temptations should be avoided when you are giving home care?

____

74. When you shop for a person, you should accurately report to the person or family the ______________________.

When you do these things, you are displaying your ______________________.

75. You should read the manufacturer's instructions before using any appliance. This shows ______________________ for the person's property.

76. When a home care agency receives Medicare funds, it must meet ______________________ requirements. This means you must meet the ______________________.

77. What questions should you ask if you are interviewing for a job in home care?

A. ______________________

B. ______________________

C. ______________________

D. ______________________

E. ______________________

F. ______________________

78. When you are in the home, what should you do if a conflict or problem occurs?

A. Make every effort ______________________

B. Explain the problem to ______________________

C. Do not ______________________. This would be very ______________________ behavior.

Independent Learning Activities

- How well do you take care of your own health? What can you do to improve your health practices?
  - Do you maintain a healthy weight by eating calories adequate for your energy needs? What can you do to improve your diet?
  - How much sleep do you get each night?
  - How do you practice good body mechanics at all times—not just at work?
  - How many hours do you exercise each week? What type of exercise do you do?
  - When did you last have your eyes checked? Do you wear glasses if they were prescribed?
  - Do you smoke? If so, how much? Have you considered any smoking cessation programs?
  - Are you taking any drugs that affect your thinking, feeling, behavior, and function? Did a doctor prescribe them, or are you self-medicating? Have you talked with your doctor about the effects of any drugs you are taking?
  - Do you drink alcohol? If so, how much? Have you been told it affects your behavior? Have you considered finding a program to help you to quit drinking alcohol?

- Have you ever applied for a job? How did you feel when you were being interviewed? After reading this chapter, how would you handle a future interview?

- Role-play a job interview with a classmate. Take turns playing the interviewer and the job applicant. Use the lists in this chapter to ask questions. Practice answers that you can use in a real interview.

- Think of three people you could use as references when applying for a job. Ask their permission to use them as references. If they agree, make a list of the people and their titles, addresses, and telephone numbers to use when you apply for a job.

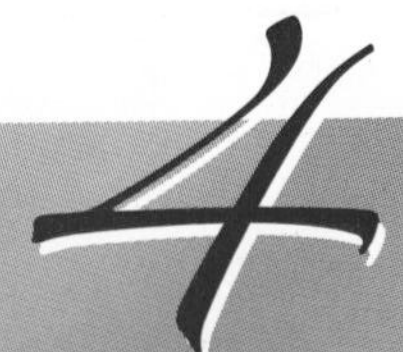

Communicating With the Health Team

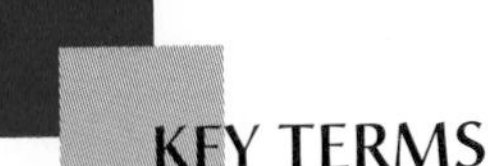

KEY TERMS

Abbreviation
Anterior
Chart
Combining vowel
Communication
Conflict
Distal
Dorsal
Kardex
Lateral
Medial
Medical record
Posterior
Prefix
Proximal
Recording
Reporting
Root
Suffix
Ventral
Word element

Fill in the Blanks: Key Terms

1. A vowel added between two roots or between a root and a suffix to make pronunciation easier is a ______________________.
2. At or toward the front of the body or body part is ventral or ______________________.
3. A ______________________ is a word element placed at the end of a root; it changes the meaning of the word.
4. At the side of the body or body part is ______________________.
5. A clash between opposing interests or ideas is ______________________.
6. An ______________________ is a shortened form of a word or phrase.
7. A part of a word is a ______________________.
8. A ______________________ is a type of card file that summarizes information found in the medical record.
9. The medical record is also called the ______________________.
10. The part nearest to the center or the point of origin is ______________________.

11. ______________________________ is the exchange of information; a message sent is received and interpreted by the intended person.

12. Another term for ventral is ______________________________.

13. A written account of a person's condition and response to treatment and care is the chart or ______________________________.

14. ______________________________ is at or toward the back of the body or body part; posterior.

15. The oral account of care and observations is ______________________________.

16. ______________________________ is the part farthest from the center or from the point of attachment.

17. A word element placed at the end of a root is the ______________________________. It changes the meaning of the word.

18. A word element containing the basic meaning of the word is the ______________________________.

19. Another word for dorsal is ______________________________.

20. ______________________________ is the written account of care and observations.

21. ______________________________ is at or near the middle or midline of the body or body part.

Circle the BEST Answer

22. When health team members communicate, they share all of this information *except*
    A. Gossip about the person and his family
    B. What was done for the person
    C. What needs to be done for the person
    D. The person's response to treatment

23. A nursing assistant tells the nurse that Mr. Jones ate a small amount of his lunch. The nurse
    A. Knows this means Mr. Jones ate one half of his meal
    B. Thinks Mr. Jones ate two or three bites of food
    C. Thinks Mr. Jones ate only 25% of his meal
    D. Asks for further information because words may have different meanings to different people

24. When giving information to another health team member
    A. Be brief and concise to reduce the omission of important details.
    B. Use terms that may or may not be familiar to others.
    C. Give many details and information that is unrelated to the information.
    D. Use general terms instead of facts.

25. The medical record or chart is
    A. A temporary record of the person
    B. Discarded when the person leaves the agency
    C. A permanent legal document
    D. Given to the person when he or she is discharged

26. Which of these is not included in the person's chart?
    A. The daily menu
    B. X-ray reports
    C. Special consents
    D. Nursing history

27. A nursing assistant
    A. May read the charts in all health care agencies
    B. Is never allowed to read a person's chart
    C. Must know the agency policy before reading the chart
    D. Is allowed to tell the person what is recorded in the chart

28. If a person asks to see his or her record, the nursing assistant
    A. Reports the request to the nurse
    B. Checks the agency policy to see whether this is allowed
    C. Gives the chart to the person's legal representative
    D. Gives the chart to the person

29. The admission sheet contains
    A. Doctors orders
    B. Name, birth date, age, and gender of the person
    C. Test results
    D. Special diet information

30. The nursing history is completed
    A. When the person is discharged
    B. When the person is admitted
    C. By the doctor
    D. By the nursing assistant

31. Information about the person's signs and symptoms are found in the
    A. Nursing history
    B. Graphic sheet
    C. Progress notes
    D. Kardex

32. Vital signs taken every shift are recorded in the
    A. Nursing history
    B. Graphic sheet
    C. Flow sheet
    D. Progress notes

33. In long-term care, OBRA requires a written summary of the person
    A. Each shift
    B. Each day
    C. Every month
    D. Every 3 months

34. A weekly care record that has boxes for each day of the week is used in
    A. Home care
    B. Hospitals
    C. Long-term care
    D. All of the above

35. The Kardex is
    A. Used to record visits by health team members
    B. A sheet used to record vital signs taken every 15 minutes
    C. A record of the person's family history
    D. Is a quick, easy source of information about the person

36. The nursing assistant reports information about the person
    A. At the end of the shift
    B. When any changes from normal happen in the person's condition
    C. Each time care is given
    D. Only in writing

37. The rules for recording include all of these *except*
    A. Always use ink in the color required by the agency.
    B. Completely erase any errors.
    C. Sign all entries with your name and title as required by the agency.
    D. Record only what you observed and did yourself.

38. If you are recording using the 24-hour clock, which of these is correct?
    A. 8:00 AM
    B. 1:00 PM
    C. 1300
    D. 5:30 PM

Choose the correct spelling of medical terms in the next five questions.

39. Slow heart rate
    A. Bradecardia
    B. Bradycardia
    C. Bradacordia
    D. Bradicardia

40. Difficulty in urinating
    A. Dysuria
    B. Dysurya
    C. Dysuira
    D. Disuria

41. Blue color or condition
    A. Cyonosis
    B. Cyinosis
    C. Cyanosis
    D. Cianosys

42. Rapid breathing
   A. Tachepnea
   B. Tachypinea
   C. Tachypnea
   D. Tachypnia

43. Opening into trachea
   A. Tracheastomy
   B. Trachiostomy
   C. Tracheostome
   D. Tracheostomy

44. If a person points to the left side of his body below the umbilicus and tells you he has pain, you will tell the nurse he has pain in the
   A. Right upper quadrant
   B. Left lower quadrant
   C. Left upper quadrant
   D. Right lower quadrant

45. When describing the position of body parts, the hands and fingers are
   A. Medial
   B. Distal
   C. Proximal
   D. Posterior

46. When you are given a computer password, you
   A. Must never change it
   B. Can share it with a co-worker
   C. Should never tell anyone your password
   D. Can use another person's password when entering the computer

47. The agency computers should *not* be used to
   A. Send messages and reports to the nursing staff
   B. Store resident records and care plans
   C. Send e-mails that require immediate reporting
   D. Monitor blood pressures, temperatures, and heart rates

48. Privacy is protected when you
   A. Log off after making an entry
   B. Prevent others from seeing what is on the screen
   C. Destroy or shred computer-printed worksheets
   D. All of the above

49. When you answer the telephone, do not put the caller on hold if
   A. The person has an emergency.
   B. The caller is a doctor.
   C. The call needs to be transferred to another unit.
   D. You are too busy to find the nurse.

50. When you answer a phone when giving home care, you should
   A. Give your name, title, and location.
   B. Simply answer with, "Hello."
   C. Explain that you are there to give care to the person who lives in the home.
   D. Hand the receiver to the person in the home and not speak to the caller.

51. If you have a conflict with a co-worker, you should
   A. Ask the nurse in charge to schedule you at different times.
   B. Ignore the person.
   C. Identify the cause of the conflict, and try to resolve it.
   D. Talk to other co-workers to explain your side of the story.

52. When a conflict occurs, what is the first step you should take?
   A. Talk with co-workers to see whether they also have a conflict with the person.
   B. Confront the person, and demand that the person meet with you.
   C. Identify the real problem.
   D. Assume the conflict will resolve itself if you ignore it.

53. Why is it important to resolve a conflict at work?
   A. Unkind words or actions may occur.
   B. The work environment becomes unpleasant.
   C. Care is affected.
   D. All of the above are true.

Matching

Match the word with the correct definition.

54. ________ Difficulty urinating
55. ________ Inflammation of kidneys
56. ________ Pertaining to blue coloration
57. ________ Caused by bacteria
58. ________ Study of the skin
59. ________ Incision into large intestine
60. ________ Instrument used to examine bronchi
61. ________ Inflammation of the tongue
62. ________ Nerve pain
63. ________ Examination of rectum with instrument
64. ________ Excision of the gallbladder
65. ________ Excision of an ovary
66. ________ Incision into the stomach
67. ________ Inflammation of the stomach
68. ________ Inflammation of the intestine

A. Bacteriogenic
B. Bronchoscope
C. Cholecystectomy
D. Colostomy
E. Cyanotic
F. Dermatology
G. Dysuria
H. Enteritis
I. Gastrostomy
J. Gastritis
K. Glossitis
L. Nephritis
M. Neuralgia
N. Oophorectomy
O. Proctoscopy

Fill in the Blanks

69. Next to each time, write the time, using the 24-hour clock.

A. _______ 11:00 AM

B. _______ 8:00 AM

C. _______ 4:00 PM

D. _______ 7:30 AM

E. _______ 6:45 PM

F. _______ 12:00 noon

G. _______ 3:00 AM

H. _______ 4:50 AM

I. _______ 5:30 PM

J. _______ 10:45 PM

K. _______ 11:55 PM

L. _______ 9:15 PM

Write the definition of each prefix.

70. auto- ________________________________

71. brady- ________________________________

72. dys- ________________________________

73. ecto- ________________________________

74. leuk- ________________________________

75. macro- ________________________________

76. neo- ______________________

77. supra- ______________________

78. uni- ______________________

Write the definition of each root word.

79. adeno ______________________

80. angio ______________________

81. broncho ______________________

82. cranio ______________________

83. duodeno ______________________

84. entero ______________________

85. gyneco ______________________

86. masto ______________________

87. pyo ______________________

Write the definition of each suffix.

88. -asis ______________________

89. -genic ______________________

90. -oma ______________________

91. -phasia ______________________

92. -ptosis ______________________

93. -plegia ______________________

94. -megaly ______________________

95. -scopy ______________________

96. -stasis ______________________

Write the correct abbreviations.

97. Before meals ______________________

98. After meals ______________________

99. With ______________________

100. Cancer ______________________

101. Discontinued ______________________

102. Lower left quadrant ______________________

103. Every day ______________________

104. Range-of-motion ______________________

Labeling

Convert the times from military to standard time and from standard to military time. Use the figure below as a guide.

105. 2:00 AM = ________

106. 10:30 AM = ________

107. 5:00 AM = ________

108. 9:30 AM = ________

109. 5:45 PM = ________

110. 10:45 PM = ________

111. 0600 hrs = ________ AM/PM

112. 1145 hrs = ________ AM/PM

113. 1800 hrs = ________ AM/PM

114. 2200 hrs = ________ AM/PM

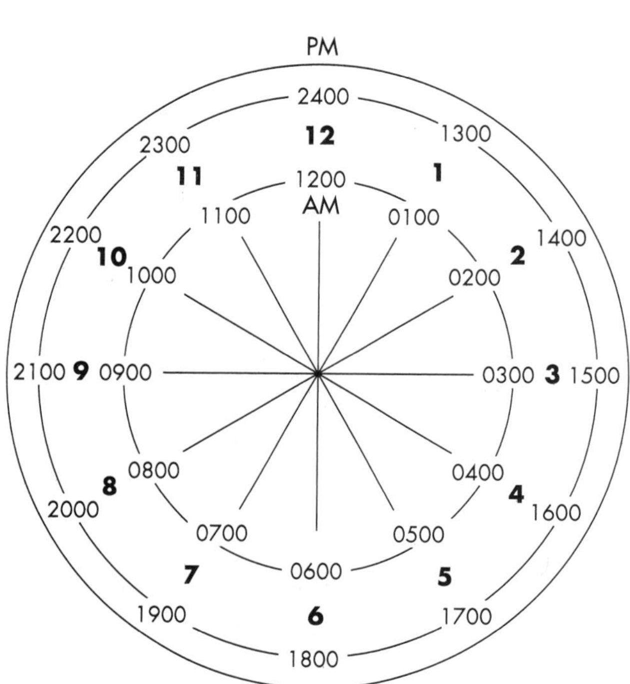

115. Label the four abdominal regions in the figure below. Use RUQ, LUQ, RLQ, and LLQ to label.

A. ______________________

B. ______________________

C. ______________________

D. ______________________

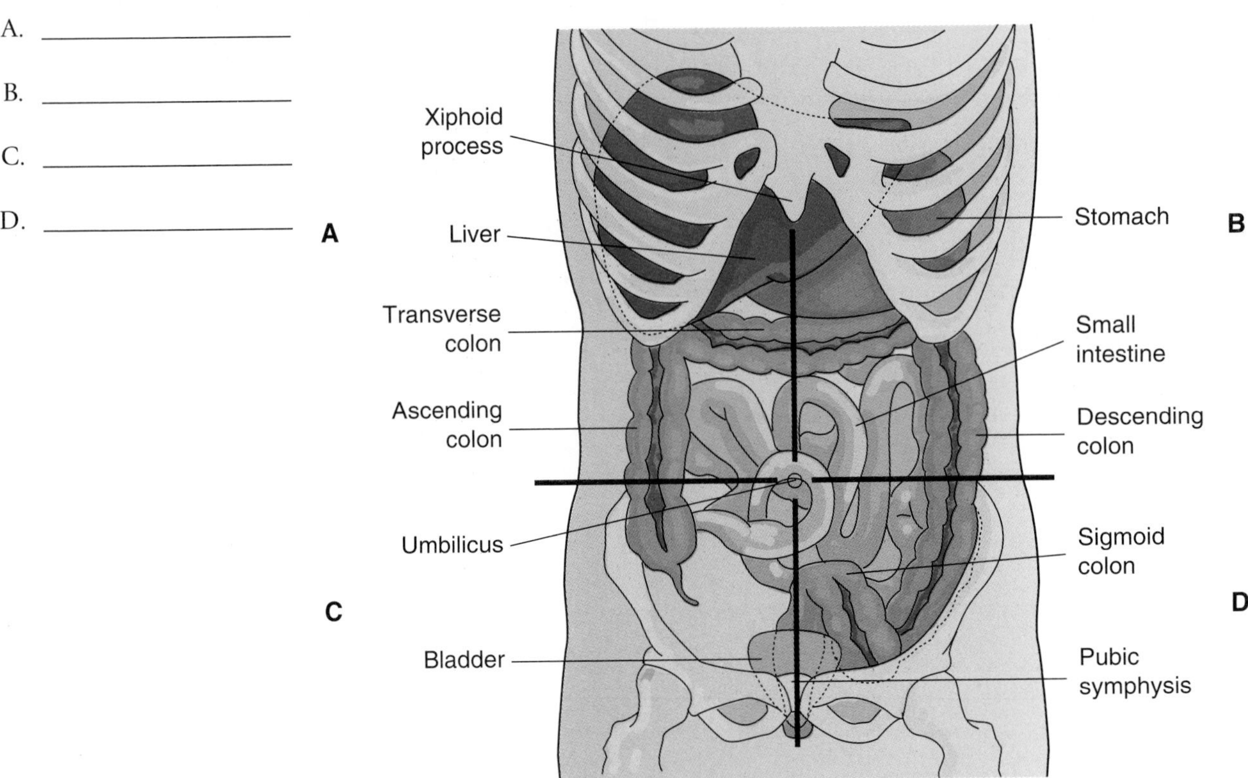

Nursing Assistant Skills Video Exercise

View the* Basic Principles *video to answer these questions.

116. Basic rules of communication are

A. ______________________

B. ______________________

C. ______________________

D. ______________________

E. ______________________

F. ______________________

117. When you communicate with the person, you should

A. ______________________

B. ______________________

C. ______________________

D. ______________________

E. ______________________

F. ______________________

118. When recording, what should you record and what rules are important?

A. ______________________

B. ______________________

C. ______________________

D. ______________________

E. ______________________

F. ______________________

G. ______________________

H. ______________________

Optional Learning Exercises

CLASS EXPERIMENT

It is often difficult to describe fluids in a clear and precise manner. Set up the following examples that imitate situations in which you need to describe intake, output, or drainage. Describe as accurately as possible what you see in terms of amounts, colors, and textures. Compare your notes with classmates to see whether you are using words that have the same meaning. What words were used that were clearly understandable? What words were used that had more than one meaning?

1. Bloody drainage: Mix a teaspoon of ketchup and a teaspoon of water. Pour onto the center of a paper napkin.
2. Urine: Pour a tablespoon of tea into the center of a paper towel.
3. Bleeding: Smear a teaspoon of red jelly in the center of a paper towel.
4. Broth: Pour 4 ounces of tea into a bowl.

CLASS EXPERIMENT

Substance	Observations
Bloody drainage	
Urine	
Bleeding	
Broth	

CASE STUDY

Mr. Larsen was admitted to a subacute care center after his abdominal surgery 1 week ago. This morning the nursing assistant gave Mr. Larsen a shower and helped him sit in a comfortable chair. The nursing assistant noticed that he sat in the chair very still and held his arms across his abdomen. He asked for a pillow and held tightly against his abdomen.

Imagine you are the patient and answer these questions.

- What would you like the nursing assistant to ask you?
- How would you communicate your feelings to the nursing assistant?
- How could you let the nursing assistant know that you had pain without telling her?

Imagine you are the nursing assistant, and answer these questions.

- As the nursing assistant, what observations would be important to make about Mr. Larsen?
- What questions could you ask Mr. Larsen?
- What nonverbal communication would give you information about Mr. Larsen?

CASE STUDY

Mrs. Miller was admitted to the health care center since you worked 3 days ago. You have just started your shift and have been assigned to Mrs. Miller.

- What information would you need to know before giving care? Why?
- What information would be important to provide to the oncoming shift?
- What methods would you use to communicate this information?

Independent Learning Activities

- Answer these questions about situations in which you may need to communicate with others.
  - When have you had a problem with communicating? Why was it difficult? How did you handle it?
  - Think about a time when you believed you communicated well. What made the communication successful? How could you use a similar technique in caring for others?
  - How would you communicate with a person who speaks a language that you do not speak or understand? What methods could you use to explain what you are going to do?
  - How would you communicate with a person from a different culture?

- Make flash cards of the prefixes, suffixes, and root words in Chapter 4.
  - Put the meaning of each one on the back of the appropriate card. Work alone or with a partner, and by looking at the cards, practice identifying the correct meaning of each term.

- The next time you or a member of your family visit the doctor and are instructed to fill a prescription, look at what the doctor has written.
  - Do you see any abbreviations that you learned in this chapter? What do they mean?
  - How did this chapter help you understand what was written?

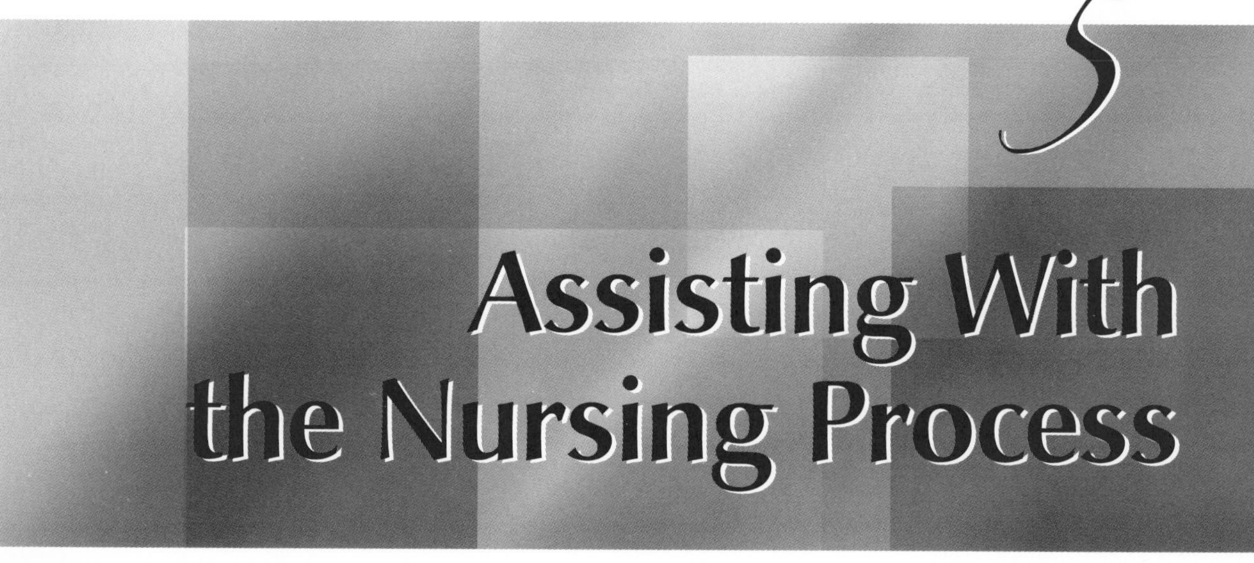

KEY TERMS

Assessment
Evaluation
Goal
Implementation
Medical diagnosis
Nursing care plan
Nursing diagnosis
Nursing intervention
Nursing process
Objective data
Observation
Planning
Signs
Subjective data
Symptoms

Fill in the Blanks: Key Terms

1. ______________________ are things a person tells you about that you cannot observe through your senses; symptoms.
2. ______________________ is to perform or carry out measures in the care plan; a step in the nursing process.
3. The method RNs use to plan and deliver nursing care is the ______________________.
4. Another name for subjective data is ______________________.
5. A written guide about the person's care is the ______________________.
6. ______________________ is collecting information about the person; a step in the nursing process.
7. Another name for objective data is ______________________.
8. The ______________________ describes a health problem that can be treated by nursing measure; a step in the nursing process.
9. Information that is seen, heard, felt, or smelled is ______________________ or signs.

10. A step in the nursing process that is used to measure when goals in the planning step were met is called ______________________________.

11. ______________________________ is the setting of priorities and goals; a step in the nursing process.

12. A ______________________________ is an action or measure taken by the nursing team to help the person reach a goal.

13. A ______________________________ is that which is desired in or by the person as a result of nursing care.

14. Using the senses of sight, hearing, touch, and smell to collect information is ______________________________.

15. The identification of a disease or condition by a doctor is a ______________________________.

Circle the BEST Answer

16. Which of these is *not* a step in the nursing process?
    A. Assessment
    B. Objective data
    C. Planning
    D. Evaluation

17. The nursing process focuses on
    A. The doctor's orders
    B. The person's nursing needs
    C. Tasks and procedures that are needed
    D. Reducing the cost of health care

18. The nursing process
    A. Stays the same from admission to discharge
    B. Is used in all health care settings
    C. Cannot be used in home care
    D. Can only be used for adults

19. When you observe by using your senses, you assist the nurse to
    A. Assess the person
    B. Plan for care
    C. Implement care for the person
    D. Evaluate the person

20. Which of these is an example of objective data you can collect?
    A. Mrs. Hewitt complains of pain and nausea.
    B. Mr. Stewart tells you he has a dull ache in his stomach.
    C. You are taking Mrs. Jensen's blood pressure, and you notice her skin is hot and moist.
    D. Mrs. Murano tells you she is tired because she could not sleep last night.

21. A minimum data set (MDS) is used in
    A. Long-term care centers
    B. All health care settings
    C. Acute care settings
    D. Home care

22. The MDS is updated
    A. At least once a year
    B. Every month
    C. On discharge
    D. All of the above

23. A nursing diagnosis
    A. Identifies a disease or condition
    B. Helps identify drugs or therapies used by the doctor
    C. Describes a health problem that can be treated by nursing measures
    D. Identifies only physical problems

24. When a nurse uses the nursing process, the person is given
    A. Only one nursing diagnosis
    B. No more than five nursing diagnoses
    C. As many nursing diagnoses as are needed
    D. Nursing diagnoses that involve only physical needs

25. Planning involves
    A. Setting priorities and goals
    B. Choosing nursing interventions to help the person reach a goal
    C. Writing the nursing care plan
    D. All of the above

26. A care conference is conducted
    A. Once a month for each person
    B. To meet agency guidelines
    C. To develop or revise a person's nursing care plan
    D. To implement the care plan

27. OBRA requires the use of resident assessment protocols (RAP). They are
    A. Conferences held to update care plans
    B. Guidelines used to develop the person's care plan
    C. Conferences held when one problem affects a person's care
    D. Conferences attended by the person, family, and health team members

28. What part of the nursing process is being carried out when you give personal care to a person?
    A. Assessing
    B. Planning
    C. Implementing
    D. Evaluating

29. Nurses will measure when goals in the planning steps are met during
    A. Assessing
    B. Planning
    C. Implementing
    D. Evaluating

Fill in the Blanks

30. When you make observations while you give care, what senses are used?
    A. ______________________
    B. ______________________
    C. ______________________
    D. ______________________

31. Name the body system or other area you are observing in each of these examples (from Box 5-1, Basic Observations).
    A. Is the abdomen firm or soft?
    ____
    B. Is the person sensitive to bright lights?
    ____
    C. Are sores or reddened areas present?
    ____
    D. What is the frequency of the person's cough?
    ____
    E. Can the person bathe without help?
    ____
    F. Can the person swallow food and fluids?
    ____
    G. What is the position of comfort?
    ____
    H. Does the person correctly answer questions?
    ____
    I. Does the person complain of stiff or painful joints?
    ____

32. An assessment and screening tool completed when the person is admitted to a long-term care facility is called ______________________.
    A. The form is updated before each ______________________.
    B. A new form is completed ______________________ and whenever ______________________.

33. When planning care, needs that are required for life and survival must be met before ______________________.

34. Name the two resident care conferences used in long-term care.
    A. The ______________________ is held regularly to develop, review, and update care plans.
    B. ______________________ are held when one problem affects a person's care.

35. The assignment sheet tells you about

A. ______________________________

B. ______________________________

C. ______________________________

D. ______________________________

Nursing Assistant Skills Video Exercise

View the* Basic Principles *video to answer these questions about the nursing process.

36. Name the part of the nursing process in the following descriptions:

A. Information is collected about the person.

____

B. Statements describe health problems that are treated by nursing measures.

____

C. Priorities and goals are identified, and the nursing care plan is developed.

____

D. Actions are performed by the nurse or delegated to the nursing team.

____

E. Reviewed to determine whether goals were met.

____

37. The written guide about the care a person needs helps ensure the same care is provided by members of the nursing team is called the ______________________________.

Optional Learning Exercises

List at least three nursing interventions for each of these nursing diagnoses and goals.

38. *Nursing diagnosis:* Feeding self
Care deficit: Related to weakness in right arm
Goal: Patient will eat 75% of each meal by (specified date).
Interventions:

A. ______________________________

B. ______________________________

C. ______________________________

39. *Nursing diagnosis:* Hygiene self
Care deficit: Related to forgetfulness
Goal: Patient will be assisted to maintain good hygiene throughout hospital stay.
Nursing interventions:

A. ______________________________

B. ______________________________

C. ______________________________

Independent Learning Activities

- Ask permission to look at the nursing care plans used at the agency where you have your clinical experience. Answer these questions about the nursing care plans.
  - How do the nurses develop the plans? What resources do they use?
  - How often are the plans reviewed and revised?
  - How do the nursing assistants use the plans?
  - How do nursing assistants help develop and revise the interventions?
  - How do the nurses communicate the information on the nursing care plan?

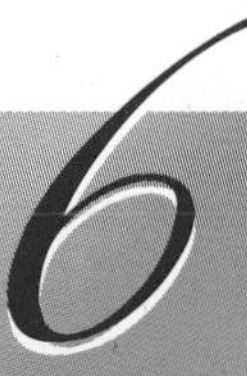

6 Understanding the Person

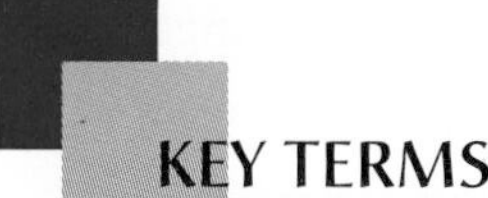

KEY TERMS

Body language
Culture
Disability
Esteem
Geriatrics
Holism
Need
Nonverbal communication
Obstetrics
Paraphrasing
Pediatrics
Psychiatry
Religion
Self-actualization
Self-esteem
Verbal communication

Fill in the Blanks: Key Terms

1. ______________________________ is the characteristics of a group of people—language, values, beliefs, habits, likes, dislikes, and customs—passed from one generation to the next.
2. Communication that uses the written or spoken word is ______________________________.
3. ______________________________ is restating the person's message in your own words.
4. The branch of medicine concerned with the problems and diseases of old age and older persons is ______________________________.
5. Messages sent through facial expressions, gestures, posture, hand and body movements, gait, eye contact, and appearance is ______________________________.
6. The worth, value, or opinion one has of a person is ______________________________.
7. ______________________________ is communication that does not use words.
8. The branch of medicine concerned with mental health problems is ______________________________.
9. Thinking well of oneself and seeing oneself as useful and having value is ______________________________.

10. ______________________________ is a concept that considers the whole person—physical, social, psychological, and spiritual parts that are woven together and cannot be separated.

11. A lost, absent, or impaired physical or mental function is a ______________________________.

12. The branch of medicine concerned with the care of women during pregnancy, labor, and childbirth, and the 6 to 8 weeks after birth is ______________________________.

13. ______________________________ is experiencing one's potential.

14. ______________________________ is the branch of medicine concerned with the growth, development, and care of children who range in age from newborn to teenagers.

15. A ____________________ is something necessary or desired for maintaining life and well-being.

16. ______________________________ is spiritual beliefs, needs, and practices.

Circle the BEST Answer

17. Who is the most important person in the health care agency?
    A. Patient or resident
    B. Doctor
    C. Director of nursing
    D. Administrator

18. You can show that you see the person as a whole person by which of these statements?
    A. "I need to give a bath to the gallbladder in 205."
    B. "The old guy in 220 needs something for pain."
    C. "Mrs. Jones is complaining of a lot of pain in her leg this morning."
    D. "Room 235 needs something for pain."

19. When you are caring for a person, you should
    A. Consider only the physical problems the person has.
    B. Treat the physical, social, psychological, and spiritual parts separately.
    C. Ignore the person's experiences, life-style, culture, joys, sorrows, and needs.
    D. Consider the person—physical, social, psychological, and spiritual parts.

20. The lowest level basic needs are
    A. Physiological or physical
    B. Safety and security
    C. Love and belonging
    D. Self-esteem

21. Oxygen, food, water, elimination, rest, and shelter needs
    A. Relate to feeling safe from harm, danger, and fear
    B. Are needed to survive
    C. Relate to love, closeness, and affection
    D. Relate to the worth, value, or opinion one has of a person

22. It is important to tell a person the reason a procedure is needed because it
    A. Helps the person feel more safe and secure
    B. Makes the person feel loved
    C. Is required by law
    D. Increases the person's self-esteem

23. You may need to repeat information many times to a person who has been admitted to a long-term care nursing center because the person
    A. May be scared and confused
    B. Is not in a secure home setting
    C. Is in a strange place with strange routines
    D. All of the above

24. Meeting love and belonging needs is important because
    A. It helps the person to think well of him or herself.
    B. Some people become weaker or die from the lack of love and belonging.
    C. The person will feel more safe and secure.
    D. It helps the person experience his or her potential.

25. A need that is rarely, if ever, totally met is
    A. Safety and security
    B. Love and belonging
    C. Self-actualization
    D. Self-esteem

26. When you are caring for a person from a different culture or religion than your own, you should
    A. Judge the person's behavior according to your own practices.
    B. Assume that the person's behavior will not be influenced by culture or religion.
    C. Give needed care, and do not worry about culture or religious beliefs.
    D. Respect and accept the person's culture and religion.

27. A culture that believes hot and cold imbalances cause disease is from
    A. Mexico
    B. England
    C. Vietnam
    D. Russia

28. If a person wants to visit with a spiritual leader while you are giving care you should
    A. Tell the spiritual leader that you must complete the care first.
    B. Provide privacy during the visit.
    C. Stay with the person during the visit.
    D. Tell the person this is not allowed while in the nursing facility.

29. When a person does not follow all beliefs and practices of his or her religion, you should
    A. Assume the person is not religious.
    B. Know that each person is unique.
    C. Call a spiritual leader to help the person follow the beliefs.
    D. Not be concerned about the person's religion when giving care.

30. You are caring for Mrs. Kim, who is foreign speaking, and she nods "yes" to all of your questions. This probably means that
    A. Mrs. Kim is a very cooperative patient.
    B. She does not understand what you are saying and is pretending to understand.
    C. In her culture, agreeing is the polite thing to do.
    D. She is concealing negative emotions.

31. When people are ill, they
    A. Feel angry, upset, and useless
    B. May fear death, disability, chronic illness, and loss of function
    C. Fear being laughed at for being afraid
    D. All of the above

32. A person who is having the appendix removed is
    A. An adult with medical problems
    B. A person having surgery
    C. A person with mental health problems
    D. A person needing subacute care or rehabilitation

33. Which of these persons would need the care of a branch of medicine called pediatrics?
    A. A woman who had a new baby today
    B. An older person with problems and diseases of old age
    C. A 7-year-old child with pneumonia
    D. A person receiving kidney dialysis

34. Which of these persons would not receive care in a long-term care center?
    A. A man who is recovering from minor surgery
    B. An alert person with a chronic illness who requires help with personal care
    C. A 25 year-old who is unable to care for himself because of injuries
    D. A person with a terminal illness

35. Which of these is part of the Patient's Bill of Rights?
    A. The person must follow all recommended treatments or plans of care.
    B. The doctor does not need to share all of the information about his or her treatment.
    C. The person should know when students and other trainees are involved in his or her care.
    D. Hospital charges are not given to the person, but only to the insurance companies.

36. Which of these would *not* help effective communication?
    A. Use words that have the same meaning to both you and the person.
    B. Communicate in a logical and orderly manner.
    C. Give specific and factual information.
    D. Use medical terminology when talking to the person.

37. When using verbal communication, a rule to follow is
    A. Ask one question at a time.
    B. Speak in a loud voice so the person can hear you.
    C. Ask several questions at a time, and then wait for the answers.
    D. Use slang words to make the person comfortable.

38. Mrs. Stevens cannot speak. How does she use verbal communication?
    A. She may use touch.
    B. Her body language sends messages.
    C. She can use gestures to communicate.
    D. She may write messages on a paper pad.

39. When you use touch to communicate, it is important to
    A. Be aware of the person's culture and practices about touch.
    B. Make sure the person likes to be touched.
    C. Follow the person' care plan.
    D. Do all of the above.

40. When you go to Mrs. Hart's room, you can tell she is not happy or not feeling well because
    A. Her hair is well groomed.
    B. She has a slumped posture.
    C. She smiles when you come in the room.
    D. She has applied her makeup.

41. All of these would show you listen effectively *except* when you
    A. Face the resident and have good eye contact.
    B. Lean back, and cross your arms.
    C. Respond to the resident by asking questions.
    D. Use words the person can understand.

42. Which of these is paraphrasing?
    A. "You don't know how long you will be here?"
    B. "Do you want to take a tub bath or a shower?"
    C. "Tell me about living on a farm."
    D. "Can you explain what you mean?"

43. When you say, "Mr. Davis, have you taken a shower this morning?" you are
    A. Paraphrasing his thoughts
    B. Asking a direct question
    C. Focusing his thoughts
    D. Asking an open-ended question

44. Responses to open-ended questions are generally
    A. Longer and give more information than direct questions
    B. "Yes" or "no" answers
    C. Able to make sure you understand the message
    D. Focused on dealing with a certain topic

45. When you do not understand the message, you may
    A. Ask the person an open-ended question.
    B. Make a statement to clarify what he is saying.
    C. Use nonverbal communication.
    D. Use silence to show you do not understand.

46. Mr. Parker often rambles and tells long stories during which his thoughts wander. You need to know if he had a bowel movement today, so you will
    A. Make a clarifying statement.
    B. Ask an open-ended question.
    C. Ask a focusing question.
    D. Paraphrase his thoughts.

47. What is best if the person takes long pauses between statements?
    A. Just being there shows you care.
    B. Try to cheer the person up by talking.
    C. Leave the room.
    D. Find another resident to talk with him.

48. A barrier to communication would be
    A. Asking a clarifying question
    B. Giving your opinion
    C. Remaining silent when the person is silent
    D. Paraphrasing the person's message

49. When you care for a person who is comatose, you should
    A. Explain everything you are going to do.
    B. Remain silent so that you do not disturb the person.
    C. Enter the room quietly so that you do not startle the person.
    D. Do all of the above.

50. Mrs. Duke has visitors and you need to give care. What would you do?
    A. Give the care while visitors are present.
    B. Politely ask the visitors to leave the room until you are finished.
    C. Ask the visitors to give the care.
    D. Tell the visitors that they must leave the nursing center.

51. When a person is admitted to a nursing center for respite care, it means the
    A. Person needs complex care.
    B. Caregivers need a break from giving care.
    C. Family no longer wants the person to live with them.
    D. Person is dying and needs terminal care.

52. When you are caring for a person who becomes angry, you should
    A. Avoid answering signal lights.
    B. Tell the person what you are going to do and when.
    C. Explain to the person why he or she should not be angry.
    D. Tell the person to stop being angry.

53. If a person hits, pinches, or bites you when you are giving care, you should
    A. Discuss the behavior with the nurse to decide how to deal with the person.
    B. Stop giving care to the person.
    C. Firmly tell the person to stop acting like that.
    D. Refuse to care for the person when he or she is assigned to you.

Fill in the Blanks

54. What are the parts of the person you consider when you use the concept of holism?

    A. ______________________________

    B. ______________________________

    C. ______________________________

    D. ______________________________

55. List the basic needs in order, starting with the lowest level.

    A. ______________________________

    B. ______________________________

    C. ______________________________

    D. ______________________________

    E. ______________________________

56. Name the culture that may follow the listed belief or custom.

    A. ______________________________—Food and medicine is given to restore the hot-cold balance.

    B. ______________________________—Folk healers called jerbero use herbs and spices to prevent or cure diseases.

    C. In Vietnam or in ____________________—Men shake hands with other men but do not shake hands with women.

    D. ______________________________—Eyes are rolled upward to express disapproval.

    E. ______________________________—Facial expressions may mean the opposite of what the person is feeling. Negative emotions may be concealed with a smile.

    F. ______________________________ and Asian cultures—Eye contact is impolite and an invasion of privacy.

    G. ______________________________—Silence is a sign of respect, particularly to an older person.

    H. ______________________________—All family members are involved in the person's care.

57. According to the Patient's Bill of Rights, what happens if a person refuses treatment or a plan of care?

    ____

    ____

    ____

58. The patient has a right to discuss and request information about

    A. ______________________________

    B. ______________________________

    C. ______________________________

    D. ______________________________

59. When you use verbal communication, words are

    ______________________________ or

    ______________________________.

60. Written words are used when a person cannot

    ______________________________ or

    ______________________________.

61. If a person can hear but cannot speak or read, ask questions that have

    ______________________________.

62. Nonverbal communication messages more accurately reflect a person's ____________________ than words do.

63. Body language is nonverbal communication that is shown with

A. ______________________

B. ______________________

C. ______________________

D. ______________________

E. ______________________

F. ______________________

G. ______________________

64. When you listen to a person, you respond by

A. ______________________

B. ______________________

C. ______________________

D. ______________________

65. When you fail to listen, you can miss complaints of ______________________.

Crossword Puzzle

Fill in the crossword puzzle on the following page by answering the clues with words from this list.

clarifying	focusing	paraphrasing
comatose	holism	silence
culture	need	touch
direct	nonverbal	verbal
esteem		

Across

2. Communication expressed with gestures, facial expressions, posture, body movements, touch, and smell
7. The worth, value, or opinion one has of a person
9. Communication in which the words are spoken or written
10. An unconscious person who cannot respond to others
11. A communication method that is useful when a person rambles or wanders in thought
12. A communication method in which you can ask the person to repeat the message, say you do not understand, or restate the message
13. The characteristics of a group of people—language, values, beliefs, habits, likes, dislikes, customs—passed from one generation to another

Down

1. Restating the person's message in your own words
3. A concept that considers the whole person—physical, social, psychological, and spiritual parts
4. A question that focuses on certain information and may require a "yes" or "no" answer or more information
5. Something necessary or desired for maintaining life and mental well-being
6. Nonverbal communication that conveys comfort, caring, loving, affection, interest, concern, and reassurance
8. Communicating by not saying anything

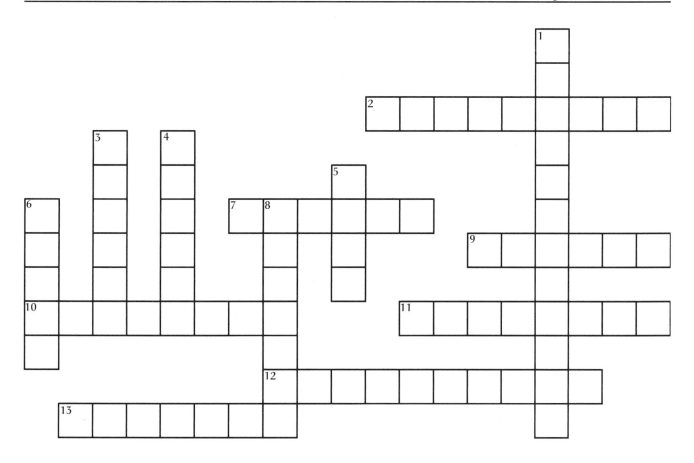

Nursing Assistant Skills Video Exercise

View the **Basic Principles** *video to answer these questions.*

66. The Patient's Bill of Rights is used in ______________________ and was developed by the ______________________.

67. The Resident's Bill of Rights is used in ______________________ and is required by ______________________.

68. When you screen a person, you are giving the person the right to ______________________.

69. When you share only information about the person, you are meeting the right to ______________________.

70. When you allow the person to choose foods to eat or clothes to wear, you are allowing the right of ______________________.

71. When you are giving care, you should use these guidelines to communicate:

    A. Avoid words ______________________.

    B. Use familiar ______________________.

    C. Be ______________________.

    D. Do not add ______________________.

    E. Stay ______________________.

    F. Present ______________________.

Optional Learning Exercises

BASIC NEEDS

Physical needs

72. What are the six physical needs required for survival?

 A. ______________________

 B. ______________________

 C. ______________________

 D. ______________________

 E. ______________________

 F. ______________________

73. The physical needs must be met before the ______________________ needs.

Safety and security

74. Safety and security needs relate to protection from

 A. ______________________

 B. ______________________

 C. ______________________

75. Why do many people feel a loss of safety and security when admitted to a nursing center?

 A. ______________________

 B. ______________________

 C. ______________________

Love and belonging

76. The need for love and belonging relates to

 A. ______________________

 B. ______________________

 C. ______________________

Self-esteem

77. Self-esteem means to

 A. Think ______________________.

 B. See ______________________.

 C. See oneself as having ______________________.

78. Why is it important to encourage residents to do as much as possible for themselves?

 ____

Self-actualization

79. What does self-actualization involve?

 A. ______________________

 B. ______________________

 C. ______________________

80. What happens if self-actualization is postponed?

 ____

CULTURE AND RELIGION PRACTICES

Religion

81. How can you help a resident observe religious practices if services are held in the nursing center?

 ____

82. What should you do if the resident wants to leave the center to attend services or have a visit from a spiritual leader?

 ____

83. If the resident wants a pastor to visit in the room, you should

 A. ______________________

 B. ______________________

 C. ______________________

Cultural health care reliefs

Mexico and the Dominican Republic

84. People from these cultures believe when hot and cold imbalances occur, it causes ______________________.

85. What are "hot" conditions?

A. ______

B. ______

C. ______

D. ______

E. ______

86. What are "cold" conditions?

A. ______

B. ______

C. ______

D. ______

E. ______

Vietnam

87. How are foods and medications given to restore hot-cold balance?

A. ______

B. ______

Cultural sick practices

88. How do Vietnamese folk practices treat these illnesses?

A. Common cold

______

B. Headache and sore throat

______

89. What illnesses do these Russian folk practices treat?

A. ______—An ointment is placed behind the ears and temples and also on the back of the neck.

B. ______—Dough made of dark rye flour and honey is placed on the spinal column.

Cultural touch practices

90. Why is touch important in Mexico and the Philippine cultures?

______

91. What nonverbal communication using touch is common in Russia?

______

92. If you are caring for a resident from India, what might you notice about his practice of shaking hands?

______

93. Residents from some countries might not like to be touched. Give two examples of these countries.

______

______

Eye contact practices

94. Why would you avoid making direct eye contact with a resident from Mexico?

______

95. If a resident from Vietnam blinks when you explain a procedure, it probably means that the message ______.

96. Direct eye contact is practiced among people from ______ and ______.

Family roles in sick care

97. You are caring for a resident from China. You might expect the family members to ______, ______, and ______ the person.

98. A man from Mexico is a resident, and his daughter says she cannot care for him when he goes home. This may be because in Mexico, women cannot give care if

_______________________________________.

Using Communication Methods

You have completed your duties for the morning and have some free time. Mr. Harry Donal is a resident in a nursing center. He rarely has visitors, and you try to spend time with him when you can. Answer the following questions about the communication techniques you use when you visit with Mr. Donal.

99. You sit in a chair next to Mr. Donal so you can see each other. This position will help you to have better _______________________________.

100. You should lean ___________________________ Mr. Donal to show interest.

101. Mr. Donal says, "I know this is the best place for me, but I miss my flower garden at home." You respond, "You miss your home?" This is an example of

_______________________________________.

102. You ask Mr. Donal, "You told me you did not sleep well last night. Can you tell me why?" He replies, "There was a lot of noise in the hall." This is an example of a

_______________________________________.

103. You say to Mr. Donal, "Tell me about your flower garden at home." This is an

_________________________________ question.

104. When you say, "Can you explain what that means," you are asking a person to

_______________________________________.

105. Mr. Donal says that he "hurts all over" and then begins to talk about the weather. You say, "Tell me more about where you hurt. You said you hurt all over." This statement helps in

_________________________________ the topic.

106. Mr. Donal begins to cry when he talks about his flower garden. How can you show caring and respect for his situation and feelings?

____

107. When Mr. Donal begins to cry, you quickly begin to talk about the activities planned this morning. Changing the subject is a

_______________________________________.

Independent Learning Activities

- Review the section in Chapter 6 that discusses basic needs to answer these questions about how well you are meeting your own needs. The answers may be shared in a discussion group or privately answered to help you understand yourself better.
  - Do you smoke? What need may be affected by smoking?
  - What kinds of foods and fluids do you eat? Is your diet meeting your basic needs for food and water?
  - How much rest and sleep do you get each day? How much do you need to feel well rested?
  - How safe do you feel at home? At school? In your community? How do your feelings affect your ability to hold a job or attend school?
  - Who are the people who make you feel loved? Who help you when you have problems?
  - What are you doing that helps you meet the need for self-actualization?

- Answer these questions about your personal health care practices.
  - What health care practices are followed in your family? How are these practices related to your cultural or religious beliefs?
  - How often do you go to the doctor? For regular checkups? Do you only go when ill?
  - When do you go to the dentist? Once or twice a year for cleaning and checkups? Only when you have a toothache?
  - When a family member is in a health care center, how does your family respond? Does someone stay with the person and provide all of the care, or do family members visit for brief periods and let health care workers provide all care? Is the family response related to any cultural or religious practices?

- Look at your answers to both sets of the previous questions.
  - How well are you meeting your basic needs? How could you improve in meeting these needs? What changes would be the most beneficial?
  - How much influence on your practices comes from cultural or religious traditions in your family? Are these influences helping or hindering you in meeting needs?

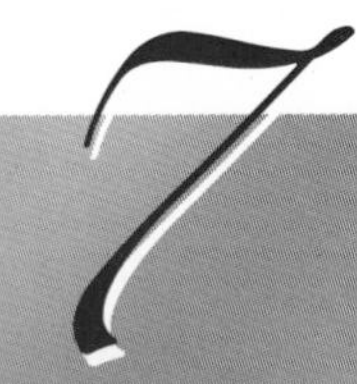

Body Structure and Function

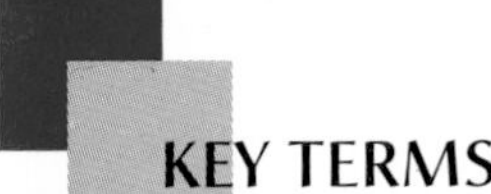

KEY TERMS

Artery
Capillary
Cell
Digestion
Hemoglobin
Hormone
Immunity
Menstruation
Metabolism
Organ
Peristalsis
Respiration
System
Tissue
Vein

Fill in the Blanks: Key Terms

1. The substance in red blood cells that carries oxygen and gives blood its color is ________________.
2. ________________ is protection against a disease or condition.
3. The process of supplying cells with oxygen and removing carbon dioxide from them is ________________.
4. The process of physically and chemically breaking down food so that it can be absorbed for use by the cells is ________________.
5. ________________ is the burning of food for heat and energy by the cells.
6. A blood vessel that carries blood away from the heart is an ________________.
7. ________________ is the involuntary muscle contractions in the digestive system that move food through the alimentary canal.
8. Organs that work together to perform special functions form a ________________.
9. The basic unit of body structure is a ________________.
10. Groups of tissues with the same function form an ________________.

11. A ______________________________ is a tiny blood vessel.

12. A group of cells with a similar function is ______________________________.

13. ______________________________ is the process in which the lining of the uterus breaks up and is discharged from the body through the vagina.

14. A chemical substance secreted by the glands into the bloodstream is a ______________________________.

15. A ______________________________ is a blood vessel that carries blood back to the heart.

Circle the BEST Answer

16. A cell is
    A. Only found in muscles
    B. The basic unit of body structure
    C. Can live without oxygen
    D. A group of tissues

17. The control center of a cell is the
    A. Membrane
    B. Protoplasm
    C. Cytoplasm
    D. Nucleus

18. Genes control
    A. Cell division
    B. Tissues
    C. Physical and chemical traits inherited by children
    D. Organs

19. Connective tissue
    A. Covers internal and external body surface
    B. Receives and carries impulses to the brain and back to the body parts
    C. Anchors, connects, and supports other body tissues
    D. Allows the body to move by stretching and contracting

20. Living cells of the epidermis contain
    A. Blood vessels and many nerves
    B. Sweat and oil glands
    C. Pigment that gives skin color
    D. Hair roots

21. Sweat glands help
    A. The body regulate temperature
    B. Keep the hair and skin soft and shiny
    C. Protect the nose from dust, insects, and other foreign objects
    D. The skin sense pleasant and unpleasant sensations

22. Long bones
    A. Allow skill and ease in movement
    B. Bear the weight of the body
    C. Protect organs
    D. Allow various degrees of movement and flexion

23. Blood cells are manufactured in
    A. The heart
    B. The liver
    C. Blood vessels
    D. Bone marrow

24. Joints move smoothly because of
    A. Cartilage
    B. Synovial fluid
    C. Muscle
    D. Ligaments

25. A joint that moves in all directions is a
    A. Ball and socket
    B. Hinge
    C. Pivot
    D. All of the above

26. Voluntary muscles are
    A. Found in the stomach and intestines
    B. Attached to bones
    C. Cardiac muscle
    D. Tendons

27. Muscles produce heat by
    A. Contracting
    B. Relaxing
    C. Maintaining posture
    D. Working automatically

28. The central nervous system consists of
    A. A myelin sheath
    B. Nerves throughout the body
    C. The brain and spinal column
    D. Cranial nerves

29. The medulla controls
   A. Muscle contraction and relaxation
   B. Heart rate, breathing, blood vessel size, and swallowing
   C. Reasoning, memory, and consciousness
   D. Hearing and vision

30. Cerebrospinal fluid
   A. Cushions shocks that could injure the structures of the brain and spinal cord
   B. Controls voluntary muscles
   C. Lubricates movement
   D. Controls involuntary muscles

31. Cranial nerves conduct impulses between the
   A. Brain and the head, neck, chest, and abdomen
   B. Brain and the skin and extremities
   C. Brain and the internal body structure
   D. Spinal cord and the lower extremities

32. When you are frightened, the ________________ nervous system is stimulated.
   A. Sympathetic
   B. Parasympathetic
   C. Central
   D. Cranial

33. Receptors for vision and nerve fibers of the optic nerve are found in the
   A. Sclera
   B. Choroids
   C. Retina
   D. Cornea

34. What structure of the ear is involved in balance?
   A. Malleus
   B. Auditory canal
   C. Tympanic membranes
   D. Semicircular canals

35. Hemoglobin in red blood cells gives blood its red color and carries
   A. Oxygen
   B. Food to cells
   C. Waste products
   D. Water

36. Red blood cells live for
   A. About 9 days
   B. 3 or 4 months
   C. 4 days
   D. A year

37. White blood cells or leukocytes
   A. Protect the body against infection
   B. Are necessary for blood clotting
   C. Carry food, hormone, chemicals, and waste products
   D. Pick up carbon dioxide

38. The left atrium of the heart
   A. Receives blood from the lungs
   B. Receives blood from the body tissues
   C. Pumps blood to the lungs
   D. Pumps blood to all parts of the body

39. Arteries
   A. Return blood to the heart
   B. Pass food, oxygen, and other substances into the cells
   C. Pick up waste products including carbon dioxide from the cells
   D. Carry blood away from the heart

40. In the lungs, oxygen and carbon dioxide are exchanged
   A. In the epiglottis
   B. Between the right bronchus and the left bronchus
   C. By the bronchioles
   D. Between the alveoli and capillaries

41. The lungs are protected by the
   A. Diaphragm
   B. Pleura
   C. Bony framework of ribs, sternum, and vertebrae
   D. Lobes

42. Food is moved through the alimentary canal (gastrointestinal [GI] tract) by
   A. Chyme
   B. Peristalsis
   C. Swallowing
   D. Bile

43. Water is absorbed from chyme in the
   A. Small intestine
   B. Stomach
   C. Esophagus
   D. Large intestine

44. Digested food is absorbed through tiny projections called
   A. Jejunum
   B. Ileum
   C. Villi
   D. Colon

45. A function of the urinary system is to
    A. Remove waste products from the blood
    B. Rid the body of solid waste
    C. Rid the body of carbon dioxide
    D. Burn food for energy

46. A person feels the need to urinate when the bladder contains about
    A. 1000 ml of urine
    B. 500 ml of urine
    C. 250 ml of urine
    D. 125 ml of urine

47. Testosterone is needed for
    A. Male secondary sex characteristics
    B. Female secondary sex characteristics
    C. Sperm to be produced
    D. Ova to be produced

48. The prostate gland lies
    A. In the scrotum
    B. In the testes
    C. Just below the bladder
    D. In the penis

49. The ovaries secrete progesterone and
    A. Estrogen
    B. Testosterone
    C. Ova
    D. Semen

50. When an ovum is released from an ovary, it travels first through the
    A. Uterus
    B. Fallopian tubes
    C. Endometrium
    D. Vagina

51. Menstruation occurs when
    A. The hymen is ruptured
    B. The ovary releases an ovum
    C. The endometrium breaks up
    D. Fertilization occurs

52. A fertilized cell implants in the
    A. Ovary
    B. Fallopian tubes
    C. Endometrium
    D. Vagina

53. The master gland is the
    A. Thyroid
    B. Parathyroid
    C. Adrenal
    D. Pituitary

54. Thyroid hormone regulates
    A. Growth
    B. Metabolism
    C. Proper functioning of nerves and muscles
    D. Energy produced during exercise

55. If too little insulin is produced by the pancreas, the person has
    A. Tetany
    B. Slow growth
    C. Diabetes mellitus
    D. Slowed metabolism

56. When antigens enter the body, they are attacked and destroyed by
    A. Antibodies
    B. Lymphocytes
    C. B cells
    D. T cells

Matching

Match the terms with the description.

Musculoskeletal System

57. ________	Connective tissue at end of long bones	A. Periosteum
58. ________	Skeletal muscle	B. Joint
59. ________	Membrane that covers bone	C. Cartilage
60. ________	Connects muscle to bone	D. Synovial fluid
61. ________	Point at which two or more bones meet	E. Striated muscle
62. ________	Heart muscle	F. Smooth muscle
63. ________	Involuntary muscle	G. Cardiac muscle
64. ________	Acts as a lubricant so the joint can move smoothly	H. Tendon

Nervous System

65. ________ Contains eustachian tubes and ossicles
66. ________ Has 12 pairs of cranial nerves and 31 pairs of spinal nerves
67. ________ White of the eye
68. ________ Outside of cerebrum; controls highest function of brain
69. ________ Inner layer of eye; receptors for vision are contained here
70. ________ Controls involuntary muscles, heart beat, blood pressure, and other functions
71. ________ Light enters eye through this structure
72. ________ Contain midbrain, pons, and medulla
73. ________ Waxy substance secreted in auditory canal
74. ________ Contains semicircular canal and cochlea

A. Sclera
B. Cornea
C. Retina
D. Cerumen
E. Middle ear
F. Inner ear
G. Brainstem
H. Cerebral cortex
I. Autonomic nervous system
J. Peripheral nervous system

Circulatory System

75. ________ Liquid part of blood
76. ________ Thin sac covering the heart
77. ________ Very tiny blood vessel
78. ________ Substance in blood that picks up oxygen
79. ________ Carries blood away from heart
80. ________ White blood cell
81. ________ Carries blood toward heart
82. ________ Red blood cell
83. ________ Thick muscular portion of heart
84. ________ Platelet; necessary for clotting
85. ________ Membrane lining inner surface of heart

A. Plasma
B. Erythrocyte
C. Hemoglobin
D. Leukocyte
E. Thrombocyte
F. Pericardium
G. Myocardium
H. Endocardium
I. Artery
J. Vein
K. Capillary

Respiratory System

86. ________	Air passes from larynx into this structure	A. Epiglottis
87. ________	A two-layered sac that covers the lungs	B. Larynx
88. ________	Piece of cartilage that acts like a lid over larynx	C. Bronchiole
89. ________	Separates the lungs from the abdominal cavity	D. Trachea
90. ________	The voice box	E. Alveolus
91. ________	Small branch (among others) that divides from the bronchus	F. Diaphragm
92. ________	Tiny one-celled air sac	G. Pleura

Digestive System

93. ________	Structure that adds more digestive juices to chyme	A. Liver
94. ________	Semiliquid food mixture formed in stomach	B. Chyme
95. ________	Portion of GI tract that absorbs food	C. Colon
96. ________	Stores bile	D. Duodenum
97. ________	Portion of GI tract that absorbs water	E. Jejunum
98. ________	Produces bile	F. Saliva
99. ________	Moistens food particles in the mouth	G. Pancreas
100. ________	Produces digestive juices	H. Gallbladder

Urinary System

101. ________	Basic working unit of the kidney	A. Bladder
102. ________	Bean-shaped structure that produces urine	B. Glomerulus
103. ________	A cluster of capillaries in Bowman's capsule	C. Kidney
104. ________	Structure that allows urine to pass from the bladder	D. Meatus
105. ________	A tube attached to the renal pelvis of the kidney	E. Nephron
106. ________	Hollow muscular sac that stores urine	F. Tubule
107. ________	Opening at the end of the urethra	G. Ureter
108. ________	Fluid and waste products form urine in this structure	H Urethra

Reproductive System

109. ________ Male or female sex organ
110. ________ Two folds of tissue on each side of the vagina
111. ________ Sac between thighs that contains testes
112. ________ External genitalia of female
113. ________ Testicles; sperm produced here
114. ________ Attached to uterus; ovum travel through this structure
115. ________ Stores sperm and produces semen
116. ________ Tissue lining the uterus

A. Scrotum
B. Testes
C. Seminal vesicle
D. Gonad
E. Fallopian tube
F. Endometrium
G. Labia
H. Vulva

Endocrine System

117. ________ Released by pancreas regulates sugar in blood
118. ________ Sex hormone secreted by testes
119. ________ Sex hormone secreted by ovaries
120. ________ Regulates metabolism
121. ________ Regulates calcium levels in the body
122. ________ Stimulates to produce energy during emergencies

A. Epinephrine
B. Estrogen
C. Insulin
D. Parathormone
E. Testosterone
F. Thyroxine

Immune System

123. ________ Normal body substances that recognize abnormal or unwanted substances
124. ________ Group of cells that destroy invading cells
125. ________ Group of white blood cells that digest and destroy microorganisms
126. ________ Group of cells that cause production of antibodies
127. ________ Abnormal or unwanted substances
128. ________ Types of white blood cells that produce antibodies

A. Antibodies
B. Antigens
C. Phagocytes
D. Lymphocytes
E. B cells
F. T cells

Labeling

129. Name the parts of the cell.

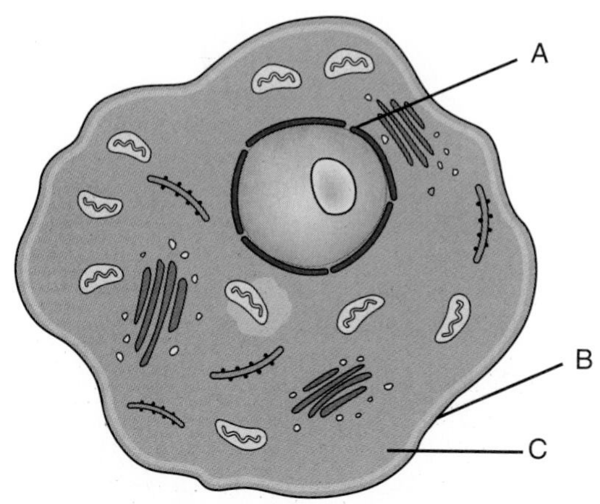

A. ______________________

B. ______________________

C. ______________________

130. Name each type of joint.

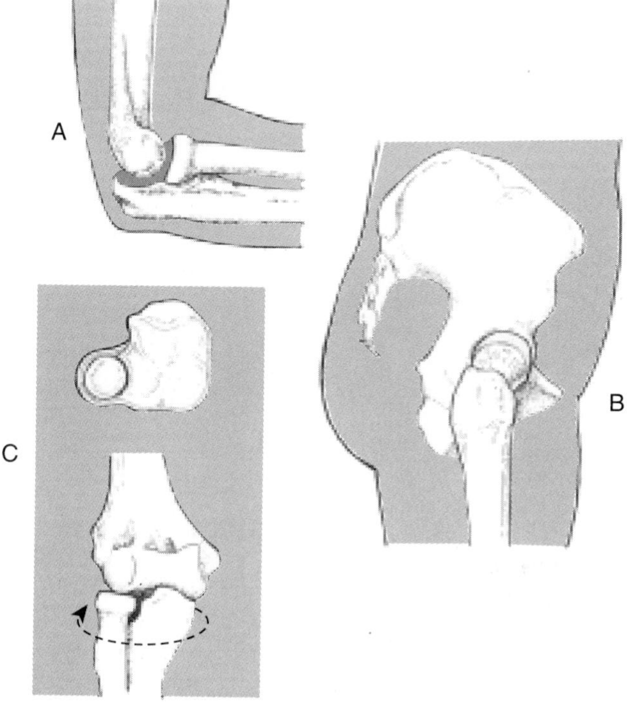

A. ______________________

B. ______________________

C. ______________________

131. Name the parts of the brain.

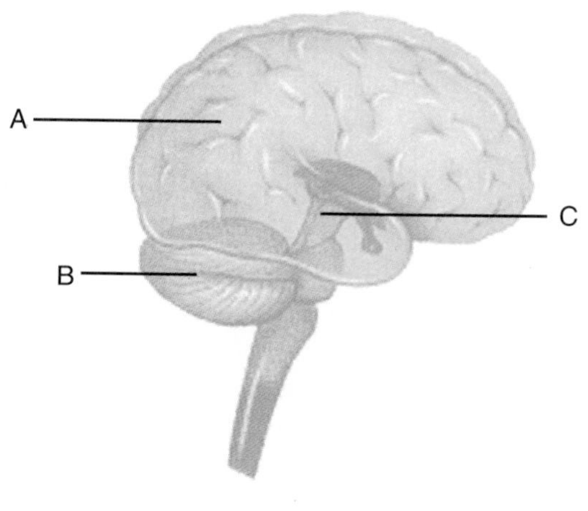

A. ______________________

B. ______________________

C. ______________________

132. Name the four chambers of the heart.

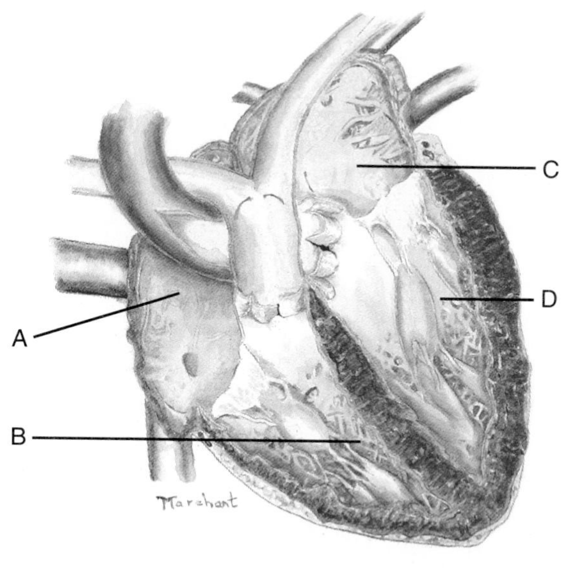

A. ______________________

B. ______________________

C. ______________________

D. ______________________

133. Name the structures of the respiratory system.

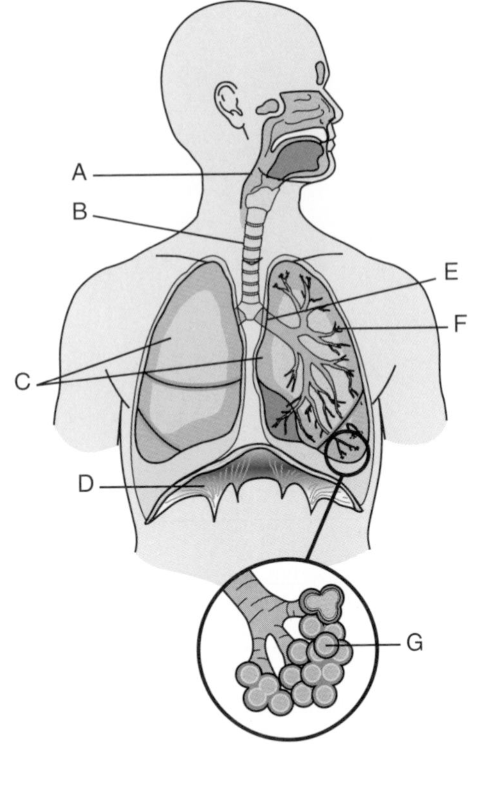

A. ______________________

B. ______________________

C. ______________________

D. ______________________

E. ______________________

F. ______________________

G. ______________________

134. Name the structures of the digestive system.

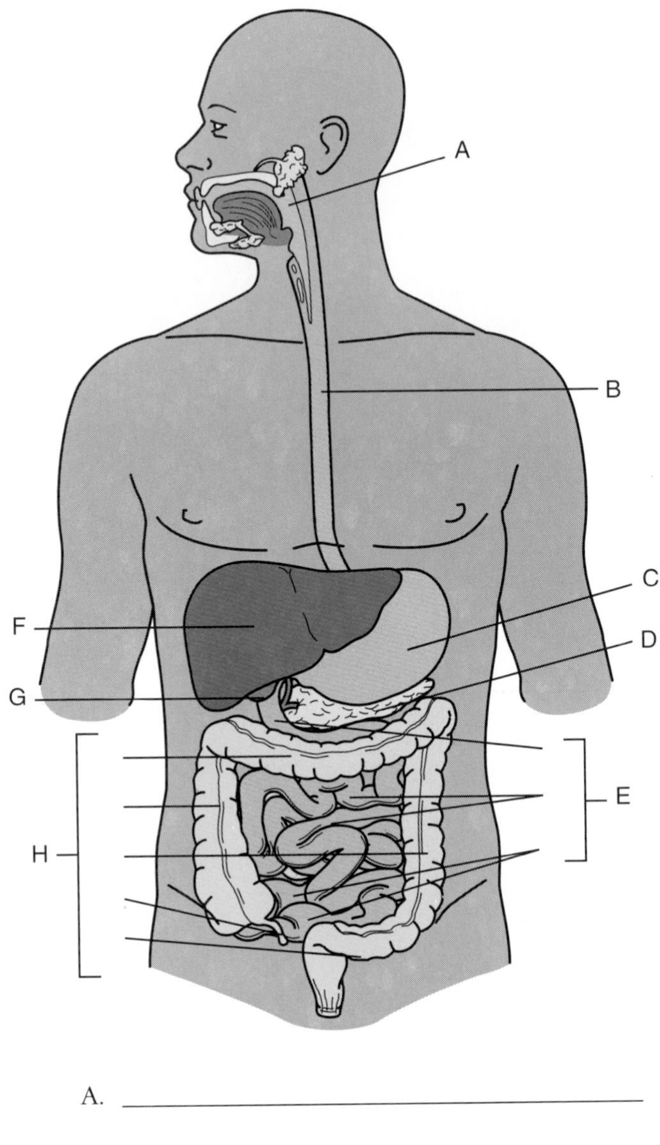

A. ______________________

B. ______________________

C. ______________________

D. ______________________

E. ______________________

F. ______________________

G. ______________________

H. ______________________

135. Name the structures of the urinary system.

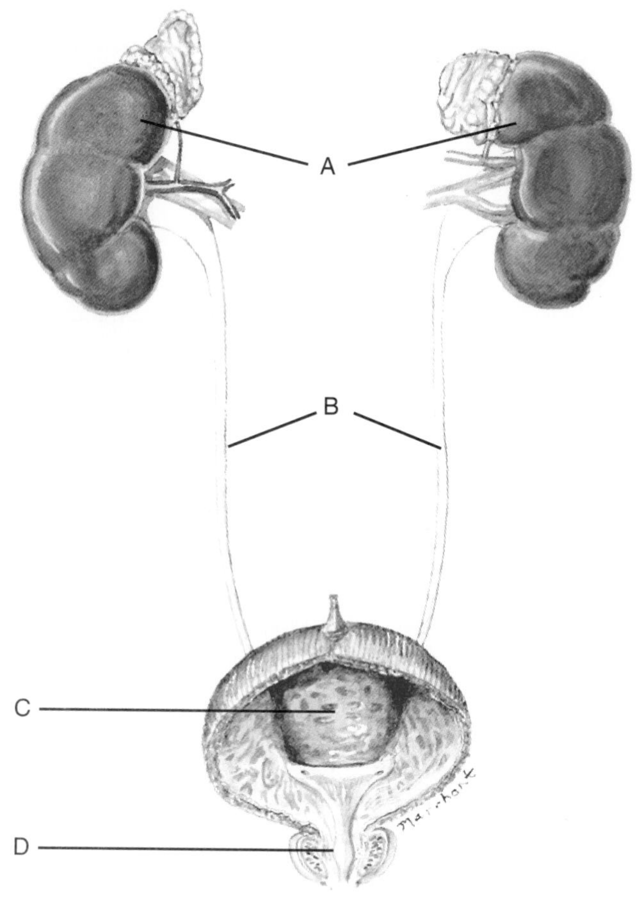

A. ______

B. ______

C. ______

D. ______

136. Name the structures of the male reproductive system.

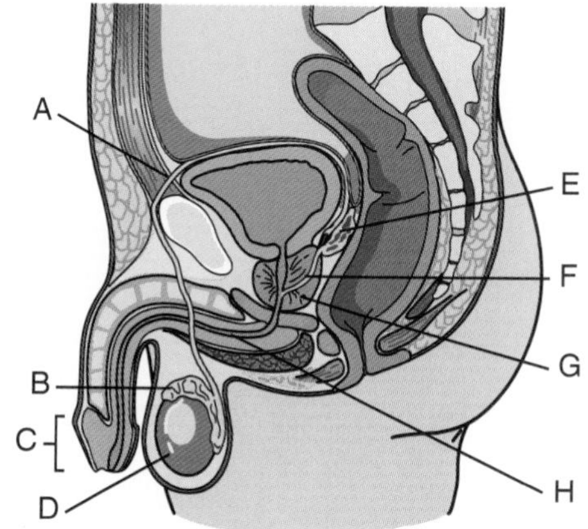

A. ______

B. ______

C. ______

D. ______

E. ______

F. ______

G. ______

H. ______

137. Name the external female genitalia.

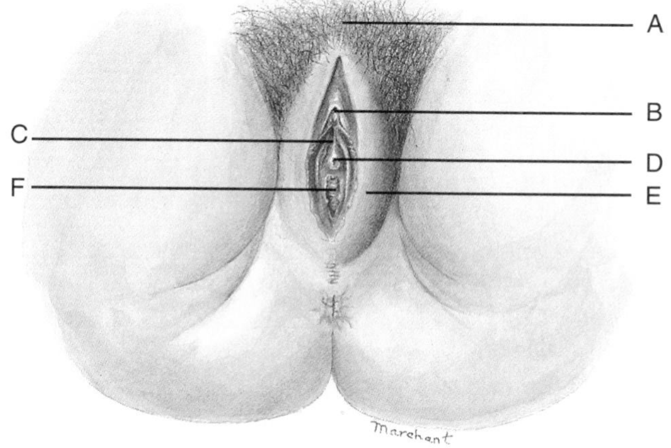

A. ______

B. ______

C. ______

D. ______

E. ______

F. ______

Optional Learning Exercises

138. Explain the function of each part of the cell

A. Cell membrane: ______

______

B. Nucleus: ______

______

C. Cytoplasm: ______

______

D. Protoplasm: ______

______

E. Chromosomes: ______

______

F. Genes: ______

______

139. List what structures are contained in the two skin layers

A. Epidermis: ______

______

B. Dermis: ______

______

140. Explain the function of each type of bone

A. Long bone: ______

______

B. Short bone: ______

______

C. Flat bone: ______

______

D. Irregular bone: ______

______

141. Describe how each type of joint moves, and give an example of each type.

A. Ball and socket: ______

______

Example: ______

B. Hinge: ______

______

Example: ______

C. Pivot: ______

______

Example: ______

142. Explain what happens when muscles contract.

______

______

______

143. Explain the function of the three main parts of the brain. Include the function of the cerebral cortex and the midbrain, pons, and medulla.

A. Cerebrum: ______

______

Cerebral cortex: ______

______

B. Cerebellum: ______

______

C. Brainstem: ______

______

Midbrain and pons: ______

______

Medulla: ______

______

144. Explain how the sympathetic and parasympathetic nervous systems balance each other.

____

____

____

145. Explain what happens to each of these structures when light enters the eye.

A. Choroid: ______________________________

____

B. Cornea: ______________________________

____

C. Lens: ______________________________

____

D. Retina: ______________________________

____

146. Explain how each of these structures help carry sound in the ear.

A. Ossicles: ______________________________

____

B. Cochlea: ______________________________

____

C. Auditory nerve: ______________________________

____

147. Where are red blood cells destroyed as they wear out?

____

____

____

148. When an infection occurs, what do white blood cells do?

____

____

____

149. Explain the function of the four chambers of the heart.

A. Right atrium: ______________________________

____

B. Left atrium: ______________________________

____

C. Right ventricle: ______________________________

____

D. Left ventricle: ______________________________

____

150. Explain where each vein carries blood.

A. Inferior vena cava: ______________________________

____

B. Superior vena cava: ______________________________

____

151. Explain what happens in the alveoli.

____

____

____

152. After food is swallowed, explain what happens in each part of the digestive tract.

A. Stomach: ______________________________

____

B. Duodenum: ______________________________

____

C. Jejunum and ileum: ______________________________

____

D. Colon: ______________________________

____

E. Rectum: ______________________________

____

F. Anus: ______________________________

____

153. Explain what happens in each structure of the kidney.

A. Glomerulus: ______________________________

____

B. Collecting tubules: ______________________________

____

C. Ureters: ______________________________

____

D. Urethra: ______________________________

____

E. Meatus: ______________________________

____

154. Sperm is produced in the testicles. What happens to the sperm in each structure?

A. Testes: ______________________________

____

B. Vas deferens: ______________________________

____

C. Seminal vesicle: ______________________________

____

D. Ejaculatory duct: ______________________________

____

E. Prostate gland: ______________________________

____

F. Urethra: ______________________________

____

155. What is the function of the endometrium?

____

____

____

156. Menstruation occurs about every __________ days.

Ovulation usually occurs on or about the day

__________ of the cycle.

157. What is the function of each pituitary hormone?

A. Growth hormone: ______________________________

____

B. Thyroid-stimulating hormone: ______________________________

____

C. Adrenocorticotropic hormone: ______________________________

____

D. Antidiuretic hormone: ____________________

____

E. Oxytocin: ____________________

____

158. What is the function of insulin?

____

____

____

What happens if too little insulin is produced?

____

____

____

159. What happens when the body senses an antigen?

____

____

____

Independent Learning Activities

- Using your own body, move joints of each type to see how they move.
  - Which joint is a ball and socket? How many ways were you able to move it?
  - Which joint moves like a hinge? How does it work differently than the ball and socket?
  - Which joint is a pivot? Compare its movement to the other two joints.
- Listen to a friend's chest with a stethoscope.
  - What sounds do you hear?
  - What body systems are making the sounds?
  - Are you able to count any of the sounds you hear? What are you counting?
- Listen to your lower abdomen with a stethoscope.
  - What sounds can you hear?
  - What causes sound in the abdomen? What body system is involved in this activity?
  - What is occurring when you hear your "stomach growl?" What is the term for this activity?
- Look at a friend's eyes in a dimly lit area, and observe the size of the pupils.
  - What size are the pupils? Are they both the same?
  - Shine a flashlight in the eye. What happens to the pupil?
  - What happens when you move the light away? If you see a change, how quickly does it occur?

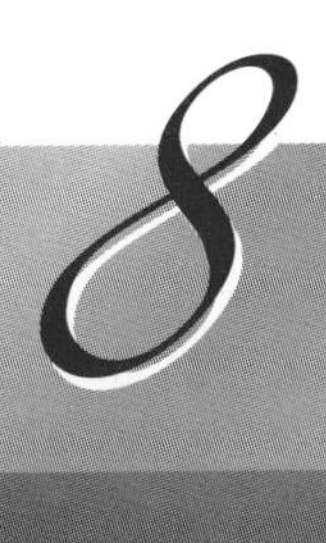

Growth and Development

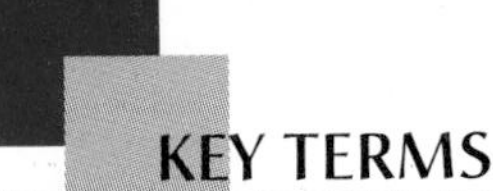

KEY TERMS

Adolescence
Development
Developmental task
Ejaculation
Growth
Infancy
Menarche
Menopause
Primary caregiver
Puberty
Reflex

Fill in the Blanks: Key Terms

1. The first menstruation and the start of menstrual cycles is ______________________________.
2. ______________________________ is the time between puberty and adulthood; a time of rapid growth and physical and social maturity.
3. The release of semen is ______________________________.
4. The period when reproductive organs begin to function and secondary sex characteristics appear is ______________________________.
5. ______________________________ is the first year of life.
6. ______________________________ is changes in mental, emotional, and social functionings.
7. An involuntary movement is a ______________________________.
8. ______________________________ is the physical changes that can be measured and that occur in a steady, orderly manner.

9. The person mainly responsible for providing or assisting with the child's basic needs is the

____.

10. A skill that must be completed during a stage of development is a

____.

11. ___________________________________ is the time when menstruation stops and menstrual cycles end.

Circle the BEST Answer

12. Growth is measured all of these ways *except*
   A. The ways a person behaves and thinks
   B. In height and weight
   C. By changes in appearance
   D. By changes in body functions

13. Growth and development begin
   A. At fertilization
   B. At birth
   C. When a baby sits up
   D. When children have growth spurts

14. The process of growth and development
   A. Occurs in a random order or pattern
   B. Progresses at a steady pace in each stage
   C. Occurs from the center of the body outward
   D. From the foot to the head

15. Movements in the newborn are uncoordinated and lack purpose because
   A. The baby has not been taught to move in a pattern.
   B. The central nervous system is not well developed.
   C. The baby moves with only reflexes.
   D. The baby has skipped a developmental task.

16. The birth weight of a newborn
   A. Doubles in the first year
   B. Triples in the first year
   C. Doubles in the first 3 months
   D. Triples in the first 6 months

17. Reflexes present in newborns
   A. Are learned behaviors
   B. Remain active through the first year
   C. Are abnormal developmental tasks
   D. Decline and then disappear as the central nervous system develops

18. Infants can play peek-a-boo by
   A. 2 to 3 months
   B. 4 to 5 months
   C. 8 to 9 months
   D. Their first birthday

19. Toddlerhood is called the "terrible twos" because the child
   A. Needs to assert independence
   B. Is more dependent on the primary caregiver
   C. Begins to walk
   D. Is not yet toilet trained

20. A major task for toddlers is
   A. Learning to walk
   B. Learning to feed themselves
   C. Learning to share toys with others
   D. Toilet training

21. Toddlers learn to feel secure when
   A. Primary caregivers are consistently present.
   B. Long periods of separation from primary caregivers are planned.
   C. Needs are not met quickly.
   D. They are allowed to be alone for long periods.

22. Three-year-old children are able to
   A. Play simple games and learn simple rules.
   B. Use a pencil to print letters, numbers, and their first names.
   C. Hop, skip, and throw and catch a ball.
   D. Be more responsible and truthful.

23. During the preschool years, children grow
   A. Much more rapidly than during infancy
   B. 2 to 3 inches per year and gain about 5 pounds per year
   C. Very slowly, if at all
   D. 6 to 7 inches per year and gain about 10 pounds per year

24. Baby teeth are lost, and permanent teeth erupt at about
   A. 2 years of age
   B. The end of the first year
   C. Around age 6
   D. At 9 or 10 years of age

25. Reading, writing, grammar, and math skills develop during
    A. Toddlerhood
    B. Preschool years
    C. School age
    D. Late childhood

26. Girls have a growth spurt during
    A. School age
    B. Late childhood
    C. Adolescence
    D. Young adulthood

27. During late childhood, children
    A. Do not accept adult standards and rules without question
    B. Increase their math and language skills
    C. Need factual sex education
    D. All of the above

28. Girls reach puberty
    A. When menarche occurs
    B. Between the ages of 12 and 16 years
    C. When they stop growing
    D. Later than boys

29. Coordination and graceful movements develop in adolescence
    A. As growth spurts occur
    B. As puberty is reached
    C. When all growth stops
    D. As muscle and bone growth even out

30. Adolescents need guidance and discipline because
    A. They need to remain dependent on parents.
    B. Judgment and reasoning are not always sound.
    C. They are just learning right from wrong.
    D. All of the above are true.

31. Teens usually do not understand why parents worry about sexual activities, pregnancy, and sexually transmitted diseases because
    A. They are emotionally unstable at this stage.
    B. Independence from adults is important.
    C. They may have trouble controlling sexual urges and considering the consequences of sexual activity.
    D. They do not have a sense of right and wrong or good and bad.

32. Development ends
    A. When puberty occurs
    B. When all physical growth is complete
    C. At young adulthood
    D. At death

33. Young adulthood includes all of these tasks *except*
    A. Adjusting to physical changes
    B. Learning to live with a partner
    C. Developing a satisfactory sex life
    D. Choosing education and a career

34. A developmental task of middle adulthood is
    A. Developing leisure-time activities
    B. Coping with a partner's death
    C. Preparing for one's own death
    D. Learning to live with a partner

Matching

Match the description with the correct reflex of a newborn.

35. ________ Occurs when legs extend and then flex
36. ________ Occurs when baby is held upright and the feet touch a surface
37. ________ Occurs when baby's mouth is guided to the nipple
38. ________ Occurs when lips are touched
39. ________ Occurs when fingers close firmly around an object

A. Moro (startle) reflex
B. Rooting reflex
C. Sucking reflex
D. Grasp (palmar) reflex
E. Step reflex

Match the developmental task with the correct age group.

40. ________ Accepting changes in body and appearance
41. ________ Developing leisure-time activities
42. ________ Gaining control of bowel and bladder functions
43. ________ Becoming independent from parents and adults
44. ________ Learning to eat solid foods
45. ________ Adjusting to decreased strength and loss of health
46. ________ Learning how to study
47. ________ Learning how to get along with peers
48. ________ Increasing ability to communicate and understand others
49. ________ Tolerating separation from primary caregiver
50. ________ Learning to live with a partner
51. ________ Developing moral or ethical behavior
52. ________ Learning basic reading, writing, and arithmetic skills
53. ________ Developing stable sleep and feeding patterns
54. ________ Performing self-care activities
55. ________ Using words to communicate with others
56. ________ Adjusting to aging parents
57. ________ Accepting male or female role appropriate for one's age
58. ________ Beginning to talk and communicate with others
59. ________ Choosing education and a career

A. Infancy (birth to 1 year)
B. Toddler (1 to 3 years)
C. Preschooler (3 to 6 years)
D. School Age (6 to 9 or 10 years)
E. Late Childhood (9 or 10 to 12 years)
F. Adolescence (12 to18 years)
G. Young Adulthood (18 to 40 years)
H. Middle Adulthood (40 to 65 years)
I. Late Adulthood (65 years and older)

Crossword Puzzle

Fill in the crossword puzzle by answering the clues with words from this list.

development	menopause	preadolescence	step
grasp	moro	puberty	sucking
growth	neonatal	rooting	

Across

1. Event that occurs to women between ages of 40 and 55
6. Time between childhood and adolescence (late childhood)
8. Reflex that occurs when the lips are touched
9. Physical changes that can be measured and that occur in a steady, orderly manner
10. Changes in mental, emotional, and social function

Down

2. Period between ages of 9 and 15 that girls reach; period between ages of 12 and 16 that boys reach
3. Reflex where the feet move up and down as in stepping motions
4. Reflex that occurs when the cheek is touched near the mouth
5. Period of infancy from birth to 1 month
7. Reflex that occurs a loud noise, a sudden movement, or the head falling back startles the baby
9. Reflex that occurs when the palm is stroked

Optional Learning Exercises

INFANCY

60. You are observing a newborn. You know that the infant
    A. Sleeps ______________ a day
    B. Can turn the head from ______________
61. When an infant is between 1 month and 1 year
    A. He or she has tears and can follow objects with the eyes at __________ months.
    B. The Moro, rooting, and grasp reflexes disappear by __________ months.
    C. The baby can roll from front to back by __________ months.
    D. He or she can learn to drink from a cup with handles by __________ months.
    E. Walking skills increase by __________ months.

TODDLERHOOD

62. During toddlerhood, the developmental tasks are
    A. ______________
    B. ______________
    C. ______________
    D. ______________
63. At 18 months, a toddler knows only ______________ words. By age 2 years, the child knows about ______________ words.

PRESCHOOL

64. What personal skills can be done by a 3 year old?
    A. Put on ______________.
    B. Manage ______________.
    C. Wash ______________.
    D. Brush ______________.
65. Four year olds prefer the primary caregiver of the ______________ sex.
66. Communication skills increase in a 5 year old.
    A. They can speak in ______________.
    B. Questions have more ______________.
    C. The child wants words ______________.

SCHOOL AGE

67. Play in school-age children has a ______________.
    A. They like household tasks such as ______________.
    B. Rewards such as ______________ are important.

LATE CHILDHOOD

68. The developmental tasks of late childhood are like those for ______________________. Preadolescents show more ______________ and ____________________ in achieving the tasks. The tasks are
    A. ______________________
    B. ______________________
    C. ______________________
    D. ______________________
    E. ______________________
    F. ______________________

ADOLESCENCE

69. The developmental tasks of adolescence are
    A. ______________________
    B. ______________________
    C. ______________________
    D. ______________________
    E. ______________________
70. During adolescence, boys grow about ______________________ inches and gain ________________ pounds.
71. Girls grow about ______________ inches and gain ________________ pounds.

YOUNG ADULTHOOD

72. During young adulthood, little physical growth occurs, but ______________________ development will continue.
73. Many factors affect the selection of a partner during young adulthood. They include
    A. ______________________
    B. ______________________
    C. ______________________
    D. ______________________
    E. ______________________
    F. ______________________
    G. ______________________

MIDDLE ADULTHOOD

74. During middle adulthood, weight control becomes a problem because ______________________.
75. People in middle adulthood may have parents who are ______________________ and ______________________. Many also deal with the ____________________ of parents.

LATE ADULTHOOD

76. The developmental tasks of late adulthood are
    A. ______________________
    B. ______________________
    C. ______________________
    D. ______________________
    E. ______________________

Independent Learning Activities

- Ask permission to observe a group of children either at home or in a day care setting. After observing them, answer these questions.
  - How many children did you observe?
  - What stages did you see?
  - List the developmental tasks you could observe in each age group.
  - How many children in each age group were meeting all of the developmental tasks?
  - How many children did you see that were not meeting developmental tasks for the age group?
  - What differences did you see in physical sizes of children in the same age groups?
  - How did physical size relate to development? For example, did the biggest children seem more or less advanced in developmental tasks?

- Look at the information in the textbook that relates to your own age and answer these questions.
  - How many developmental tasks have been met? Were these tasks met during the stage you are in or at an earlier stage?
  - How many developmental tasks have not been met? Are these the tasks that you are now working toward? What steps are you taking to meet these tasks?

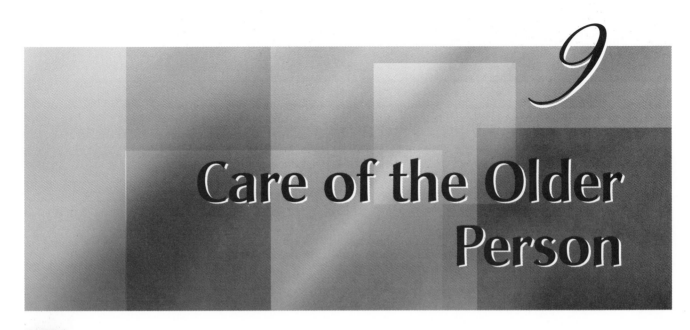

9 Care of the Older Person

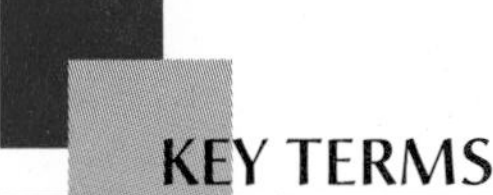

KEY TERMS

Geriatrics
Gerontology
Involuntary seclusion
Old
Old-old
Ombudsman
Young-old

Fill in the Blanks: Key Terms

1. Persons 85 years of age and older are ________________.
2. ________________ is separating a person from others against his or her will; keeping the person confined to a certain area or away from his or her room without consent.
3. Persons between 65 and 74 years of age are ________________.
4. ________________ is the care of aging people.
5. Persons between 75 and 84 years of age are ________________.
6. The study of the aging process is ________________.
7. An ________________ is someone who supports or promotes the needs and interests of another person.

Circle the BEST Answer

8. How many people are currently over 65?
   A. 1 in 10
   B. 1 in 100
   C. 1 in 8
   D. 1 in 4
9. Most older people live
   A. In a nursing center
   B. Alone
   C. In a family setting
   D. With non-relatives

10. The old-old age range is
    A. 65 to 74 years
    B. 75 to 84 years
    C. 60 to 65 years
    D. 85 years and older

11. As aging occurs
    A. Disability always results.
    B. Changes are gradual.
    C. Most people adapt poorly.
    D. All of the above occur.

12. Social changes of aging include
    A. Graying hair
    B. Disabilities
    C. Retirement and deaths of loved ones
    D. Decreased physical strength

13. All of these are benefits of retiring *except*
    A. The person can do whatever he or she wants.
    B. Travel and leisure time activities are possible.
    C. The person can relax and enjoy life.
    D. The person may have poor health and medical bills.

14. Money problems can result with retirement because
    A. Income is reduced.
    B. Expenses increase.
    C. The person is unable to work.
    D. The person planned for retirement.

15. Reduced income may force life-style changes such as
    A. Buying cheaper food
    B. Avoiding buying needed drugs
    C. Relying on family for money
    D. All of the above

16. Loneliness may be a bigger problem for foreign-born persons because
    A. Families from other cultures do not care about older persons.
    B. Native-born persons do not accept the person.
    C. They may not have anyone to talk to in their native language.
    D. They have more chronic illnesses.

17. An older person can adjust to social relationship changes by doing all of these *except*
    A. Stay at home alone to save money.
    B. Find new friends.
    C. Develop hobbies and attend church and community activities.
    D. Maintain regular contact with family.

18. A benefit when children care for older parents may be
    A. The older person may feel unwanted and useless.
    B. The older person may feel more secure.
    C. Tension may develop among the children and the family.
    D. Parents and children change roles.

19. When a partner dies, the older person
    A. Accepts this as part of life
    B. May develop serious physical and mental problems
    C. Easily forms new friendships
    D. Usually has prepared for this change

20. What causes wrinkles to appear on an older person?
    A. Decreases in oil and sweat gland secretions
    B. Fewer nerve endings
    C. Loss of elasticity, strength, and fatty tissue layer
    D. Poor circulation

21. Healing in older people is delayed as a result of
    A. Poor nutrition
    B. Decreased number of blood vessels
    C. Fewer nerve endings
    D. Loss of fatty tissue

22. Hot water bottles and heating pads are not used with older persons because
    A. Older persons generally complain that they are too warm.
    B. The skin is dry.
    C. Burns are a risk because of decreased sensitivity to heat and cold.
    D. Blood vessels decrease in number.

23. Older persons can prevent bone loss and loss of muscle strength by
    A. Participating in activities and exercise and maintaining a good diet
    B. Taking hormones
    C. Resting with feet elevated
    D. Taking vitamins

24. Bones may break easily because
    A. Joints become stiff and painful.
    B. Joints become slightly flexed.
    C. Bones lose strength and become brittle.
    D. Vertebrae shorten.

25. Dizziness may increase in older people because
    A. They have difficulty sleeping.
    B. Blood flow to the brain is decreased.
    C. Nerve cells are lost.
    D. Brain cells are lost.

26. Older persons
    A. Have longer memories
    B. Often remember events from long ago better than recent events
    C. May remember more recent events better than events of long ago
    D. Always become confused as aging progresses

27. Painful injuries and disease may go unnoticed because
    A. The person is confused.
    B. Touch and sensitivity to pain are reduced.
    C. Memory is shorter.
    D. The blood flow is reduced.

28. Older people often complain that food has no taste because
    A. Memory loss has occurred.
    B. The appetite decreases.
    C. Taste buds decrease in number.
    D. They cannot sense heat and cold.

29. Eyes become easily irritated because
    A. The lens yellows.
    B. The eye takes longer to adjust to changes in light.
    C. Tear secretion is less.
    D. The person becomes farsighted.

30. When severe circulatory changes occur, the person
    A. May be encouraged to walk long distances
    B. May need rest periods during the day
    C. May not do any kind of exercise
    D. Should only exercise once a week

31. When a person has difficulty breathing, it is easier to breathe when
    A. Lying flat in bed
    B. Covered with heavy bed linens
    C. Allowed to be on bedrest
    D. Resting in the semi-Fowler's position

32. Dulled taste and smell decreases
    A. Peristalsis
    B. Appetite
    C. Saliva
    D. Swallowing

33. Older persons need
    A. Fewer calories
    B. Less fluids
    C. More calories
    D. Low protein diets

34. Many older persons have to urinate several times during the night because
    A. Bladder infections are common.
    B. Urine is more concentrated.
    C. The bladder size decreases.
    D. Urinary incontinence may occur.

35. Having a side-by-side refrigerator or an elevated dishwasher may help an older person who has
    A. Poor eyesight
    B. Limited reach
    C. Limited flexibility
    D. A hearing loss

36. An elevated toilet seat and shower seat is helpful for the person with
    A. Limited reach
    B. Poor eyesight
    C. Limited flexibility and lifting
    D. A hearing loss

37. Therapies to regain or maintain the highest level of functioning may be given in the home by
    A. Homemaker services
    B. Rehabilitation services
    C. A case manager
    D. Home health care

38. All of these are advantages of an older person living with family *except*
    A. It provides companionship.
    B. The family can provide care.
    C. They can share living expenses.
    D. Sleep arrangements may need to change.

39. Adult day care centers
    A. Provide meals, supervision, and activities for older persons
    B. Only accept self-care persons and those who can walk without help
    C. Provide complete care
    D. Provide respite care

40. Living in apartment allows persons to
    A. Remain independent
    B. Share common meals with others
    C. Enjoy gardening and yard work
    D. Repair appliances and maintain the property

41. A housing option that is a group of apartments for people of the same age is
    A. An accessory apartment
    B. Congregate housing
    C. Homesharing
    D. Assisted living

42. Assisted living facilities provide the following *except*
    A. Nursing care
    B. Help with meals
    C. Health care
    D. Social contact with other residents

43. Continuing care retirement communities (CCRC)
    A. Have independent living units
    B. Have food service and help nearby
    C. Add services, as the person's needs change
    D. All of the above

44. Nursing centers are housing options for older persons who
    A. Need only companionship
    B. Cannot care for themselves
    C. Need care during the daytime while family members work
    D. Are developmentally disabled

45. A quality nursing center must meet OBRA requirements to
    A. Be approved by the medical society
    B. Receive Medicare and Medicaid funds
    C. Give care
    D. Be licensed by the local health department

46. A quality nursing center would *not* be required to have
    A. An activity area for resident's use
    B. Halls wide enough to allow two wheelchairs to pass with ease
    C. Toilet facilities that can be accessed with wheelchairs
    D. An area where residents may have a private garden

47. Sufficient space and equipment requirements by OBRA include
    A. Halls with handrails and other safety needs
    B. Private bathrooms for each resident
    C. Expectation of residents to provide furniture for their rooms
    D. Tablecloths and cloth napkins in dining room

48. Quality of life requirements of OBRA include all of these *except*
    A. Acceptable noise level
    B. Individual televisions for each resident
    C. Paint or wallpaper that is appealing to residents
    D. Clean, soft, adequate linens for residents

49. Under OBRA, a resident has all of the following rights *except* the right to
    A. Personally choose what to wear and how to spend their time
    B. A private room in which to live
    C. Personal privacy
    D. Refuse treatment

50. Under OBRA, if a resident is incompetent (not able) to exercise his or her rights, who can exercise these rights for him or her?
    A. The doctor
    B. Spouse or adult child
    C. The charge nurse
    D. A neighbor

51. If a resident refuses treatment, what should you do?
    A. Avoid giving any care to the person, and go on to other duties.
    B. Report the refusal to the nurse.
    C. Tell the resident that the treatment must be done, and continue to carry out the treatment.
    D. Tell his family so they can make him take the treatment.

52. A student wants to observe a treatment, but the resident does not want him or her to be present. What is the correct action?
    A. The student cannot watch because doing so violates the resident's right to privacy.
    B. The student may observe from the doorway where the resident cannot see him or her.
    C. The staff nurse tells the resident that he or she must allow the student to watch.
    D. The nurse calls the resident's spouse to get permission.

53. The resident should be given the personal choice whenever it
    A. Is safely possible
    B. Does not interfere with scheduled activities
    C. Is approved by the director of nursing
    D. Is ordered by the doctor

54. If a resident voices concerns about the care and the center promptly tries to correct the situation, this action meets the resident's right to
    A. Participate in a resident group
    B. Voice a dispute or grievance
    C. Personal choice
    D. Freedom from abuse, mistreatment, and neglect

55. A resident volunteers to take care of house plants at the center. This activity is acceptable as part of all of the following *except*
    A. The care plan
    B. A requirement to receive care or care items
    C. The resident's regular activity
    D. Rehabilitation

56. When the resident and family plan activities together, this meets the resident's right to
    A. Privacy
    B. Freedom from restraint
    C. Freedom from mistreatment
    D. Participate in resident and family groups

57. The resident you are caring for has many old holiday decorations covering her nightstand. If you throw away these items without her permission, you are denying her right to
    A. Privacy
    B. Work
    C. Care and security of personal possessions
    D. Freedom from abuse

58. A staff member tells a resident that he cannot leave his room because he talks too much. This action denies the resident
    A. Freedom from involuntary seclusion
    B. Freedom from restraint
    C. Care and security of personal possessions
    D. Personal choice

59. When a resident is given certain drugs that affect mood, behavior, or mental function, it may deny the resident's right to
    A. Freedom from abuse, mistreatment, and neglect
    B. Personal choice
    C. Privacy
    D. Freedom from restraint

60. Which of these actions is part of giving courteous and dignified care?
    A. Calling the resident by a nickname he or she does not choose
    B. Assisting with dressing the person in clothing appropriate to the time of day
    C. Changing the resident's hairstyle without his or her permission
    D. Leaving the bathroom door open so you can see the person

61. You ask a resident if you may touch him or her. This is an example of
    A. Providing courteous and dignified interaction
    B. Providing courteous and dignified care
    C. Providing privacy and self-determination
    D. Maintaining personal choice and independence

62. Assisting a resident to ambulate without interfering with his or her independence is an example of
    A. Providing courteous and dignified interaction
    B. Providing courteous and dignified care
    C. Providing privacy and self-determination
    D. Maintaining personal choice and independence

63. You provide privacy and self-determination for a resident when you
    A. Knock on the door before entering and wait to be asked in.
    B. Allow the resident to smoke in designated areas.
    C. Listen with interest to what the person is saying.
    D. Groom his beard as he wishes.

64. You allow the resident to maintain personal choice and independence when you
    A. Obtain his or her attention before interacting with him or her.
    B. Provide extra clothing for warmth such as a sweater or lap robe.
    C. Assist the resident to take part in activities according to his or her interests.
    D. Use curtains or screens during personal care and procedures.

65. An ombudsman carries out which of these activities?
    A. Organize activities for a group of residents.
    B. Accompany residents to a religious service at a house of worship.
    C. Investigate and resolve complaints made by a resident.
    D. Assist the resident to choose friends.

Matching

Match physical changes during the aging process with the body system affected.

66. ________ Reduced blood flow to kidneys
67. ________ Arteries narrow and are less elastic
68. ________ Forgetfulness
69. ________ Gradual loss of height
70. ________ Decreased strength for coughing
71. ________ Decreased secretion of oil and sweat glands
72. ________ Difficulty digesting fried and fatty foods
73. ________ Heart pumps with less force
74. ________ Bladder muscles weaken
75. ________ Difficulty seeing green and blue colors
76. ________ Difficulty swallowing
77. ________ Less elastic lung tissue
78. ________ Bone mass decreases
79. ________ Facial hair in some women

A. Integumentary
B. Musculoskeletal
C. Nervous
D. Cardiovascular
E. Respiratory
F. Digestive
G. Urinary

Optional Learning Exercises

80. When bathing an older person, what kind of soap should be used?

    ____

    ____

    Often no soap is used on the ______________.

81. What can happen if a nick or cut occurs on the feet?

    ____

    ____

    Why can this happen?

    ____

    ____

82. When bone mass decreases, why is it important to turn an older person carefully?

    ____

    ____

83. Why does an older person often have a gradual loss of height?

    ____

    ____

84. What types of exercise help prevent bone loss and loss of muscle strength?

    ____

    ____

85. Older people have changes in the nervous system. When the following changes happen, what physical problems occur?

    A. Nerve conduction and reflexes are slower:

    ____

    ____

    B. Blood flow to brain is reduced:

    ____

    ____

    C. Progressive loss of brain cells:

    ____

    ____

86. When you are eating with an older person, you notice she puts salt on vegetables that taste fine to you. What may be a reason she does this?

    ____

    ____

    ____

87. A female nurse has a high-pitched voice, and several residents seem to have difficulty hearing her. They do not complain about hearing the male charge nurse. What may be a reason for the difference?

    ____

    ____

    ____

88. What exercises will help a person who must stay in bed with circulation changes?

    ____

    ____

    ____

89. What can the nursing assistant do to prevent respiratory complications from bed rest?

    ____

    ____

    ____

90. The stomach and colon empty slower, and flatulence and constipation are common in the older person. What causes these problems?

    ____

    ____

    ____

91. How does good oral hygiene and denture care improves food intake?

    ____

    ____

    ____

92. How can a nursing assistant help prevent urinary tract infections in an older person?

    ____

    ____

    ____

93. Why should you plan to give most fluids to the older person before 1700 (5:00 PM)?

    ____

    ____

    ____

Independent Learning Activities

- Interview an older person who lives independently. Use these questions to find what concerns the person has about remaining independent.
  - What physical problems does the person have, if any?
  - What activities are more difficult than they were when the person was younger?
  - What does the person use to provide safety (walkers, canes, alarms, daily phone calls)?
  - What comfort measures are needed to decrease pain or to help the person sleep?
  - What are the person's transportation needs? Does the person drive? How does the person grocery shop? Visit with family, friends? Attend social functions?
  - How are social needs met? How often does the person go to social events? How often does the person have visitors?

- Interview an older person and talk about life when the person was younger.
  - Observe facial expression and tone of voice when the person talks about events remembered. What changes do you see?
  - Compare how well the person remembers events of long ago with those that happened more recently.
  - How do you feel differently about the person after hearing about the person's youth?

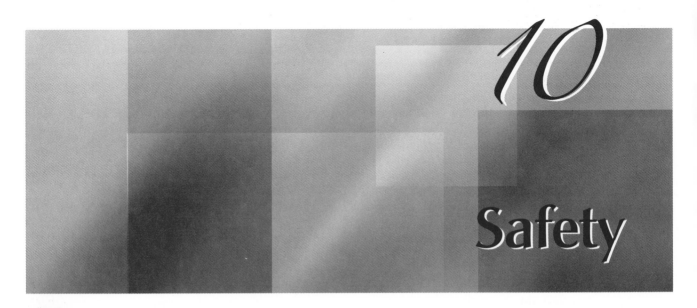

10 Safety

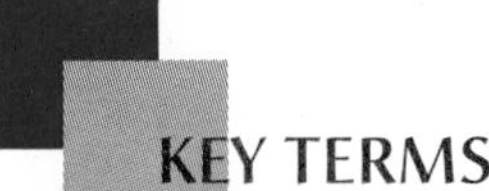

KEY TERMS

Coma
Disaster
Electrical shock
Ground
Hazardous substance
Hemiplegia
Paraplegia
Quadriplegia
Suffocation
Workplace violence

Fill in the Blanks: Key Terms

1. ______________________ are violent acts (including assault or threat of assault) directed toward persons at work or while on duty.
2. Paralysis from the neck down is ______________________.
3. ______________________ is any chemical that presents a physical hazard or a health hazard in the workplace.
4. A ______________________ is a sudden catastrophic event in which many people are injured and killed and property is destroyed.
5. ______________________ occurs when breathing stops from the lack of oxygen.
6. Paralysis on one side of the body is ______________________.
7. A ________ is a state of being unaware of one's surroundings and being unable to react or respond to people, places, or things.
8. That which carries leaking electricity to the earth and away from an electrical appliance is a ______________________.
9. ______________________ is paralysis from the waist down.
10. ______________________ occurs when electrical current passes through the body.

Circle the BEST Answer

11. To protect the person from harm you need to
    A. Use restraints.
    B. Follow the person's care plan.
    C. Limit mobility.
    D. Lock all doors.

12. Impaired vision may increase risk of injury by
    A. Leading to falls over objects
    B. Causing disorientation
    C. Preventing the person from hearing explanations and instructions
    D. Decreasing the pain sense

13. Drugs can be an accident risk factor because they
    A. Affect hearing
    B. Reduce ability to sense heat and cold
    C. Can cause loss of balance or lack of coordination
    D. Can cause hemiplegia

14. Children are at risk of injury because they
    A. Have not learned the difference between safety and danger
    B. Have not learned right from wrong
    C. Have problems sensing heat and cold
    D. Have poor vision

15. All of these are safety measures to use with young children *except*
    A. Prop the baby bottle on a rolled towel or blanket to feed a baby.
    B. Children between 4 and 8 years of age should use booster seats with a lap and shoulder belt in a vehicle.
    C. Remove drawstrings from jackets, coats, sweaters, and other clothing.
    D. Do not let children play with toys that make loud, sharp, or shrill noises.

16. Accident risk factors in older persons are all of the following *except*
    A. They may have poor vision or hearing problems.
    B. Balance is affected, and they fall easily.
    C. They are less sensitive to heat and cold.
    D. They are more sensitive to hazardous materials.

17. Identifying persons is most important because
    A. You need to give the right care to the right person.
    B. Visitors may ask your help to find someone.
    C. You need to call the person by the right name.
    D. You will have to give care to two people if you give it to the wrong person first.

18. Which of these is not a reliable way to identify the person?
    A. Check the identification bracelet.
    B. Use the person's picture to compare with the person.
    C. If person is alert and oriented, follow the center policy to identify.
    D. Call the person by name.

19. Falls may occur at shift change because
    A. People become restless when new caregivers come on duty.
    B. Confusion can occur about who is giving care and answering signal lights.
    C. People require more care at that time.
    D. No staff members are available at that time.

20. Which of these is *not* a factor that increases the risks of falling?
    A. Medication side effects
    B. Dizziness on standing
    C. Elimination needs
    D. High blood pressure

21. You will find a list of measures for the person's specific risk factors of falls in the
    A. Nurse's notes
    B. Flow sheet
    C. Care plan
    D. Doctor's orders

22. Bed rails
    A. Are used for all persons
    B. Are safe for confused and disoriented persons
    C. Are raised when the nurse and the care plan tells you
    D. Can be used when you think the person needs them

23. Gaps should be 4 inches or less
    A. Between the mattress and the headboard
    B. Between the bed rail and the mattress
    C. From the bed controls to the bed rails
    D. Between the mattress and the footboard

24. Bed rails cannot be used
    A. When the bed is in the lowest position
    B. When the bed is in the highest position
    C. Unless the person or the legal representative gives consent for raised bed rails
    D. When the person is alert

25. If you raise the bed and the person does not use bed rails, you should
    A. Raise the far bed rail if you are working alone.
    B. Raise both rails if you leave the bedside.
    C. Tell the person to lie still if you need to leave the bedside.
    D. Ask a co-worker to stand on the far side of the bed.

26. Which of these would be a safety measure to prevent falls?
    A. Allow the person to walk to the bathroom in his or her socks.
    B. Place a scatter rug next to the bed.
    C. Securely tie the person's robe belt.
    D. Turn out all lights at night.

27. When checking a crib for safety, two adult fingers should fit between the
    A. Crib rail slats
    B. Top of the crib rail and the mattress
    C. Crib rail and the mattress
    D. The baby's head and the space around the mattress

28. Handrails or grab bars
    A. Provide support for persons who are weak or unsteady when walking
    B. Provide support sitting down or getting up from a toilet
    C. Are used in getting in and out of a tub
    D. All of the above

29. Wheels on beds, wheelchairs, or stretchers are locked to
    A. Keep the equipment properly positioned.
    B. Prevent injury to you or the person.
    C. Keep the person from moving the furniture.
    D. Keep your body in alignment.

30. A leading cause of death, especially among children and older persons, is
    A. Falls
    B. Burns
    C. Accidental poisoning
    D. Suffocation

31. When children are in the kitchen
    A. Use the stove's back burners.
    B. Turn pot and pan handles so they point outward.
    C. Let children help you cook at the stove.
    D. Leave cooking utensils in pots and pans.

32. Oven mitts and potholders are kept dry because
    A. They conduct heat better.
    B. Water conducts heat and can cause burns.
    C. Moisture allows bacteria to move through the cloth.
    D. All of the above are true.

33. Accidental poisoning can occur when
    A. Harmful products are kept in their original containers.
    B. Harmful substances are labeled and stored in high, locked areas.
    C. Drugs are carried in purses, backpacks, and briefcases.
    D. Safety latches are used on kitchen, bathroom, garage, basement, and workshop cabinets.

34. Poison warning stickers should be placed on common poisons such as
    A. Drugs and vitamins
    B. Detergents, sprays, window cleaners, and paint thinner
    C. Fertilizers, insecticides, and bug sprays
    D. All of the above

35. A choking hazard for older persons can be
    A. Loose teeth or dentures
    B. Sitting up in a wheelchair to eat
    C. Food that is cut into small, bite-size pieces
    D. Making sure the person is properly positioned in bed

36. Which of these would prevent choking in children?
    A. Position infants on their stomachs for sleep.
    B. Use Mylar balloons instead of latex ones.
    C. Give the child food such as hot dogs, peanuts, or popcorn.
    D. Place an infant on a soft pillow or comforter to sleep.

37. A gas that can cause suffocation is
    A. Oxygen
    B. Carbon dioxide
    C. Carbon monoxide
    D. Nitrogen

38. If you find a piece of equipment that is damaged, take it to the
    A. Nurse
    B. Maintenance department
    C. Fire department
    D. Director of nursing

39. When using electrical items, you should
    A. Use a three-pronged plug.
    B. Touch the equipment even if you are wet.
    C. Unplug the equipment before turning it off.
    D. Use water to put out an electrical fire.

40. An electrical shock is especially dangerous because it can
    A. Start a fire
    B. Damage equipment
    C. Affect the heart and cause death
    D. Violate OBRA regulations

41. If you are shocked by electric equipment, you should
    A. Report the shock at once.
    B. Try to see what is wrong with the equipment.
    C. Make sure it has a ground prong.
    D. Test the equipment in a different outlet.

42. Wheelchair brakes should be locked when
    A. Transporting the person
    B. Taking a wheelchair up or down stairs
    C. Transferring a person to or from the wheelchair
    D. Storing the wheelchair

43. When moving a person on a stretcher, all of these practices are correct *except*
    A. Use safety straps only when the person is confused.
    B. Lock the stretcher before transferring the person.
    C. Do not leave the person unattended.
    D. Stand at the head of the stretcher. Your co-worker stands at the foot.

44. ____________________ requires that health care employees understand the risks of hazardous substances and how to handle them safely.
    A. OBRA
    B. Occupational Safety and Health Administration (OSHA)
    C. Joint Commission on Accreditation of Healthcare Organizations (JCAHO)
    D. Material safety data sheets (MSDS)

45. Warning labels may include all of these *except*
    A. Physical hazards and health hazards
    B. What protective equipment to wear
    C. The telephone number of the local emergency system
    D. Storage and disposal information

46. Where would you find the MSDS for hazardous materials?
    A. Attached to the substance
    B. In the administrator's office
    C. In a binder at a specified location on each unit
    D. On the Internet

47. All of these things are needed for a fire *except*
    A. Spark or flame
    B. Electrical equipment
    C. Materials that will burn
    D. Oxygen

48. If a person is receiving oxygen, he or she is at special risk for
    A. Burns
    B. Suffocation
    C. Poisoning
    D. Electrical shock

49. When a person is receiving oxygen, which of these is allowed in the room?
    A. Smoking by visitors but not by the person receiving oxygen
    B. Wool blankets and fabrics that may cause static electricity
    C. Electrical items that are in good working order
    D. Oil, grease, alcohol, and nail polish remover

50. If a fire occurs, what should you do first?
    A. Rescue people in immediate danger.
    B. Sound the nearest fire alarm, and call the switchboard operator.
    C. Close doors and windows to confine the fire.
    D. Use a fire extinguisher on a small fire that has not spread to a larger area.

51. If evacuation is necessary, persons who are
    A. Closest to the outside door are rescued first
    B. Able to walk are rescued last
    C. Closest to the danger are evacuated first
    D. Helpless are rescued last

52. If a space heater is used in a home, a safety practice is to
    A. Place the heater in doorways or on stairs.
    B. Keep heater 3 feet away from curtains, drapes, and furniture.
    C. Store fuel near the heater.
    D. Fill the heater when it is hot or running.

53. If you are in an apartment building and a fire occurs
    A. Use the fire alarm system and yell, "Fire!"
    B. Quickly take the elevator to the ground floor.
    C. Make sure you know one escape route.
    D. Go back into the building to help others.

54. If there is a disaster, you
    A. Are expected to go to your agency immediately
    B. May be called into work if you are off duty
    C. Should stay away or leave to get out of the way
    D. May go home to check on your family

55. Why do more assaults occur in health care settings than in other industries?
    A. Patients may be persons who are arrested or convicted of crimes.
    B. Acutely disturbed and violent persons may seek health care.
    C. Agency pharmacies are a source of drugs and therefore a target for robberies.
    D. All of the above are true.

56. Which of these would *not* be effective to prevent or control workplace violence?
    A. Stand away from the person.
    B. Know where to find panic buttons, call bells, and alarms.
    C. Sit quietly with the person in his or her room. Hold the person's hand to calm him or her.
    D. Tell the person you will get a nurse to speak to him or her.

57. You can help prevent workplace violence by doing all of these *except*
    A. Wearing long hair up and off the collar
    B. Making sure shoes have good soles that do not slip
    C. Wearing necklaces, bracelets, and earrings
    D. Wearing uniforms that fit well

58. If you are uncomfortable or threatened in a home setting, you should
    A. Report the matter to the nurse.
    B. Stay at the home and try to resolve the matter.
    C. Confront the person who is making you uncomfortable.
    D. Ignore the situation, and continue to give care.

59. When you are filling out a valuables list or envelope, which of these would be the best description?
    A. "Diamond in a gold setting"
    B. "One-carat diamond in a 14-carat gold setting"
    C. "White stone in a yellow setting"
    D. "White diamond-like stone in a gold-like setting"

Matching

Match each safety measure with the risk of injury it prevents.

60. ________ Do not use electric blankets.
61. ________ Keep person's room free of clutter.
62. ________ Ensure that people smoke only in smoking areas.
63. ________ Keep electrical items away from water.
64. ________ Assist persons with elimination needs at regular times and whenever a request is made.
65. ________ Do not give a person a shower or tub bath when there is an electrical storm.
66. ________ Never leave a person unattended in the bathtub.
67. ________ Report loose teeth or dentures to the nurse.
68. ________ Use correct equipment to move and transfer persons from bed and chair.
69. ________ Do not touch a person who is experiencing an electrical shock.
70. ________ Move all persons from the area if you smell gas or smoke.
71. ________ Do not allow smoking near oxygen tanks or concentrators.

A. Burns
B. Suffocation
C. Falls
D. Equipment

Optional Learning Exercises

72. What does RACE mean when a fire occurs?

A. R: ________________________________

B. A: ________________________________

C. C: ________________________________

D. E: ________________________________

What safety measures for infants and children is being followed in each example (Box 10-1)?

73. The babysitter makes sure she can see the child when she goes to answer the telephone.

____

____

74. You replace the bottle cap on the floor cleaner after you use it.

____

____

75. The 5 year-old sleeps in the bottom bunk, and the 8-year-old sleeps in the top bunk.

____

____

76. The primary caregiver keeps the hair dryer in the bedroom, not in the bathroom.

____

____

77. The furniture in the living room is arranged so that no furniture is under the window.

____

____

78. When visiting the community pool with children, the mother brings her cell phone.

____

____

79. When you finish cleaning the floor, you empty the bucket and turn it upside down for storage.

____

____

80. The parents decide to get a new car safety seat for an infant instead of using the seat they used for their 11-year-old child.

____

____

81. The mother takes away her necklace from the child, even though it makes the child cry.

____

____

82. When the mother buys a kid's meal at a fast-food restaurant, she reads the toy package before giving it to her 3 year old.

____

____

83. When you are helping the primary caregiver set the table for dinner, she tells you not to use the placemats.

____

____

Certain factors increase the risk for falls. List the risk in each example (Box 10-2).

84. The person is wearing bedroom slippers that are a size too big.

____

____

85. The person falls when he or she tries to go to the bathroom without assistance.

____

____

86. The person is lying in bed, stands up too quickly, and falls.

____

____

87. A person who was recently admitted to the agency gets out of bed and trips when going the wrong direction to the bathroom.

____

____

88. The person cannot find his or her glasses and falls over a chair.

____

____

89. The person trips on his intravenous (IV) pole while walking down the hall.

____

____

Which safety measure is practiced to prevent falls in each example (Box 10-3)?

90. The nursing assistant picks up newspapers that are lying next to the bed.

____

____

91. A bathmat is placed in the tub.

____

____

92. The person wears rubber-soled shoes with Velcro closures.

____

____

93. The nursing assistant takes the person to the bathroom at 8 AM, 10 AM, and 2 AM.

____

____

94. The nursing assistant gives the person a back massage and a warm drink at bedtime.

____

____

95. The nursing assistant checks the name label on the walker before giving it to the person.

____

____

96. The nursing assistant notices the signal light has fallen on the floor after visitors leave.

____

____

Read the following examples, and write the related safety measure (Box 10-4).

97. Matches are kept on the top shelf of the cupboard.

____

____

98. When getting ready to cook, the cook takes off a bulky sweater.

____

____

99. Before picking up her baby, the mother sets her coffee cup on the table.

____

____

100. Before putting a young child in the bathtub, the primary caregiver reaches in and stirs the water.

____

____

101. The nursing assistant takes the heating pad out of the bed before the person goes to bed for the night.

____

____

102. The nursing assistant sits with the confused person while he or she smokes.

____

____

Read the following examples, and write the related safety measure (Boxes 10-5 and 10-6).

103. Dates on harmful substances stored in the home are checked.

____

____

104. You ask a visitor to your home to put her purse out of reach from your children.

____

____

105. You notice the person you are caring for has dentures that are poorly fitted. You notify the nurse because

____

____

106. A crib has only a sheet with a light blanket to cover the baby while he or she sleeps.

Read the following examples and write the related safety measure (Boxes 10-7 and 10-8).

107. The nursing assistant tells the person his or her shower will be delayed until the storm passes.

108. The nursing assistant tells the nurse that he or she has never used the portable footbath before.

109. The nursing assistant carefully dries his or her hands before plugging in a razor.

110. An electric fan will not work, and the staff member follows the correct procedure to have it repaired.

111. The nursing assistant moves an electrical cord that is lying across a heat vent.

112. The nursing assistant makes sure the person has both feet on the wheelchair footrests.

113. The nursing assistant notices one wheel is flat on a wheelchair and reports it to the nurse.

114. The nursing assistant locks the wheelchair when the person is sitting in it next to his or her bed.

When handling hazardous materials, what should you do in these situations (Box 10-9)?

115. When cleaning up a hazardous material, how do you know what equipment to wear?

116. When a spill occurs, what is the correct way to wipe it up?

117. The nurse tells the nursing assistant the person is having an x-ray taken in her room.

118. The nurse tells you to open the windows in a room where you are cleaning up a hazardous material.

What fire prevention measure is being practiced in each example (Box 10-10)?

119. The person is taken to the smoking area in his or her wheelchair.

120. When cleaning a smoking area, the staff uses a metal can partially filled with sand.

____

____

121. When heating food for a person, the nursing assistant remains in the kitchen.

____

____

What measures in these examples (Box 10-11) are used or should be used to prevent or control workplace violence?

122. What types of jewelry can serve as a weapon?

____

____

123. Why is long hair worn up?

____

____

124. Why are pictures, vases, and other items removed from certain areas?

____

____

125. What type of glass protects nurses' stations, reception areas, and admitting areas?

____

____

126. What clothing items should be worn by staff to allow the ability to run?

____

____

List personal safety practices that apply in these situations (Box 10-12).

127. Why should you park your car in a parking garage?

____

____

128. What items should you keep in the car for safety?

____

____

129. Why is a "dry run" important?

____

____

130. If you think someone is following you, what should you do?

____

____

131. If someone wants your wallet or purse, what should you do?

____

____

132. How can you use your car keys as a weapon?

____

____

133. How can you use your thumbs as a weapon?

____

____

134. What part of the body can you attack on either a man or woman?

____

____

Independent Learning Activities

- Safety is important to everyone and needs to be practiced at all times. Check the following items or areas in your own home to determine whether it is safe.
  - What areas are adequately lighted for safety? What areas need improved lighting?
  - Check electrical cords and plugs on appliances and lamps. How many have frayed cords? Ungrounded plugs? Other problems that make them unsafe to use?
  - How many smoke detectors do you have in your home? When were the batteries last replaced? How can you check the smoke detector to make sure it is working correctly?
  - How many scatter rugs are used on slippery surfaces? How many have some type of backing to prevent slipping?
  - Where are hazardous materials (medications, cleaning solutions, painting supplies) stored? Which of these could be reached by children? What could be done to store them more safely?
  - Make a list of good safety practices in your home. Make a list of safety practices that could be improved.

- Develop a plan for your home and family that helps everyone know how to escape if a fire occurs.
  - Make sure every person knows at least two escape routes form the sleeping area.
  - Practice how to check a door for heat before opening.
  - Arrange a place to meet once you are outside the building.

11

Restraint Alternatives and Safe Restraint Use

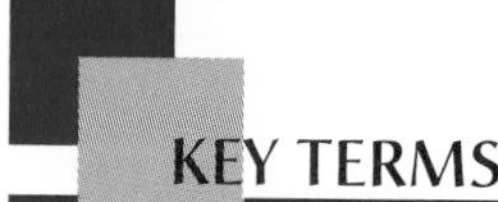

KEY TERMS

Active physical restraint
Passive physical restraint
Restraint

Fill in the Blanks: Key Terms

1. Any item, object, device, garment, material, or drug that limits or restricts a person's freedom of movement or access to one's body is a ______________________________.
2. An ______________________________ is a restraint attached to the person's body and to a fixed (non-movable) object.
3. A ______________________________ is a restraint near but not directly attached to the person's body; it does not totally restrict freedom of movement and allows access to certain body parts.

Circle the BEST Answer

4. Restraints are used
   A. Whenever the nurse feels they are necessary
   B. Only as a last resort to protect persons from harming themselves or others
   C. To ensure the person does not fall
   D. To decrease work for the staff
5. The decision to use restraints is made when the
   A. Nurse uses the nursing process to determine the person's safety needs.
   B. Doctor determines they are needed.
   C. Family requests restraints for the person.
   D. Nursing assistants providing care request the restraints.
6. Research shows that restraints
   A. Prevent falls
   B. Cause falls
   C. Are used whenever the nurse decides
   D. Are not effective
7. A person's harmful behaviors may be caused by
   A. Being afraid of a new setting
   B. Being too hot or too cold
   C. Being hungry or thirsty
   D. All of the above

8. Guidelines about using restraints are part of the resident rights in
   A. Centers for Disease Control and Prevention (CDC) regulations
   B. OSHA rules
   C. OBRA, Food and Drug Administration (FDA), and Centers for Medicare & Medicaid Assistance (CMS) regulations
   D. JCAHO recommendations

9. Restraints are *not* used to
   A. Prevent harm to the person
   B. Control the person's behaviors
   C. Prevent a person from pulling at a wound or dressing
   D. Keep an IV from being pulled out

10. Which of these is a type of restraint?
   A. Soft chair with a footstool to elevate the feet
   B. Bed without bed rails
   C. Geriatric (Geri) chair with a tray
   D. Drug that helps a person function at his or her highest level

11. The most serious risk from restraints
   A. Are cuts, bruises, and fractures
   B. Is death from strangulation
   C. Are falls
   D. Are depression, anger, and agitation

12. After receiving instructions about the proper use of a restraint, you should
   A. Ask for help to apply it to a person.
   B. Demonstrate proper application to the nurse before using it on a person.
   C. Watch someone else apply it to a person.
   D. Independently apply it to the person.

13. Which of these is *not* a physical restraint?
   A. Vest restraint
   B. Chair with an attached tray
   C. Drug that affects the person's mental function
   D. Sheets tucked in so tightly that they restrict movement

14. To use a restraint, the nurse must
   A. Get permission from the family.
   B. Obtain a doctor's order.
   C. Get permission from the interdisciplinary health team.
   D. Receive OBRA permission.

15. Which of these is an active physical restraint?
   A. Vest
   B. Bedrail
   C. Wedge cushion
   D. Pillow

16. Using a restraint requires informed consent. This consent is obtained by the
   A. Person's legal representative
   B. Doctor or nurse
   C. Person
   D. Nursing assistant

17. When restraining a combative and agitated person, it should be done
   A. Slowly by only one person
   B. Only after explaining to the person what will be done
   C. With enough staff to complete the task safely and efficiently
   D. In a public area so the person is distracted

18. The person who is restrained must be observed every
   A. 5 minutes
   B. 15 minutes
   C. 1 hour
   D. 2 hours

19. When a person is restrained, every 2 hours you should
   A. Check the person.
   B. Remove the restraints, reposition the person, and meet basic needs.
   C. Make sure the restraints are secure.
   D. Remove the restraints until the next shift.

20. Wrist restraints are used when a person
   A. Tries to get out of bed
   B. Moves his or her wheelchair without permission
   C. Pulls at tubes used in medical treatments
   D. Easily slides out of a chair

21. A belt restraint
   A. Is more restrictive than other restraints
   B. Allows the person to turn from side to side
   C. Must be released by the staff
   D. Can only be used in bed

22. The straps of vest and jacket restraints
   A. Always cross in the front
   B. Are applied next to the skin under clothing
   C. Must be secured very tightly to be safe
   D. May cross in the back

23. Elbow restraints are used
   A. To prevent older persons from pulling at tubes
   B. For children to limit movements and prevent scratching and touching incisions
   C. On only one arm at a time
   D. To prevent injury to the staff by a confused person

24. When applying wrist restraints
    A. Tie the straps to the bed rail.
    B. Tie firm knots in the straps.
    C. Place the restraints over clothing.
    D. Place the soft part toward the skin.

25. If you are using padded mitts restraints, you should
    A. Give the person a hand roll to hold.
    B. Pad the mitt with soft material.
    C. Make sure the person's hands are clean and dry.
    D. Tie the straps to the bed rails.

26. A belt restraint should be
    A. Used only when the person is in a chair or wheelchair
    B. Tightly secured with no slack in the straps
    C. Checked to ensure that the person is comfortable and in good body alignment
    D. Applied next to the skin

27. When using a vest restraint in bed
    A. The straps are secured to the bed frame at waist level out of the person's reach.
    B. The straps are secured to the bed rail.
    C. The vest crosses in the back.
    D. The person can turn over.

28. When you check a person in a vest, jacket, or belt restraint, report at once if
    A. The skin is slightly reddened under the restraint.
    B. The person needs to urinate.
    C. The person is not breathing or is having difficulty breathing.
    D. You need to reposition the person.

Matching

Match the safety guidelines with the correct example.

29. ________ Injuries and deaths have occurred from improper restraint and poor observation.
30. ________ A restraint is used only when it is the best safety precaution for the person.
31. ________ The nurse gives you the printed instructions about safely applying and securing the restraint.
32. ________ Restrained persons need repeated explanations and reassurance.
33. ________ The doctor gives the reason for the restraint, which restraint to use, and how long to use the restraint.
34. ________ Persons in immediate danger of harming themselves or others are quickly restrained.
35. ________ Because they are the least restrictive, passive physical restraints should be used when possible.
36. ________ The goal of this guideline is to meet a person's need to use as little restraint as possible.
37. ________ If told to apply a restraint, you must clearly understand the need.
38. ________ When the restraint is removed, range-of-motion exercises are performed or the person is ambulated.
39. ________ The care plan must include measures to protect the person and to prevent the person from harming others.
40. ________ The person must understand the reason for the restraints.
41. ________ The person must be comfortable and able to move the restrained part to a limited and safe extent. Food, fluid, comfort, safety, exercise, and elimination needs must be met.

A. Restraints are used to protect the person. They are not used for staff convenience or to discipline a person.
B. Restraints require a doctor's order.
C. The least restrictive method of restraint is used.
D. Restraints are used only after trying other methods to protect the person.
E. Unnecessary restraint is false imprisonment.
F. Informed consent is required for restraint use.
G. The manufacturer's instructions are followed.
H. The person's basic needs must be met.
I. Restraints are applied with enough help to protect the person and staff from injury.
J. Restraints can increase a person's confusion and agitation.
K. Quality of life must be protected.
L. The person is observed at least every 15 minutes or more often as required by the care plan.
M. The restraint is removed, the person repositioned, and basic needs are met at least every 2 hours.

Fill in the Blanks

42. When using restraints, what information is reported and recorded?

A. ______________________

B. ______________________

C. ______________________

D. ______________________

E. ______________________

F. ______________________

G. ______________________

H. ______________________

I. ______________________

J. ______________________

43. When you check the restrained person's circulation every 15 minutes, tell the nurse at once if you observe these signs or symptoms.

A. ______________________

B. ______________________

C. ______________________

D. ______________________

44. When you remove the restraints every 2 hours, what are the basic needs that should be met?

A. ______________________

B. ______________________

C. ______________________

D. ______________________

E. ______________________

45. Persons restrained in a supine position must be monitored constantly because they are a great risk for ______________________.

46. You should carry scissors with you because in an emergency ______________________.

47. When you are asked to apply restraints, what information do you need from the nurse and the care plan?

A. ______________________

B. ______________________

C. ______________________

D. ______________________

E. ______________________

F. ______________________

G. ______________________

H. ______________________

I. ______________________

J. ______________________

K. ______________________

Labeling

48. Explain what is being done in the below figure.

____

____

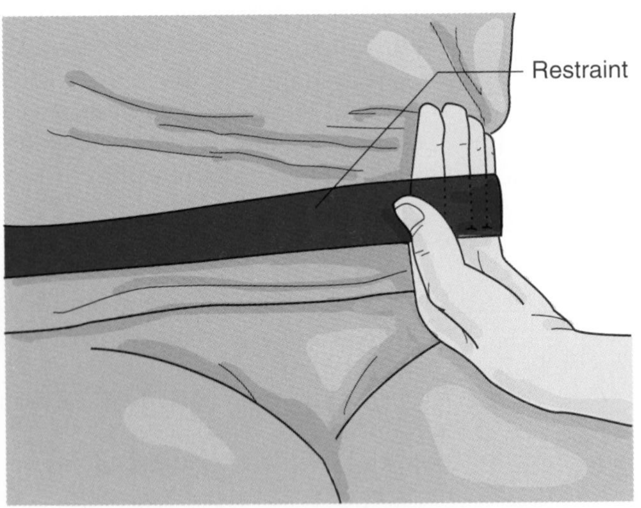

49. Draw a belt restraint applied correctly on the person in the below figure. What is the correct angle for this belt?

____

____

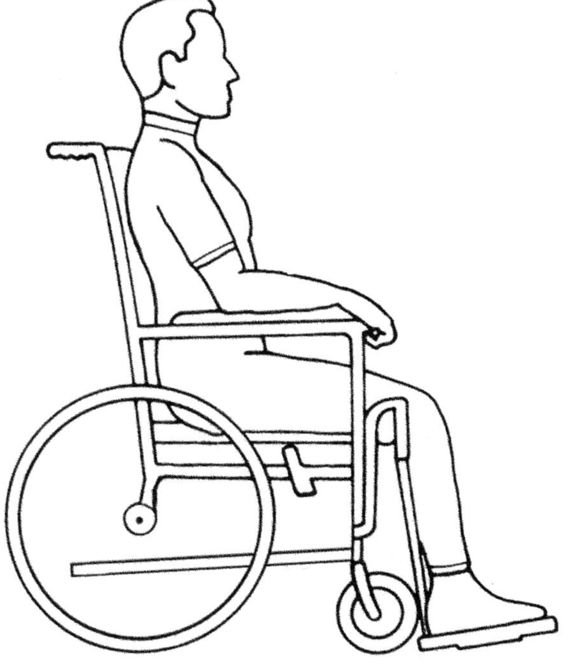

Nursing Assistant Skills Video Exercise

View the **Safety and Restraints** *video to answer these questions.*

50. Where is information about the procedure guidelines obtained?

____

____

51. How do you check to make sure a vest restraint is properly applied to allow breathing?

____

____

52. Where is a vest restraint secured on the bed to prevent sliding?

____

____

53. How do you check a wrist restraint to make sure it is properly applied?

____

____

54. After the restraints are applied, what procedure guidelines are followed?

A. ______________________________

B. ______________________________

C. ______________________________

D. ______________________________

55. If the person wearing a vest restraint has respiratory difficulty you should call ______________________________.

56. If the person wearing a wrist restraint has no pulse and the fingers are cold, blue, or pale, you should ______________________________.

57. What information is recorded and reported?

A. ______________________________

B. ______________________________

C. ______________________________

D. ______________________________

E. ______________________________

F. ______________________________

Optional Learning Exercises

58. How can a drug be considered a restraint?

A. ______________________________

B. ______________________________

C. ______________________________

59. How does a restraint increase incontinence?

____

____

60. What lifelong habits and routines could be included in the nursing care plan as alternatives to restraints?

____

____

61. Why would a person in restraints be at risk for dehydration?

____

____

62. Why would videotapes of family and friends or visiting with family be good alternatives to restraints?

____

____

63. What is the purpose of padded hip protectors and floor cushions?

____

____

Independent Learning Activities

Set up a role-play scenario in which one person is a nursing assistant and one is a person who is restrained. An active physical restraint is applied as the person sits in a chair or wheelchair. When the restraint is in place, the nursing assistant leaves and does not return for 15 minutes. Discuss the following questions with each other after the experiment.

- How did the person feel when the restraints were applied? What did the nursing assistant tell the person about the restraints?
- Did the nursing assistant ask the person if toileting was needed? If the person was thirsty?
- Was the chair comfortable? Was there any padding? Did the nursing assistant check for wrinkles? Could the person move around to reposition his or her body for comfort?
- How was the person able to get help during the 15 minutes of being alone?
- What diversions were offered while the person was restrained? Television or radio? Reading materials? A window with a pleasant view? If any of these were provided, who chose the channel, station, book, or view?
- Was the person told someone would return in 15 minutes? Was a clock or watch available to see the time? How long did it seem?
- What was learned from this experience by both people?

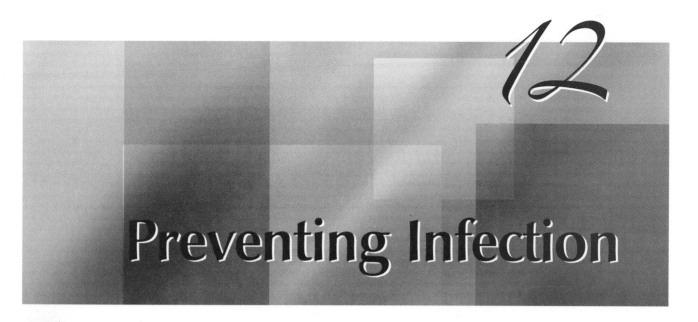

KEY TERMS

Asepsis
Biohazardous waste
Carrier
Clean technique
Communicable disease
Contagious disease
Contamination
Disinfection
Germicide
Immunity
Infection
Medical asepsis
Microbe
Microorganism
Nonpathogen
Normal flora
Nosocomial infection
Pathogen
Reservoir
Spore
Sterile
Sterile field
Sterile technique
Sterilization
Surgical asepsis
Vaccination
Vaccine

Fill in the Blanks: Key Terms

1. A human or animal that is a reservoir for microbes but does not have signs and symptoms of infection is a ______________________.
2. A ______________________ is a small living plant or animal seen only with a microscope; a microbe.
3. Protection against a certain disease is ______________________.
4. A preparation containing dead or weakened microbes is a ______________________.
5. A work area free of all pathogens and nonpathogens is a ______________________.
6. ______________________ are items contaminated with blood, body fluids, secretions, and excretions that may be harmful to others.
7. ______________________ are the practices used to remove or destroy pathogens and to prevent their spread from one person or place to another person or place; clean technique.

8. A communicable disease is also called a ______________________________.

9. An ______________________________ is a disease state resulting from the invasion and growth of microorganisms in the body.

10. ______________________________ is the practices that keep equipment and supplies free of all microbes; sterile technique.

11. A ______________________________ is a disease caused by pathogens that spread easily; contagious disease.

12. The process of destroying pathogens is ______________________________.

13. A ______________________________ is an infection acquired during a stay in a health care agency.

14. ______________________________ is being free of disease-producing microbes.

15. Another name for a microorganism is a ______________________________.

16. The environment in which microbes live and grow is a ______________________________.

17. Medical asepsis is also called ______________________________.

18. The process of becoming unclean is ______________________________.

19. The absence of all microbes is ______________________________.

20. Surgical asepsis is also called ______________________________.

21. A bacterium protected by a hard shell is a ______________________________.

22. ______________________________ are microbes that usually live and grow in a certain area.

23. A disinfectant applied to skin, tissue, or non-living objects is a ______________________________.

24. A microbe that does not usually cause an infection is a ______________________________.

25. ______________________________ is the process of destroying all microbes.

26. A microbe that is harmful and can cause an infection is a ______________________________.

27. The administration of a vaccine to produce immunity against an infectious disease is ______________________________.

Circle the BEST Answer

28. Germs are a type of microbe called
    A. Protozoa
    B. Fungi
    C. Viruses
    D. Bacteria

29. Rickettsiae are transmitted to humans by
    A. Plants
    B. Other humans
    C. Insect bites
    D. One-celled animals

30. To live and grow, all microbes require
    A. Oxygen
    B. A reservoir
    C. A hot environment
    D. Plenty of light

31. Normal flora
    A. Are always pathogens
    B. Are always nonpathogens
    C. Become pathogens when transmitted from their natural site to another site
    D. Cause signs and symptoms of an infection

32. Which of these is *not* a sign or symptom of infection?
    A. Rash
    B. Fatigue and loss of energy
    C. Constipation
    D. Sores on mucous membranes

33. An older person may not show the signs or symptoms of an infection because of changes in the
    A. Diet
    B. Immune system
    C. Mobility of the person
    D. Confusion and delirium

34. The source of infection is
    A. A break in the skin
    B. A human or animal
    C. Nutritional status
    D. A pathogen

35. In the chain of infection, a portal of exit can be
    A. Blood
    B. Human and animals
    C. General health
    D. A carrier

36. Nosocomial infections occur when
    A. Insects are present.
    B. Hand hygiene technique is poor.
    C. Medical asepsis is correctly used.
    D. A person is in isolation.

37. The practice that keeps equipment and supplies free of all microbes is
    A. Medical asepsis
    B. Clean technique
    C. Contamination
    D. Surgical asepsis

38. What is the easiest and most important way to prevent the spread of infection?
    A. Sterilize all equipment.
    B. Use only disposable equipment.
    C. Keep all residents in isolation.
    D. Practice good hand hygiene technique.

39. When washing hands you should
    A. Use hot water.
    B. Keep hands lower than the elbows.
    C. Turn off faucets after lathering.
    D. Keep hands higher than elbows.

40. Clean under the fingernails by rubbing your fingers against your palms
    A. Each time you wash your hands
    B. If you have long nails
    C. Only for the first handwashing of the day
    D. For at least 10 seconds

41. To avoid contaminating your hands, turn off the faucets
    A. After soap is applied
    B. Before drying hands
    C. With clean paper towels
    D. With your elbows

42. An alcohol-based hand rub may be used to decontaminate your hands
    A. When the hands are visibly dirty or soiled with blood, body fluids, or secretions and excretions
    B. After using the restroom
    C. After contact with the intact skin
    D. Before eating

43. You can prevent the spread of microbes in the home by
    A. Thawing frozen foods at room temperature
    B. Emptying garbage at least once a day
    C. Refreezing food items that have partially thawed
    D. Wiping cutting boards with a dry paper towel after use

44. Older persons with dementia rely on others to protect them from infection because they
    A. Do not understand aseptic practices
    B. Are more susceptible to infection
    C. Resist handwashing and other aseptic practices
    D. Never learned good hygiene practices

45. When cleaning dirty equipment
    A. Wear protective equipment.
    B. Rinse in hot water.
    C. Use the clean utility room.
    D. Remove any organic materials with a paper towel.

46. Reusable items are disinfected with
    A. Soap and water
    B. An autoclave
    C. A germicide such as alcohol
    D. High temperatures

47. A good, cheap disinfectant to use in the home is
   A. Chlorine bleach
   B. Ammonia
   C. Vinegar solution
   D. Soap and water

48. If you use boiling water to sterilize items in the home, you should
   A. Pour the water over the items in a sink.
   B. Boil the items for at least 15 minutes.
   C. Boil the items 30 to 45 minutes.
   D. Place the items in the water, bring the water to a boil, and turn the burner off.

49. Standard precautions are used for
   A. A person with a respiratory infection
   B. A person with a wound infection
   C. A person with tuberculosis
   D. All persons

50. Gloves worn in standard precautions
   A. Do not need to be changed when performing several tasks for the same person
   B. Can be worn until they tear or are punctured
   C. Should be removed before going to another person
   D. Are worn only if the person has an infection

51. When you are working in a room with isolation precautions, use paper towels to
   A. Handle contaminated items.
   B. Turn faucets on and off.
   C. Open the door to the person's room.
   D. All of the above are correct uses.

52. Decontaminate your hands
   A. After removing gloves
   B. Only when you leave the isolation area
   C. Only when moving between residents
   D. Only if gloves were not worn

53. If you are allergic to latex gloves, you should
   A. Practice hand hygiene technique each time you remove the gloves.
   B. Make sure the gloves have powder inside.
   C. Wear latex-free gloves.
   D. Never wear any gloves.

54. If you must handle used needles you should
   A. Remove needles from disposable syringes by hand.
   B. Place used disposable syringes and needles in plastic bags to discard.
   C. Recap used needles.
   D. Place used syringes and other sharp items in a puncture-resistant container.

55. A person placed in airborne precautions may have
   A. Meningitis, pneumonia, or influenza
   B. A wound infection
   C. Mumps, rubella, or pertussis
   D. Measles, chickenpox, or tuberculosis

56. You do not need to wear a mask when the person has measles or chickenpox if
   A. They no longer have skin lesions.
   B. You are immune to the disease.
   C. They are not sneezing or coughing.
   D. The skin lesions are covered.

57. A gown is worn when entering a room
   A. Isolated for airborne precautions
   B. Isolated for droplet precautions
   C. Isolated for standard precautions
   D. Where you will have substantial contact with a person in contact precautions

58. Which of these statements about wearing gloves is true?
   A. The inside of the glove is contaminated.
   B. Slightly used gloves can be saved and reused.
   C. You may need more than one pair of gloves for a task.
   D. Gloves are easier to put on when hands are damp.

59. When removing gloves
   A. Touch only the outside of the gloves with the other glove.
   B. Pull the gloves off by the fingers.
   C. Reach inside the glove with the gloved hand to pull it off.
   D. Hold the discarded gloves tightly in your hand.

60. When removing a mask, only the ties are touched because
   A. The front of the mask is contaminated.
   B. The front of the mask is sterile.
   C. Your gloves are contaminated.
   D. Your hands are contaminated.

61. When donning a gown, which of these is done first?
   A. Tie the strings at the back of the neck.
   B. Tie the waist strings at the back.
   C. Put on the gloves.
   D. It does not matter.

62. When removing protective apparel, which of these is done first?
   A. Remove the facemask.
   B. Remove and discard the gloves.
   C. Remove the gown.
   D. Untie the waist strings of the gown.

63. If you wear reusable eyewear and it is contaminated
   A. It should be discarded.
   B. It should be autoclaved.
   C. Wash it with soap and water and then with a disinfectant.
   D. Rinse in cool running water.

64. How are contaminated items identified when sent to the laundry or trash collection?
   A. Bags are transparent, so materials are visible.
   B. Items are labeled as "contaminated."
   C. Items are always double bagged.
   D. Items are labeled with BIOHAZARD symbol.

65. How are specimens collected in a contaminated room handled?
   A. Place specimen container in a BIOHAZARD specimen bag.
   B. It depends on center policy.
   C. Testing must be performed in the room.
   D. Special containers are needed.

66. If a resident in isolation precautions must be transported to another area, all of these would be done *except*
   A. The person wears a mask for all types of isolation precautions.
   B. The staff wears gown, mask, and gloves as required.
   C. The staff members in the receiving area are alerted so they can wear protective equipment as needed.
   D. The wheelchair or stretcher is disinfected after use.

67. Which of these will not help a person in isolation meet the need for love, belonging, and self esteem?
   A. Avoid the room so you do not disturb the person.
   B. Say, "Hello" from the doorway often.
   C. Encourage the person to telephone family and friends.
   D. Provide reading materials.

68. When a child is in isolation, it may be helpful if
   A. Favorite toys or blankets are brought from home.
   B. Personal protective equipment is put on before entering the room.
   C. The child is given a mask, eyewear, and a gown to touch and play with.
   D. The room is avoided so that the child is not upset.

69. You can help a person with poor vision, confusion, or dementia to tolerate isolation by
   A. Putting on personal protective equipment outside the room
   B. Keeping the door open so they can see people in the hall
   C. Letting the person see your face, stating your name, and explaining what you are doing
   D. Not wearing a mask when in the room

70. What viruses are bloodborne pathogens?
   A. Influenza and pneumococcus
   B. Measles and chickenpox
   C. Acquired immunodeficiency syndrome (AIDS) (or human immunodeficiency virus [HIV]) and hepatitis B virus (HBV)
   D. Staphylococcus and streptococcus

71. Which of these items can transmit bloodborne pathogens?
   A. Suction equipment
   B. Dressings
   C. Needles
   D. All of the above

72. How do staff members know what to do if exposed to a bloodborne pathogen?
   A. Employers provide training upon employment and annually.
   B. Information is provided on the Internet.
   C. They may attend classes offered at colleges or hospitals.
   D. The nurse tells them what they need to know.

73. The HBV vaccine
   A. Requires only one vaccination
   B. Must be given every year
   C. Involves three injections
   D. Is required by law

74. Which of these is *not* a work practice control to reduce exposure risks?
   A. Discard contaminated needles and sharp instruments in containers that are closable, puncture resistant, and leak proof.
   B. Do not store food or drinks where blood or potential infectious materials are kept.
   C. Break contaminated needles before discarding.
   D. Practice hand hygiene after removing gloves.

75. Personal protective equipment
   A. Is free to employees
   B. Is purchased by staff members
   C. Must be worn by all employees instead of regular uniforms
   D. Is paid for by deducting the cost from the employee's paycheck

76. Broken glass is cleaned up by
    A. Carefully picking it up with gloved hands
    B. Using a brush and dustpan or tongs
    C. Asking a person specially trained to remove biohazardous materials
    D. Wiping it up with wet paper towels

77. When discarding regulated waste, the containers are
    A. Plastic bags that are specially labeled
    B. Labeled as "contaminated" in red letters
    C. Melt-away bags
    D. Closable, puncture resistant, and leak proof

78. If you are working in a home and need to dispose of "sharps," you should
    A. Place needles, syringes, and other sharp items into hard plastic or metal containers.
    B. Take them with you at the end of each shift.
    C. Place them in a plastic bag labeled with the BIOHAZARD symbol.
    D. Discard with the regular trash each day.

79. If an exposure incident occurs
    A. Report it at once.
    B. You can receive a free medical evaluation and follow-up examination.
    C. You will receive a written opinion of the medical evaluation.
    D. All of the above are true.

80. If a sterile item touches a clean item
    A. It can still be used.
    B. It is contaminated.
    C. It should be handled with sterile gloves.
    D. It can be placed in the sterile field.

81. When working with a sterile field, you should
    A. Always wear a mask.
    B. Keep items within your vision and above your waist.
    C. Keep the door open.
    D. Wear clean gloves.

82. When arranging the inner package of sterile gloves
    A. Have the right glove on the left and the left glove on the right.
    B. Have the fingers pointing toward you.
    C. Have the right glove on the right and the left glove on the left.
    D. Straighten the gloves to remove the cuff.

83. When picking up the first glove
    A. Grasp it by the cuff, touching only the inside.
    B. Reach under the cuff with your fingers.
    C. Grasp the edge of the cuff with your hand.
    D. Slide your hand into the glove without touching it with the other hand.

Matching

Match the kind of asepsis being used with each example.

84. ________ An item is placed in an autoclave.

85. ________ Each person has his or her own toothbrush, towel, washcloth, and other personal care items.

86. ________ Hands are washed before preparing food.

87. ________ Contaminated items are boiled in water for 15 minutes.

88. ________ Single-use or multi-use disposable items reduce the spread of infection.

89. ________ Liquid or gas chemicals are used to destroy microbes.

90. ________ Hands are washed every time you use the bathroom.

A. Medical asepsis (clean technique)

B. Surgical asepsis (sterile technique)

Match the aseptic measures used to control the related chain of infection with the step in the chain.

91. ________ Provide the person with tissues to use when coughing or sneezing.
92. ________ Make sure linens are dry and wrinkle-free to protect the skin.
93. ________ Use leak-proof plastic bags for soiled tissues, linens, and other materials.
94. ________ Wear personal protective equipment.
95. ________ Hold equipment and linens away from your uniform.
96. ________ Assist with cleaning or clean the genital area after elimination.
97. ________ Clean from cleanest area to the dirtiest.
98. ________ Label bottles with person's name and date that it was opened.
99. ________ Follow the care plan to meet the person's nutritional and fluid needs.
100. ________ Make sure drainage tubes are properly connected.
101. ________ Do not use items that are on the floor.
102. ________ Assist the person with cough and deep-breathing exercises as directed.
103. ________ Avoid sitting on a person's bed. You will pick up microorganisms and transfer them.

A. Reservoir (host)
B. Portal of exit
C. Method of transmission
D. Portal of entry
E. Susceptible host

Match the practices with the correct principles for surgical asepsis.

104. ________ Consider any item as contaminated if it touches a clean item.
105. ________ Wear a mask if you need to talk during the procedure.
106. ________ Place all sterile items inside the 1-inch margin of the sterile field.
107. ________ Do not turn your back on a sterile field.
108. ________ Prevent drafts by closing the door and avoiding extra movements.
109. ________ Avoid spilling and splashing when pouring sterile fluids into sterile containers.
110. ________ If you cannot see an item, it is contaminated.
111. ________ You report to the nurse that contaminated an item or a field.
112. ________ Hold wet items down.

A. A sterile item can only touch another sterile item.
B. Sterile items or a sterile field are always kept within your vision and above your waist.
C. Airborne microbes can contaminate sterile items or a sterile field.
D. Fluid flows down, in the direction of gravity.
E. The sterile field is kept dry, unless the area below it is sterile.
F. The edges of a sterile field are contaminated.
G. Honesty is essential to sterile technique.

Labeling

113. This figure shows how to remove gloves. List the steps of the procedure shown in each drawing.

A. (1) ______________________________

____

(2) ______________________________

____

B. (1) ______________________________

____

C. (1) ______________________________

____

(2) ______________________________

____

D. (1) ______________________________

____

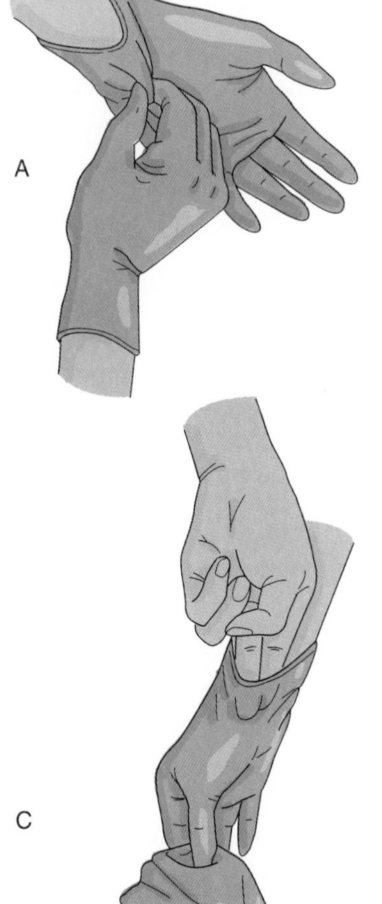

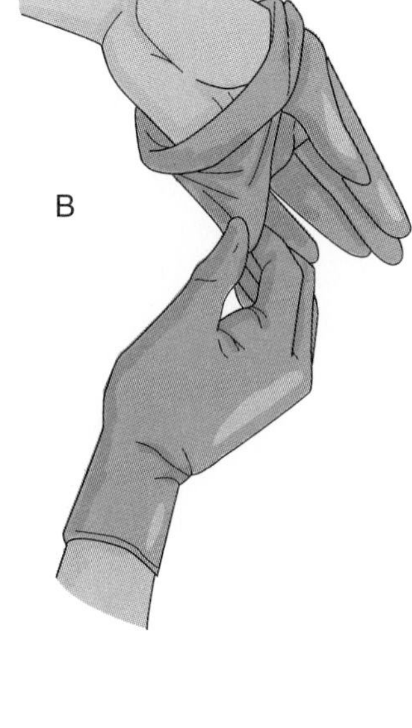

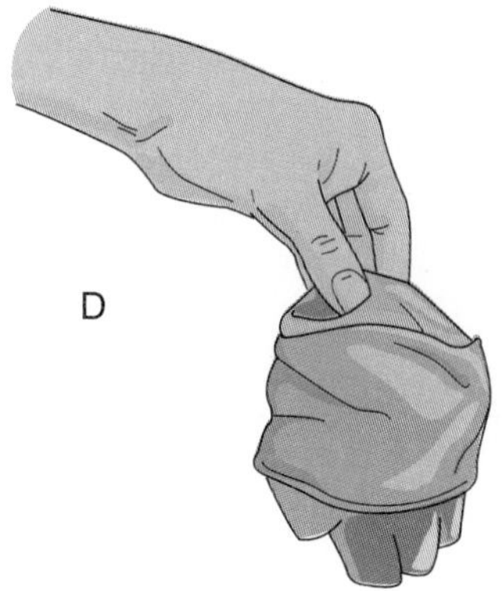

114. Color the part of the sterile field at right that would not be sterile. How wide is this space? ______________

Crossword Puzzle

Fill in the crossword puzzle by answering the clues with words from this list.

asepsis	HBV	parenteral	sharps
autoclave	HIV	PPE	sterilize
bacteria	isolation	protozoa	viruses
fungi	OPIM	Rickettsiae	

Across

1. One-celled animals; can infect the blood, brain, intestines, and other body areas
2. Any object, such as needles, scalpels, broken glass, and broken capillary tubes, that can penetrate the skin
4. Grows in living cells; causes many diseases such as the common cold, herpes, and hepatitis
8. Found in fleas, lice, ticks, and other insects; spread to humans by insect bites
10. A pressure-steam sterilizer
13. Plant life that multiplies rapidly; germs
14. Plants that live on other plants or animals; can infect the mouth, vagina, skin, feet, and other body areas

Down

1. Piercing mucous membranes or the skin barrier through such events as needle sticks, human bites, cuts, and abrasions
3. Clothing or equipment worn by an employee for protection against a hazard
5. The use of physical or chemical procedure designed to destroy all microbial life, including highly resistant bacterial spores
6. Human immunodeficiency virus
7. Barriers that prevent the escape of pathogens to other areas; usually this area is the person's room
9. Being free of disease-producing microbes
11. Other potentially infection materials; human body fluids, any tissue or organ from a human, HIV-containing cell or tissue cultures
12. Hepatitis B virus

Nursing Assistant Skills Video Exercise

View the* Basic Principles *video to answer these questions.

115. When should hands be washed?

____

____

116. How do you get a good lather when washing hands?

____

____

117. To clean the fingernails, rub them against the _______________, and clean under them with _______________.

118. When you dry the hands you should start with _______________.

Optional Learning Exercises

119. Compare medical asepsis to surgical asepsis. Medical asepsis is

____

_______________.

Surgical asepsis is

____

_______________.

120. Why are hands and forearms kept lower than elbows in handwashing?

____

____

121. What is the least time you should wash your hands?

____

____

122. Why is lotion applied after handwashing?

____

____

123. When are gloves worn in standard precautions?

____

____

124. Masks, eye protections, and face shields are worn during _______________.

125. What information does the nursing assistant need from the nurse or care plan when the resident requires transmission-based precautions?

A. _______________

B. _______________

C. _______________

D. _______________

126. If a person has measles and you are susceptible, what should you do?

____

____

127. Why is it especially important to keep the door closed with airborne precautions?

____

____

128. If a person who is in airborne precautions must leave the room, the person must wear a _______________.

129. How is preventing the spread of infection an important part of your job?

____

____

130. How does wearing gloves protect you and the person? It protects you

_______________________________________.

It protects the person

_______________________________________.

131. Why is the gown turned inside out as you remove it?

____

____

132. If you are wearing gloves, gown, and mask, in what order are they donned?

____

____

133. When you remove gloves, gown, and mask, in what order are they taken off?

____

____

134. Why is a moist mask or gown changed?

____

____

135. What basic needs may not be met when a person is in isolation?

____

____

136. In addition to blood, what body fluids are potentially infectious materials?

____

____

137. What information is included in training about bloodborne pathogens?

A. _______________________________________

B. _______________________________________

C. _______________________________________

D. _______________________________________

E. _______________________________________

F. _______________________________________

G. _______________________________________

H. _______________________________________

I. _______________________________________

J. _______________________________________

138. How are containers used to discard needles and sharp instruments identified?

____

____

139. OSHA requires these measures for safely handling and using personal protective equipment.

A. _______________________________________

B. _______________________________________

C. _______________________________________

D. _______________________________________

E. _______________________________________

F. _______________________________________

G. _______________________________________

H. _______________________________________

140. If you are asked to assist with a sterile procedure, what information do you need before beginning?

A. ______________________________

B. ______________________________

C. ______________________________

D. ______________________________

E. ______________________________

Independent Learning Activities

Handwashing practices are important to use wherever you are to prevent the spread of infection. Use this exercise to make yourself aware of your own habits.

- Make a list of when you washed your hands for 1 day.
  - How did you wash your hands? Did you use the method taught in the chapter?
  - How many times did you wash your hands at work? At home?
  - How many times did you realize you had forgotten to wash your hands? What was the reason you forgot?

- How can you improve your handwashing practices? What will you change after studying this chapter?

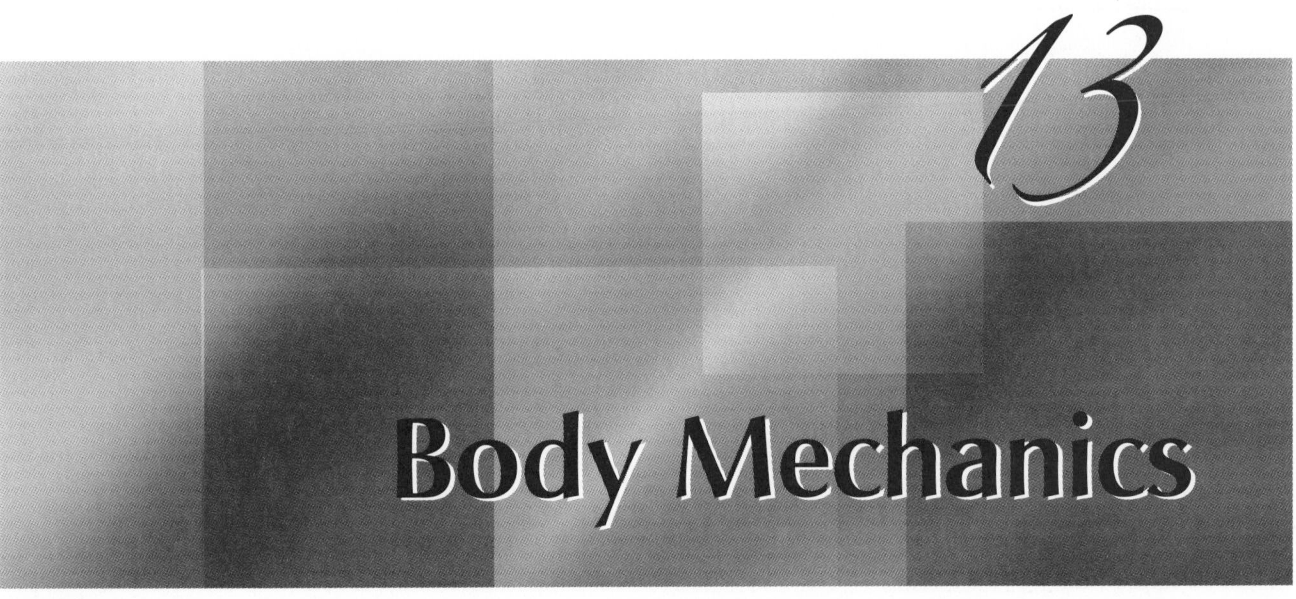

13 Body Mechanics

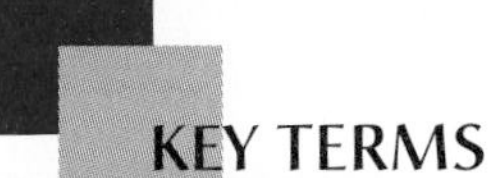

KEY TERMS

Base of support
Body alignment
Body mechanics
Dorsal recumbent position
Ergonomics
Fowler's position
Friction
Gait belt
Lateral position
Logrolling
Posture
Prone position
Shearing
Side-lying position
Sims' position
Supine position
Transfer belt

Fill in the Blanks: Key Terms

1. Another name for the lateral position is ______________________.
2. The way in which the head, trunk, arms, and legs are aligned with one another is ______________________ or posture.
3. A ______________________ is used to hold onto a person during a transfer or when walking with the person. It is also called a gait belt.
4. The ______________________ is also called the side-lying position.
5. Another name for a transfer or safety belt is a ______________________.
6. The ______________________ is the same as the back-lying or supine position.
7. ______________________ occurs when skin sticks to a surface and muscles slide in the direction the body is moving.
8. The area on which an object rests is the ______________________.
9. Turning the person as a unit, in alignment, with one motion is ______________________.
10. ______________________ is a left side-lying position in which the upper leg is sharply flexed so that it is not on the lower leg and the lower arm is behind the person.

11. A semi-sitting position with the head of the bed elevated 45 to 90 degrees is ______________________________.

12. Lying on the abdomen with the head turned to one side is ______________________________.

13. ______________________________ is using the body in an efficient and careful way.

14. The back-lying or dorsal recumbent position is also called the ______________________________.

15. ______________________________ or body alignment is the way in which body parts are aligned with one another.

16. The rubbing of one surface against another is ______________________________.

17. ______________________________ is the science of designing the job to fit the worker.

Circle the BEST Answer

18. Using good body mechanics will
    A. Prevent good posture
    B. Cause back injuries
    C. Reduce fatigue, muscle strain, and injury
    D. Cause muscle injury

19. For a wider base of support and more balance
    A. Bend your knees and squat to pick up heavy objects.
    B. Align the head, trunk, arms, and legs with one another.
    C. Stand with your feet apart.
    D. Make sure you are in good physical condition.

20. When you bend your knees and squat to lift a heavy object, you are
    A. Using poor body mechanics
    B. In danger of injury
    C. Likely to strain your back
    D. Using good body mechanics

21. If you have pain when standing or rising from a seated position, you
    A. May have a back injury
    B. Are using poor body mechanics
    C. Have worked too many hours
    D. Should exercise more

22. Which of these will help prevent back injury?
    A. Reposition a person in bed or on a chair.
    B. Transfer a person from a wheelchair to the toilet.
    C. Weigh a person.
    D. Have a co-worker help you lift, move, turn, or transfer a person.

23. How many people are needed to move a person?
    A. At least one person
    B. Two or three people
    C. One person with a mechanic lift
    D. As many as needed to move the person safely

24. How can you reduce friction and shearing?
    A. Raise the head of the bed to a sitting position.
    B. Roll or lift the person to reposition.
    C. Pull the person up in bed.
    D. Massage the skin.

25. If a resident with dementia resists your effort to move him or her, you
    A. Should get help from co-workers
    B. Should proceed calmly and slowly
    C. Let the person stay in the position that he or she likes
    D. Tell him firmly he or she must let you move him

26. Before lifting or moving a person, you need to know the following information *except*
    A. Whether special equipment is needed
    B. Whether any limits exist in the person's ability to move or be repositioned
    C. Whether the person is awake
    D. The number staff members needed to lift and move the person safety

27. For safety and efficiency, you should
    A. Decide how you will move the person before starting the procedure.
    B. Try to move the person alone at first.
    C. Ask for help only after trying to move the person alone.
    D. Always use a mechanical lift.

28. Beds are raised when moving a person to
    A. Allow the person to get out of bed with ease
    B. Allow you to use good body mechanics
    C. Prevent injury to the person
    D. Allow the person to breathe more easily

29. When raising an older person's head and shoulders
    A. You can always do this alone.
    B. A mechanical lift is needed.
    C. It is best to have help to prevent pain and injury.
    D. A transfer belt will be needed.

30. When raising the person's head and shoulders
    A. Both hands are placed under the person's back.
    B. Use a lift sheet to raise the person up.
    C. Put the person's near arm under your near arm and behind your shoulder.
    D. Rest your free arm on the edge of the bed.

31. When assisting a person to move up in bed
    A. You may move lightweight adults up in bed if they use a trapeze.
    B. You must always use two people to move any person.
    C. Two people grasp the person under the arms and pull the person up in bed as he or she remains still.
    D. You should use a mechanical lift to avoid injury to yourself and the person.

32. When moving a person up in bed, the head of the bed should be
    A. In the Fowler's position
    B. In the semi-Fowler's position
    C. As flat as possible for the person
    D. As upright as possible for the person

33. When moving the person up in bed, the pillow is placed
    A. On the bedside table
    B. Against the headboard if the person can be without it
    C. Under the knees to help the person push up
    D. Against the bedrail

34. When moving a person, you move
    A. On the count of "2"
    B. On the count of "3"
    C. When the person says he is ready
    D. As soon as everyone is in position

35. A lift sheet is used to move persons who are
    A. Older and those with arthritis and bone or joint injuries
    B. Unconscious or paralyzed
    C. Recovering from spinal cord surgery
    D. All of the above

36. When using a lift sheet to move a person
    A. The bed must be completely flat.
    B. The sheet is placed under the person from the head to above the knees.
    C. One person may work alone to the move the person.
    D. The sheet is placed under the person from the hips to the knees.

37. A person is moved to the side of the bed before turning to
    A. Ensure the person is in the middle of the bed after turning on his side.
    B. Make it easier to turn him.
    C. Prevent injury to the person.
    D. Prevent skin injuries.

38. If you are moving the person in segments, which of these would be incorrect?
    A. Start the movement with hips first, then move the shoulders and legs.
    B. Place your arms under the person's neck and shoulders, and then move the upper part toward you.
    C. Place one arm under the person's waist and the other under the thighs, then rock backward.
    D. Rock backward with your arms under the person's thighs and calves.

39. When using a lift sheet to move a person to the side of the bed, you should support the
    A. Back
    B. Knees
    C. Head
    D. Hips

40. After a person is turned for repositioning, the person
    A. Should be given good personal care
    B. Must be positioned in good body alignment
    C. Needs to have the head of the bed elevated
    D. Is at risk for friction or shearing

41. When directed to turn a person, you need to know all of the following *except*
    A. How much help the person needs
    B. Which procedure to use
    C. What supportive devices are needed for positioning
    D. Whether the doctor has ordered turning

42. When a person is turned on his side, he or she lays
    A. On the side of the bed with his or her back against the bedrail
    B. On the side of the bed with his or her face close to the bedrail
    C. In the middle of the bed
    D. In whatever position he or she is comfortable

43. To prevent musculoskeletal injuries, skin breakdown, or pressure ulcers when a person is turned, the person must be in
    A. A special bed
    B. Good body alignment
    C. Good body mechanics
    D. All of the above

44. How do you decide whether to turn a person toward you or away from you?
    A. Check the doctor's orders.
    B. It depends on the person's condition. Check the care plan.
    C. Ask the person which he or she prefers.
    D. Use the method you like best.

45. When turning the person away from you
    A. One hand is placed on the person's far shoulder, and the other is placed on the far buttock.
    B. One hand is placed on the person's near shoulder, and the other is placed on the near buttock.
    C. One hand is placed on the back near the shoulders, and the other is placed at the waist.
    D. One hand is placed on the back, and the other is placed at the knees.

46. When you position the person on the side, commonly you will do all of these *except*
    A. Have the person lie on his shoulder and arm.
    B. Position a pillow against the back.
    C. Flex the upper leg in front of the lower leg.
    D. Place a pillow under the head and neck.

47. Logrolling is used to turn
    A. Older persons with arthritic spines or knees
    B. Persons with spinal cord injuries
    C. Persons recovering from hip fractures
    D. All of the above

48. When logrolling, all of these would be correct *except*
    A. One person can work alone to logroll a person.
    B. Two or three staff members are needed to logroll a person.
    C. A turning sheet is sometimes used.
    D. The spine is kept straight throughout the move.

49. When preparing to logroll the person, a pillow is placed
    A. At the head of the bed
    B. Between the knees
    C. Under the head
    D. Under the shoulders

50. What information do you need before dangling a person?
    A. The person's diagnosis
    B. Any areas of weakness
    C. Whether the person likes to dangle
    D. When the person ate last

51. When you have a person sit on the side of the bed (dangle) and the person complains of dizziness, you should
    A. Call the nurse.
    B. Talk to the person to distract him or her.
    C. Help the person lie down in bed.
    D. Offer the person a drink of water.

52. When preparing to dangle a person, the head of the bed should be
    A. Flat
    B. Slightly raised
    C. In a sitting position
    D. At a comfortable height for the person

53. When preparing to transfer a person, you should
    A. Arrange the room to ensure enough space for a safe transfer.
    B. Keep furniture in the position the resident desires.
    C. Remove all furniture from the room.
    D. Take the person to another area if you cannot transfer in the room.

54. Nonskid footwear is used to
    A. Protect the person from falling.
    B. Allow the person to bend the foot more easily.
    C. Promote comfort for the person.
    D. Keep the feet warm.

55. When applying a gait belt, which of these is *incorrect?*
    A. Apply the belt over clothing.
    B. Tighten the belt so you can slide four fingers between the person and the belt.
    C. Place the buckle over the spine.
    D. Make sure a woman's breast is not caught under the belt.

56. When helping a person out of bed to transfer, the person should
    A. Get out of bed on the weak side.
    B. Get out of bed on the strong side.
    C. Get out of bed on the left side.
    D. Get out of bed on the right side.

57. When transferring a person, the nurse may ask you to take the
    A. Blood pressure before and after the transfer
    B. Pulse before and after the transfer
    C. Respirations before and after the transfer
    D. Temperature before and after the transfer

58. When using a transfer belt, grasp it
    A. At each side
    B. In the front
    C. By the buckle
    D. At the back

59. When transferring without a transfer belt, your hands are placed
    A. On the person's waist
    B. Under the person's arms and around the shoulder blades
    C. On the person's wrists
    D. On the person's elbows

60. When transferring a person who is weak on one side back to bed from a chair
    A. Transfer the person into the same side of the bed from which the person transferred out of bed.
    B. Transfer the person onto the opposite side of the bed from which the person transferred out of bed.
    C. Always use a mechanical lift.
    D. Always have another staff member to help.

61. Which of these is *not* a factor when the nurse decides a person will be lifted without a mechanical device?
    A. The person's height and weight
    B. The skills and strength of the staff members
    C. The height and weight of the staff members
    D. The amount of room for the transfer

62. If you are standing behind the wheelchair to transfer a person without a mechanical lift, how do you grasp the person?
    A. Grasp the person by the upper arms.
    B. Place your hands under the person's buttocks.
    C. Place your arms under the person's arms, and grasp the person's forearms.
    D. Lift the person under the axilla.

63. When using a mechanical lift
    A. You may work by yourself.
    B. At least two staff members are needed.
    C. You know that all lifts are the same and do not require special training.
    D. The person's weight is not considered because the lifts are designed to lift any person.

64. As you lift a person in the sling of a mechanical lift, the person
    A. May hold the swivel bar
    B. May hold the straps or chains
    C. Must keep the arms crossed
    D. Should keep the leg outstretched to prevent injury

65. When transferring a person from a wheelchair to the toilet
    A. The toilet should have an elevated seat.
    B. The toilet seat should be removed.
    C. Always position the wheelchair next to the toilet so that the person's strong side is near the toilet.
    D. Unlock the wheelchair wheels to allow movement during the transfer.

66. Before transferring a person from a wheelchair to the toilet you need to check
    A. The doctor's order
    B. To ensure the grab bars are secure
    C. Whether the person has soiled the bed
    D. The amount of urine voided the last time the person used the toilet

67. When moving the person to the stretcher, which of these is *not* needed?
    A. A drawsheet or lift sheet
    B. A stretcher with safety straps and side rails
    C. A transfer belt
    D. At least three workers to move the person

68. When moving the person from the bed to the stretcher, you
    A. Have two workers stand behind the stretcher.
    B. Have two workers stand beside the bed.
    C. Grab the edges of the lift sheet, and spread it across the stretcher.
    D. Loosen the bed sheets before beginning.

69. How often does a person need to be repositioned?
    A. Once a shift
    B. At least every 2 hours
    C. Once a day
    D. Every 4 hours

70. When repositioning a person, you may also be delegated to
    A. Ambulate the person.
    B. Assist the person to the bathroom.
    C. Perform skin care measures.
    D. Perform all of the above.

71. Persons with heart and respiratory disorders usually can breathe more easily in the
    A. Fowler's position
    B. Semi-Fowler's position
    C. Supine position
    D. Prone position

72. Most older persons cannot tolerate the ________ position.
    A. Lateral
    B. Sims'
    C. Fowler's
    D. Prone

73. When positioning a person in the supine position, the nurse may ask you to place a pillow under the person's lower leg to
    A. Improve the circulation.
    B. Assist the person to breathe easier.
    C. Lift the heels off of the bed to prevent them from rubbing on the sheets.
    D. Prevent swelling of the legs and feet.

74. You usually place a pillow against the person's back when the person is positioned in the ___________ position.
    A. Lateral
    B. Prone
    C. Supine
    D. Semi-Fowler's

75. In the chair position, a pillow is not used
    A. To position paralyzed arms
    B. To support the feet
    C. Under the upper arm and hand
    D. Behind the back if restraints are used

76. When moving a person who cannot help up in the wheelchair, which of these steps would be *incorrect?*
    A. Have the tallest worker stand behind the wheelchair.
    B. A worker stands in front of the person and places the hands and arms under the person's knees.
    C. The person uses his arms and legs to push up on the count of "3."
    D. Lock the wheelchair wheels.

Fill in the Blanks

77. Where are strong, large muscles located that are used to lift and move heavy objects?

    A. ______________________________

    B. ______________________________

    C. ______________________________

    D. ______________________________

78. Back injuries are a major risk when lifting. Good body mechanics involve

    A. ______________________________

    B. ______________________________

79. What are three quality-of-life actions that should be taken before performing procedures?

    A. ______________________________

    B. ______________________________

    C. ______________________________

80. Many procedures for lifting and moving include the same pre-procedure guidelines. These are:

A. Follow ________________________________.

B. Ask ________________________________.

C. Wash ________________________________.

D. Identify ________________________________.

E. Explain ________________________________.

F. Provide ________________________________.

G. Lock ________________________________.

H. Raise ________________________________.

81. Many procedures for lifting and moving include the same post-procedure guidelines. These are:

A. Provide ________________________________.

B. Place ________________________________.

C. Raise ________________________________.

D. Lower ________________________________.

E. Unscreen ________________________________.

F. Wash ________________________________.

G. Report ________________________________.

82. After transferring a person, you should report and record

A. ________________________________

B. ________________________________

C. ________________________________

D. ________________________________

83. What is the purpose of the paper or sheet you collect when getting ready to transfer a person to a chair or wheelchair?

____

____

84. If your center has a "no-lift" policy, you must use

________________________________.

Labeling

85. Label the positions in each of the drawings.

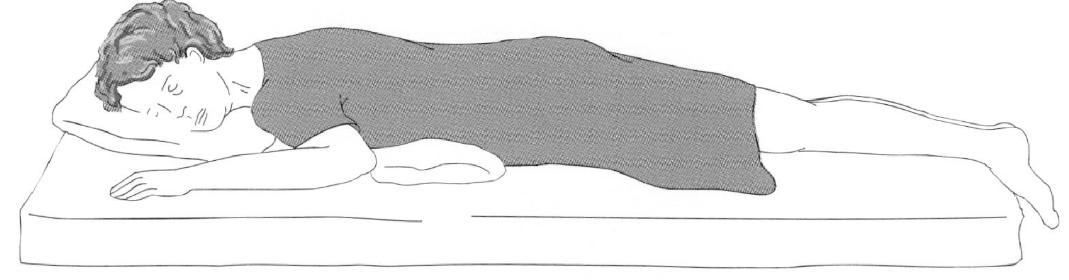

A. ________________________________

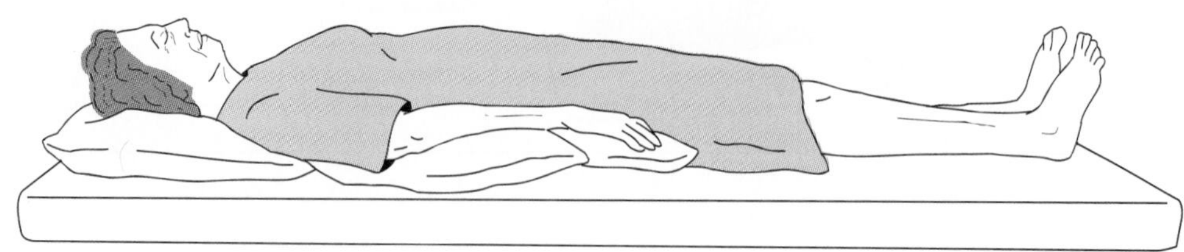

B. ________________________________

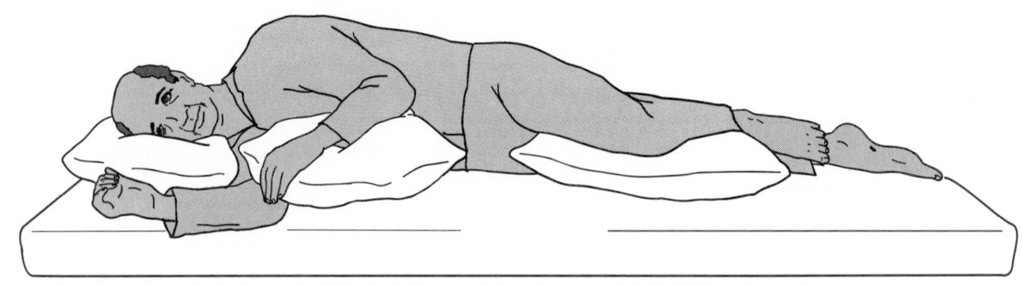

C. ______________________________

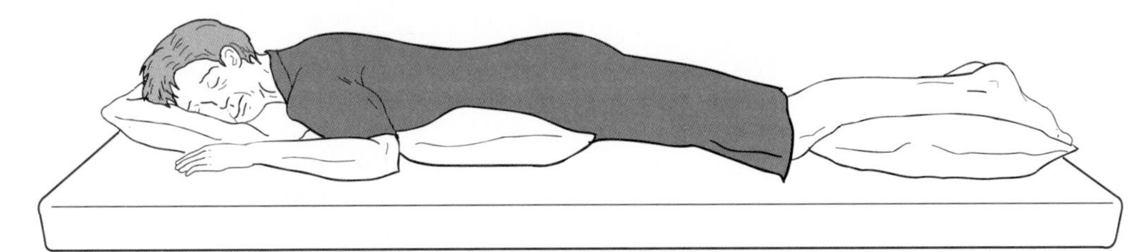

D. ______________________________

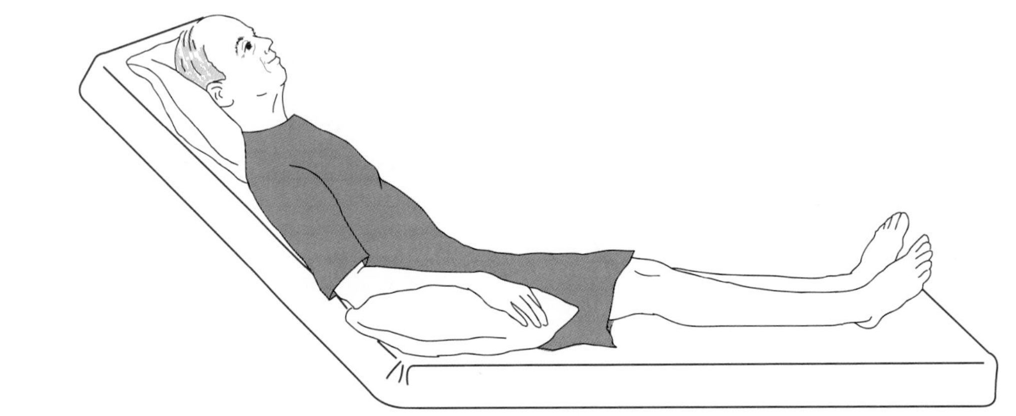

E. ______________________________

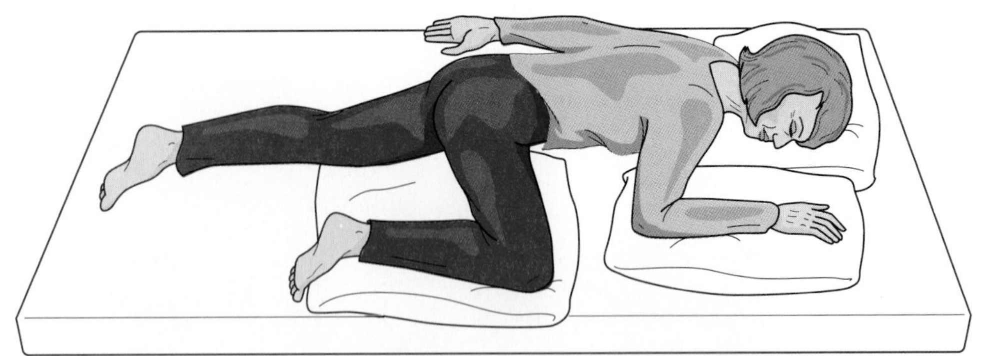

F. ______________________________

Nursing Assistant Skills Video Exercise

View the first part of the **Body Mechanics and Exercise** *video to answer these questions.*

86. What are the three principles of body mechanics that should be used when performing lifting and moving procedures?

    A. ______________________

    B. ______________________

    C. ______________________

87. When you are standing correctly, what body parts make up the base of support?

    ____

    ____

88. When lifting and moving, when do you decide how to move the person and get help?

    ____

    ____

89. How do you provide privacy for the person?

    ____

    ____

90. What four muscles do you use when moving a person up in bed?

    ____

    ____

    ____

    ____

91. When turning a person, after moving the person closer to your side, the near leg is ______________________.

92. Where do you place your arms to position a person to dangle?

    ____

    ____

93. Place the wheelchair even with the ______________________ when preparing to transfer a person from the bed to a wheelchair.

94. As the person stands to transfer from the bed to the wheelchair, how do you brace and block the person's feet?

    ____

    ____

95. After the person is sitting in the wheelchair, where do you position the chair?

    ____

    ____

96. What observations are reported after transferring a person to the wheelchair?

    A. ______________________

    B. ______________________

    C. ______________________

    D. ______________________

Optional Learning Exercises

97. According to OSHA, certain activities are associated with back injuries. Read the following examples, and list the activity that could cause a back injury in each example.

    A. The nursing assistant does not raise the level of the bed when changing linens.

    ____

    ____

    B. While you are walking with Mr. Smith he slips and starts to fall.

    ____

    ____

    C. Mrs. Tippett slides down in bed and looks uncomfortable.

    ____

    ____

D. You are giving a complete bed bath to Mrs. Miller, and she needs to be turned.

____

____

E. You find Mrs. Watson lying on the floor.

____

____

F. Mr. Brooks needs help to use the toilet. He is in a wheelchair.

____

____

98. When a person has been logrolled and is being positioned in good alignment, where would you place pillows?

A. ______________________________

B. ______________________________

C. ______________________________

D. ______________________________

99. Why is it important to provide support when a person is dangling on the side of the bed?

____

____

100. Regular position changes and good body alignment promotes:

A. ______________________________

B. ______________________________

C. ______________________________

D. ______________________________

These prevent

E. ______________________________

F. ______________________________

101. Pressure ulcers occur when the person lays or sits

______________________________.

They may also occur when linens are

______________________________.

102. Contractures can be prevented by

______________________________.

Independent Learning Activities

After learning about using good body mechanics in this chapter, think about how well you practice body mechanics in your daily life and answer these questions.

- How much do the books that you carry with you each day weigh? How do you carry them? When carrying them, where is your base of support? Is your body in good alignment?
- Do you have small children that you pick up? How do you lift them? What methods listed in the chapter do you use?
- When carrying groceries into the house, do you hold them close to the body? How well are you using good body mechanics?
- At the end of the day, how do you feel? How could using good body mechanics help you avoid any discomfort?

14 The Person's Unit

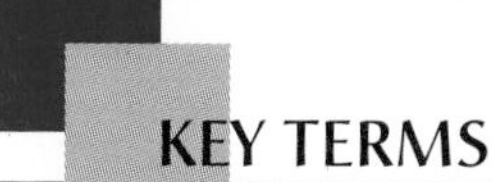

KEY TERMS

Fowler's position
Full visual privacy
Reverse Trendelenburg's position
Semi-Fowler's position
Trendelenburg's position

Fill in the Blanks: Key Terms

1. In ______________________, the head of the bed is raised 30 degrees, and the knee portion is raised 15 degrees; or the head of the bed is raised 30 degrees.
2. ______________________ is a semi-sitting position; the head of the bed is raised 45 to 90 degrees.
3. The head of the bed is raised, and the foot of the bed is lowered in ______________________.
4. In ______________________, the head of the bed is lowered, and the foot of the bed is raised.
5. The person has the means to be completely free from public view while in bed when they have ______________________.

Circle the BEST Answer

6. When people share a room
   A. You may rearrange items and furniture in the room as needed.
   B. Each person has a private area.
   C. They may use each other's belongings.
   D. They generally share furniture such as a dresser.

7. OBRA requires that nursing centers maintain a temperature range of
   A. 68° to 74° F
   B. 61° to 71° F
   C. 71° to 81° F
   D. 78° to 85° F

8. Infants, older persons, and those who are ill
   A. Need cooler room temperatures
   B. Need warmer room temperatures
   C. Are insensitive to changes in room temperature
   D. Need a warmer room at night

9. The nursing staff cannot control which one of the following factors that affects comfort?
   A. Illness
   B. Temperature
   C. Noise
   D. Odors

10. You may best protect a person who is sensitive to drafts by
    A. Putting the person to bed
    B. Giving the person a hot shower or bath
    C. Offering a lap robe or a warm sweater to wear
    D. Pulling the privacy curtain around the person

11. Older persons are sensitive to cold because they
    A. Have poor circulation and less fatty tissue
    B. Are often confused about their surroundings
    C. Are more active
    D. Are used to wearing heavier clothes

12. If unpleasant odors occur, do all of these *except*
    A. Use spray deodorizers around persons with breathing problems.
    B. Provide good personal hygiene for persons.
    C. Change and dispose of soiled linens and clothing.
    D. Empty and clean bedpans, commodes, urinals, and kidney basins promptly.

13. Noises in a health care agency may keep a person from meeting the need for
    A. Love and belonging
    B. Self-esteem
    C. Rest
    D. Safety and security

14. Which of these measures will not reduce noises in a health care agency?
    A. Have drapes in the rooms.
    B. Use only metal equipment.
    C. Promptly answer the telephone.
    D. Oil the wheels on the equipment.

15. Bright lighting is helpful for all of these *except*
    A. Persons with poor vision
    B. Helping the staff perform procedures
    C. Making the room more cheerful
    D. Helping persons rest and relax

16. Beds are kept at the lowest horizontal position to
    A. Give care
    B. Let the person get out of bed with ease
    C. Transfer persons to a stretcher
    D. Maintain good body alignment

17. Cranks on manual beds are kept down when not in use to
    A. Prevent persons from operating the bed
    B. Prevent anyone walking past the crank from bumping into it
    C. Keep the bed in the correct position
    D. Make sure they are ready to use at all times

18. How can the staff prevent a person from adjusting an electric bed to unsafe positions?
    A. Lock the bed into a position.
    B. Unplug the bed.
    C. Put the person in a bed that cannot be repositioned.
    D. Keep reminding the person not to change the position.

19. What bed position raises the head of the bed and the knee portion?
    A. Fowler's
    B. Semi-Fowler's
    C. Trendelenburg's
    D. Reverse Trendelenburg's

20. The bed wheels are locked
    A. Only when giving care
    B. When the person is not using bed rails
    C. At all times except when moving the bed
    D. When the person requests it

21. What items should not be placed on the overbed table?
    A. Meals
    B. Personal care items
    C. Writing and reading materials
    D. Bedpans, urinals, and soiled linens

22. Where are the bedpan and urinal kept in the bedside table?
    A. Wherever the person wants
    B. On the top shelf
    C. On the bottom shelf
    D. In the top drawer

23. Privacy curtains
    A. Are sometimes used in rooms with more than one bed
    B. Are always pulled completely around the bed when giving care
    C. Can block sounds and conversations
    D. May be open when giving personal care

24. Full visual privacy as required by OBRA can be achieved by
    A. Closing a privacy curtain
    B. Placing a movable screen around the person
    C. Closing the door
    D. All of the above

25. Personal care items
    A. May be supplied by the agency
    B. Must be supplied by the person
    C. Are supplied when ordered by the doctor
    D. Cannot be brought into the agency by the person

26. When the person is weak on the left side, the call bell is
    A. Placed on the left side
    B. Removed from the room
    C. Placed on the right side
    D. Replaced by an intercom

27. If a confused person cannot use a call bell
    A. Explain often how to use the call bell.
    B. Use an intercom instead.
    C. Remove the call bell.
    D. Check the person often.

28. Elevated toilet seats
    A. Help persons with joint problems
    B. Make wheelchair transfers more difficult
    C. Help when transferring the person with a mechanical lift
    D. Are used if the person is very tall

29. When a person uses a bathroom call bell
    A. It flashes above the room door and at the nurse's station.
    B. It makes the same sound as the room call bell.
    C. It activates the intercom.
    D. All of the above occur.

30. Closet and drawer space
    A. Is shared by persons in a room with more than one person
    B. Can be cleaned out by a staff member
    C. Can be searched without the person's permission
    D. Must have free access for the person

31. In long-term care centers, a person can bring some furniture and personal items to use in the room as long as the choices
    A. Do not interfere with the rights of others
    B. Match the color and decoration in the room
    C. Can be cared for by the person or the family
    D. Do not need to be attached to the wall

32. Which of these is *not* a responsibility when maintaining the person's unit?
    A. Throw away extra papers and other items that may clutter the room.
    B. Arrange personal items as the person prefers.
    C. Empty the wastebasket as least once a day.
    D. Explain the causes of strange noises.

Labeling

33. In this figure

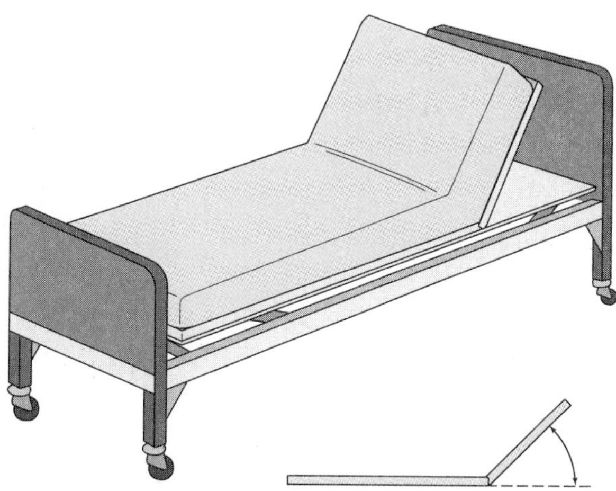

A. What is the bed position called?

____

B. What is the angle of the head of the bed?

____

34. In this figure

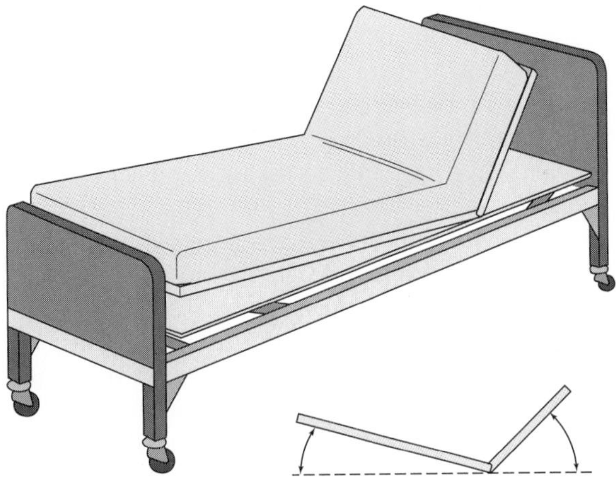

A. What is the bed position called?

____

B. What is the angle of the head of the bed?

____

C. What is the angle of the foot of the bed?

____

35. In this figure

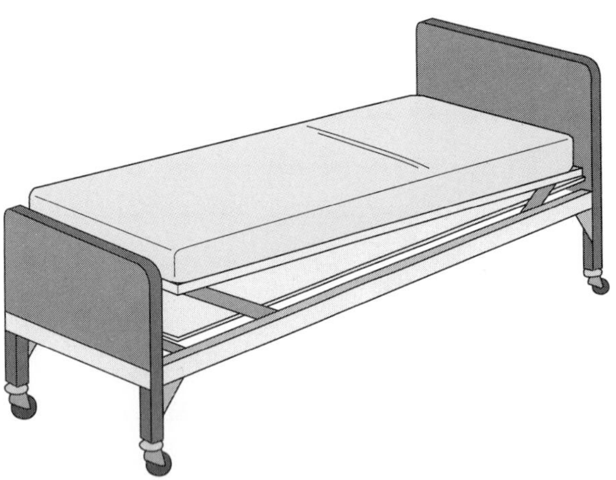

A. What is the bed position called?

____

B. What is the position of the head of the bed and the foot of the bed?

____

C. Who decides this position is to be used?

____

36. In this figure

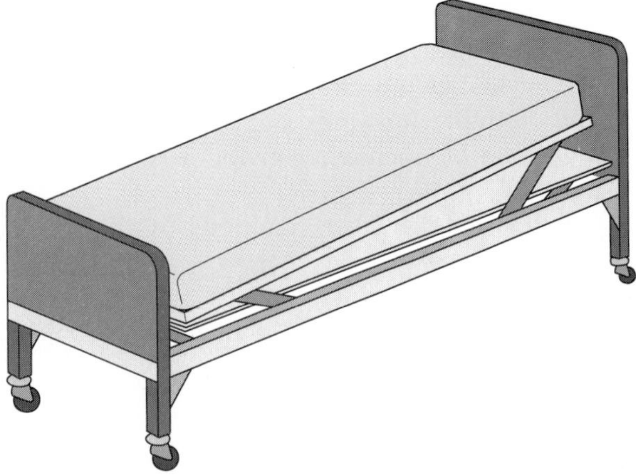

A. What is the bed position called?

____

B. What is the position of the head of the bed and the foot of the bed?

____

C. Who decides this position is to be used?

____

Optional Learning Exercises

37. Comfort is affected by three factors that cannot be controlled. These factors are

A. _______________

B. _______________

C. _______________

38. List four factors that can be controlled to increase comfort.

A. _______________

B. _______________

C. _______________

D. _______________

39. In these situations, how would you protect a person from drafts?

    A. The person is dressing for the day.

    ____

    B. The person is sitting in a wheelchair.

    ____

    C. You are assisting a person who is going to bed for the night.

    ____

    D. You are giving personal care to the person.

    ____

40. How can you help to eliminate odors in these situations?

    A. You are caring for a person who is frequently incontinent.

    ____

    B. The person is vomiting and has wound drainage.

    ____

    C. The person changes his own ostomy drainage bag in his bathroom.

    ____

    D. The person keeps a urinal at his bedside and uses it himself during the day.

    ____

41. When the staff talks loudly and laughs in the hallways, some persons may think that ______________________________________.

42. How can the staff reduce noises and increase person comfort?

    A. Control ______________________________.

    B. Handle ______________________________.

    C. Keep ______________________________.

    D. Answer ______________________________.

43. What are two times when bright lights are helpful for a person with poor vision?

    A. ______________________________

    B. ______________________________

44. What does OBRA require for furniture and equipment listed?

    A. Closet space ______________________________

    ____

    B. Bedding ______________________________

    ____

    C. Chair ______________________________

    ____

    D. Bed position ______________________________

    ____

    E. Toilet seat ______________________________

    ____

    F. Number of persons in a room ______________

    ____

    G. Windows ______________________________

    ____

    H. Call system ______________________________

    ____

I. Odors, noise, lighting ______________________

____

J. Handrails, bedrails ______________________

____

45. The bed in the flat position is used for

A. ______________________

B. ______________________

46. Semi-Fowler's position has two different definitions. They are

A. ______________________

B. ______________________

47. How do you know which of the ways in #46 to position the bed when semi-Fowler's position is ordered?

____

____

48. What two methods are used to raise the foot of the bed with Trendelenburg's position?

A. ______________________

B. ______________________

49. How can you place a person in Fowler's or semi-Fowler's position if the person has a regular bed?

____

____

____

50. When the nursing team uses the overbed table as a work area, what are the only items that can be placed on it?

____

____

51. What are your responsibilities in these situations regarding the call bell?

A. The person is sitting in a chair next to the bed.

____

B. The person is weak on the right side.

____

C. The person calls out instead of using the call bell.

____

D. The person is embarrassed because she soiled the bed after signaling for assistance.

____

E. The call bell in a bathroom rings while you are busy in another room.

____

52. The person is allowed to bring personal items to make his or her space as homelike as possible. The health team must make sure the person's choices

A. ______________________

B. ______________________

C. ______________________

Independent Learning Activities

When you are in the health care center as a student, find an empty room and practice using the equipment. Answer these questions about the equipment.

- Where are the controls for the bed?
  - How do you operate the head of the bed?
  - How do you operate the knee control of the bed?
  - How do you adjust the height of the bed?
- Where is the call bell located?
- Where are controls for the television and radio?
- Does the center have an intercom system? How is it used?

Ask the staff these questions about the call bells.

- How does the staff know when a person turns on the call bell?
- When a person uses a bathroom call bell, how does the staff know the difference?

Think about what temperature is comfortable for you and answer these questions. This exercise will help you understand the importance of individual preferences for persons in the health care center.

- What is the usual temperature of your home?
- Who decides what the temperature will be in your home? Partner, spouse, roommate, children?
- Would the temperature you prefer be comfortable for an infant? An older person? Why or why not?

Think about the noises in your home and how they affect you. This exercise will help you understand why noise levels in the nursing center can affect persons.

- When you study, do you turn on the television or radio? Listen to music? Prefer complete silence?
- What noises do you like when going to sleep? Television? Radio? Soft music?
- Does everyone in your household agree on how loud or soft to play a radio or TV? How are conflicts about noise levels resolved?
- If you are in noisy surroundings that is unacceptable, how do you react? How does it affect your ability to think? To rest? To study? How does it affect your relationship with others?

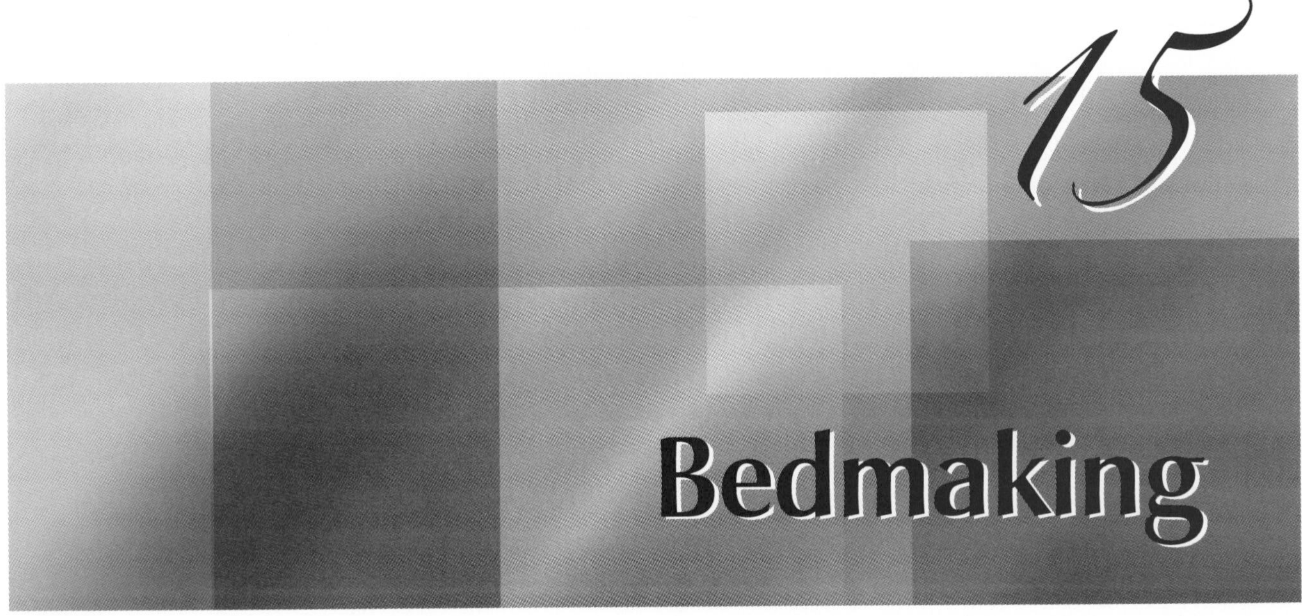

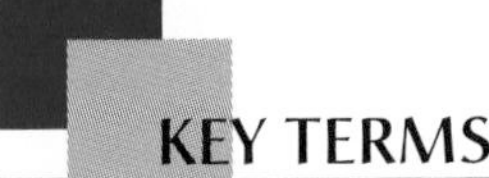

KEY TERMS

Drawsheet
Plastic drawsheet

Fill in the Blanks: Key Terms

1. A drawsheet placed between the bottom sheet and cotton drawsheet to keep the mattress and bottom linens clean and dry is a ______________________.

2. A ______________________ is a small sheet placed over the middle of the bottom sheet; it helps to keep the mattress and bottom linens dry and clean.

Circle the BEST Answer

3. In nursing centers, a complete linen change is usually done
   - A. Only when the linens are wet or soiled
   - B. Every day
   - C. On the person's bath or shower day
   - D. Once a week

4. Making the bed every day
   - A. Increases comfort
   - B. Prevents skin breakdown
   - C. Prevents pressure ulcers
   - D. All of the above

5. A closed bed is
   - A. Not in use
   - B. Made with the top linens fan-folded back to make it easier for the person to get in to bed
   - C. Made with the person in it
   - D. Made to transfer a person from a stretcher to the bed

6. An open bed is
   - A. In use. The bed is made with the person in it.
   - B. In use. The top linens are folded back so that the person can get into bed.
   - C. Not in use until bedtime. The top linens are not folded back.
   - D. In use. It is made to transfer a person from a stretcher to the bed.

7. When making a bed, medical asepsis is practiced by
   A. Putting clean or dirty linens on the floor
   B. Shaking the linens as you place them on the bed
   C. Raising the bed to a comfortable height to prevent injury to the nursing assistant
   D. Holding the linens away from your uniform

8. If extra clean linens are brought to a person's room, you should
   A. Return the unused linens to the linen room.
   B. Store the extra linens in the person's closet.
   C. Put the unused linens in the dirty laundry.
   D. Use the linens for a person in the next room.

9. Which of these linens will be collected first when making a closed bed?
   A. Bath towel
   B. Bath blanket
   C. Mattress pad
   D. Top sheet

10. When you remove dirty linens, which of these actions is incorrect?
    A. Gather all the dirty linens in one large roll.
    B. Roll each piece away from you.
    C. Top and bottom sheets, drawsheets, and pillowcases are always changed.
    D. The blanket and bedspread may be reused for the same person.

11. In a long-term nursing center, linens are changed
    A. Every morning
    B. Every other day
    C. Usually weekly, unless they are wet, damp, soiled, or very wrinkled
    D. As often as the person requests a linen change

12. The person is given the right of personal choice when you
    A. Allow the person to use bed linens from home.
    B. Decide which linens will look best in the room.
    C. Tell the person you will make the bed at 9 AM.
    D. Choose the pillows and blanket the person needs for comfort.

13. When caring for a person in the home, the linens are changed
    A. Once a day
    B. Twice a week
    C. Only if the person gives you permission
    D. Once a week or more often if the person asks you to do so

14. A plastic drawsheet can
    A. Cause discomfort and skin breakdown
    B. Be hard to keep tight and wrinkle free
    C. Keep the mattress and bottom linens clean and dry
    D. All of the above

15. When caring for a person at home, the mattress and linens may be protected with a
    A. Flat sheet folded in half to serve as a cotton drawsheet
    B. Plastic trash bag
    C. Dry cleaning bag
    D. Plastic mattress protector

16. When you are delegated to make a bed, why do you need to know the person's schedule for treatments, therapies, and activities?
    A. You need to make sure the bed is flat.
    B. It is best to change linens after treatment or when the person is out of the room.
    C. You need to unlock beds that have been locked in a certain position.
    D. You will know what type of bed to make.

17. When assigned to make an occupied bed, which of these is *not* information you need from the nurse or care plan?
    A. What linens are needed for this person
    B. If the person uses bed rails
    C. When the bed was changed last
    D. How to position the person and the needed positioning devices

18. When making a bed in the home, you should
    A. Always follow the person's wishes.
    B. Only make the bed as stated in the care plan.
    C. Follow the person's wishes unless they ask you to do something unsafe.
    D. Use your own methods to make the bed.

19. When treating stains on linens in the home, you should *not*
    A. Use a stain-removing agent supplied by the person.
    B. Mix ammonia with bleach or other chemicals.
    C. Mix ammonia and liquid dishwashing detergent in water.
    D. Rinse the item in cool water after soaking.

20. When making beds for children, it is important to
    A. Make sure bumper pads fit snugly against the slats.
    B. Make sure the mattress is at least 26 inches lower than the top of the crib rails.
    C. Tell the nurse if more than two fingers fit between the mattress and crib sides.
    D. All of the above are important.

21. When making a bed, you use good body mechanics when you
    A. Bend from the waist to remove and replace linens.
    B. Stretch across the bed to smooth linens.
    C. Raise the bed to a comfortable height to work.
    D. Lock the wheels.

22. When a person is discharged, what is done in addition to changing the bed?
    A. New pillows are placed on the bed.
    B. The bed frame and mattress are cleaned according to center policy.
    C. The bed is sterilized.
    D. The bedspread and blanket may be reused.

23. When making a bed, position the bottom sheet with
    A. The lower edge even with the top of the mattress
    B. The hem stitching facing downward
    C. The large hem at the bottom and the small hem at the top
    D. All of the above

24. When the top sheet, blanket, and bedspread are in place on the bed
    A. Each one is separately tucked under the mattress.
    B. The sheet and blanket are tucked together, and the bedspread is allowed to hang loose over them.
    C. All three are tucked together under the foot of the bed, and the corners are mitered.
    D. All three are allowed to hang loose over the foot of the bed.

25. The pillow is placed on the bed with
    A. The open end away from the door.
    B. The seam of the pillowcase toward the foot of the bed.
    C. The pillow leaning against the head of the bed.
    D. The open end toward the door.

26. An open bed is made
    A. With the linens fanfolded to one side
    B. The same as a closed bed with the top linens folded back
    C. With the person in the bed
    D. When the room is unoccupied

27. When you change the linens for a comatose person, it is important to
    A. Keep the bed in the low position.
    B. Unlock the wheels.
    C. Use special linens.
    D. Explain each step of the procedure to the person before it is done.

28. When making an occupied bed, a bath blanket is used to
    A. Protect the person while he or she is being bathed.
    B. Cover the person for warmth and privacy.
    C. Protect the bed linens.
    D. Protect the person from dirty linens.

29. When making an occupied bed for a person who does not use bed rails, you should
    A. Have a co-worker work on the other side of the bed.
    B. Push the bed against the wall.
    C. Always keep one hand on the person while you are making the bed.
    D. Only change linens when the person is out of the bed for tests or therapies.

30. When making an occupied bed
    A. First remove all the dirty linens from the bed.
    B. Ask the person to roll from side to side for each piece of the bottom linens.
    C. Fanfold all linens one piece at a time toward the person.
    D. Ask the person to raise the hips so that you can push the linens under the buttocks.

31. Which of these steps is *not* done when making a surgical bed?
    A. Tuck all top linens under the mattress together and make a mitered corner.
    B. Remove all linens from the bed.
    C. Put a mattress pad on the mattress.
    D. Place the bottom sheet with the lower edge even with the bottom of the mattress.

Fill in the Blanks

32. Number this list from 1 to 13 in the order you would collect the linens to make a bed.
    _____ Pillowcase(s)
    _____ Top sheet
    _____ Gown
    _____ Bottom sheet (flat or fitted)
    _____ Mattress pad
    _____ Bedspread
    _____ Plastic drawsheet, waterproof drawsheet, or waterproof pad
    _____ Bath blanket
    _____ Hand towel
    _____ Cotton drawsheet
    _____ Bath towel(s)
    _____ Blanket
    _____ Washcloth

Nursing Assistant Skills Video Exercise

View the Bedmaking *video to answer these questions.*

33. There are six basic principles of bedmaking. List the two missing basic principles.

    (1) Protect privacy and confidentiality.

    (2) Prevent infection.

    (3) Promote comfort and safety.

    (4) Select appropriate equipment.

    (5) ______________________________

    (6) ______________________________

34. As part of the procedure guidelines you should use Standard Precautions and ______________________________ standards.

35. Gloves are worn when ____________________.

36. If the blanket and bedspread are to be reused, they should be ______________________________.

37. Before removing the dirty top sheet, cover the person with a ______________________________ to provide warmth and privacy.

38. When you have removed all of the dirty linens, you should remove ____________________ and wash ______________________________.

39. After the person rolls over the fanfolded linens, what does the worker on the second side of the bed remove?

    ____

    ____

40. When you put the top sheet on the bed, the hemstitching should be

    ______________________________.

41. When do you remove the bath blanket that covers the person while the linens are changed?

    ____

    ____

Optional Learning Exercises

42. How often is a complete linen change made in a nursing center?

    ____

    How often are linens changed in a hospital?

    ____

    Why are linen changes done less often in a nursing center?

    ____

43. Beds are made every day to increase

    ____

    and to prevent ______________________________

    and ______________________________.

44. Even when a complete linen change is not scheduled, you should do the following to keep beds neat and clean:

    A. ______________________________

    B. ______________________________

    C. ______________________________

    D. ______________________________

    E. ______________________________

45. When handling linens, practice medical asepsis. Explain why each of the following actions would be poor medical asepsis.

    A. Holding the linens close to your body and uniform

    ____

    B. Shaking the linens to straighten

    ____

C. Placing the dirty linens on the floor

____

46. The mattress pad, plastic drawsheet, blanket, and bedspread are reused for the same person unless they are _______________.

47. If you were making a bed in a home, how would you use a twin sheet for a drawsheet?

____

48. When giving care in a home, what should you tell a family member who suggests using a plastic trash bag to protect the linens and mattress?

A. _______________

B. _______________

C. _______________

49. When working in a home, you may make an ammonia solution to remove stains from linen. This solution contains

A. _______________

B. _______________

C. _______________

50. Explain the safety concern with each of these examples.

A. A soft crib

____

B. A crib mattress that allows more than two adult fingers to fit between the mattress and the crib

____

C. A mattress that is 20 inches below the top of the crib

____

D. Bumper pads that do not fit snugly against the

____

51. When you are making beds, you should wear gloves when _______________ linens.

Why?

____

Independent Learning Activities

- When you make beds at home this week, practice the methods you learned in this chapter.
  - What linens did you collect? What was the order of the linens?
  - Did you remember to make as much of one side of the bed as possible before moving to the other side?
  - What step could not be carried out at home that would have helped you to use good body mechanics?
  - Think about the methods you used to change your bed before reading this chapter. How did you change your bed-making practices now that you have studied this chapter?

- Practice with a classmate, and take turns as a resident who must have an occupied bed made. Ask these questions about your feelings.
  - In what ways was your privacy protected?
  - Did the caregiver offer you any choices before making your bed? What were these choices?
  - Did you feel safe at all times? If not, what made you feel unsafe?
  - What was uncomfortable during the bed change?
  - How were you positioned after the bed was made?

- It is sometimes difficult for a new nursing assistant to remember the order in which to collect linens. If you have difficulty with this, make a list in a pocket notebook or on a 3 × 5 index card. Carry it with you when you are working.

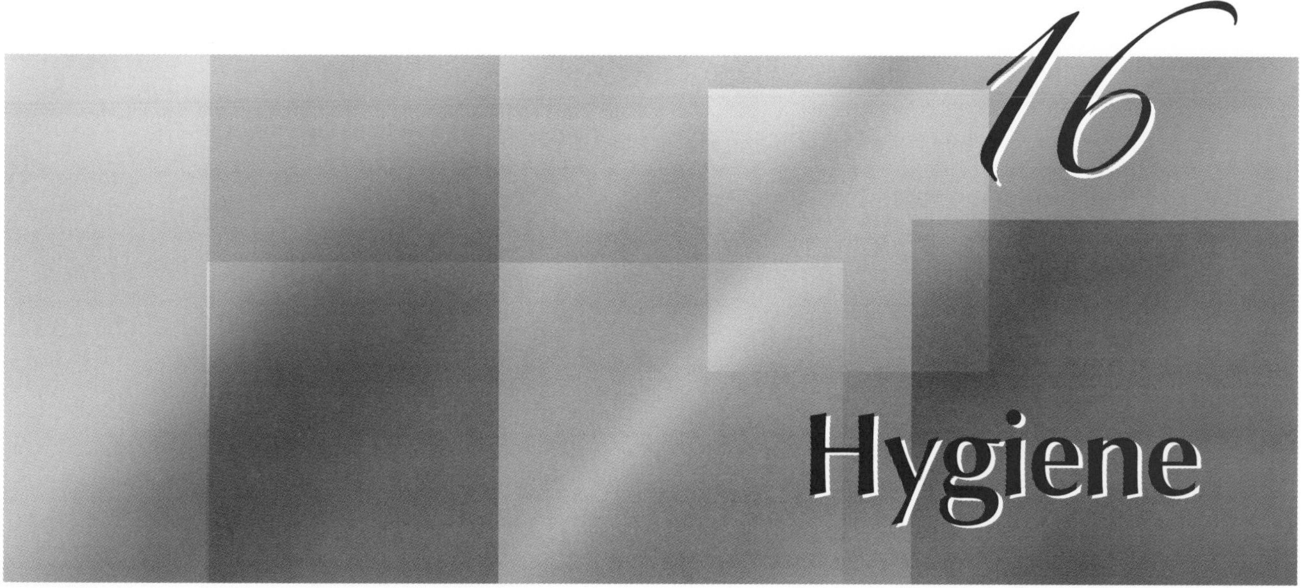

KEY TERMS

AM care
Aspiration
Early morning care
Evening care
HS care
Morning care
Oral hygiene
Pericare
Perineal care
Plaque
PM care
Tartar

Fill in the Blanks: Key Terms

1. Another name for HS care or PM care is

    ____.

2. ________________________________, or pericare, is the cleansing of the genital and anal areas.

3. Sometimes HS care or evening care is called

    ____.

4. Routine care performed before breakfast or early morning care is called

    ____.

5. ____ is mouth care or measures that keep the mouth and teeth clean.

6. Hardened plaque on teeth is

    ____.

7. ____ occurs when breathing fluid or an object into the lungs.

8. Care given after breakfast when cleanliness and skin care are more thorough is called

    ____.

9. Another name for perineal care is

    ____.

10. ____ is a thin film that sticks to the teeth. It contains saliva, microorganisms, and other substances.

11. Another name for AM care is

________________________________.

12. Care given in the evening at bedtime is

________________________________.

It is also called evening care or PM care.

Circle the BEST Answer

13. If a person needs help with personal hygiene, you can find out what needs they have by
    A. Looking at the care plan
    B. Asking the family
    C. Asking other staff members
    D. Making your own decisions

14. You should assist a person with personal hygiene
    A. Only when the person asks
    B. Only in the morning
    C. Whenever necessary
    D. Only when it is your assignment

15. When giving personal hygiene, you need to remember to protect the person's right to
    A. Privacy and personal choice
    B. Care and security of personal possessions
    C. Activities
    D. Environment

16. Which of these hygiene measures is *not* done before breakfast?
    A. Assisting with elimination
    B. Straightening units, including making beds
    C. Assisting with personal hygiene by bathing and giving a back massage and perineal care
    D. Assisting with oral hygiene

17. Which of these is performed every time you offer hygiene measures throughout the day?
    A. Assist with dressing and hair care.
    B. Wash face and hands.
    C. Assist with activity.
    D. Help the person change into sleepwear.

18. If good oral hygiene is not done regularly, the person may develop periodontal disease. This disease can lead to
    A. Dry mouth
    B. Tartar buildup
    C. Tooth loss
    D. Cavities

19. All of these health team members may assess the person's need for mouth care *except* the
    A. Speech and language pathologist
    B. Physical therapist
    C. Nurse
    D. Dietician

20. After the first baby teeth erupt, you can help prevent "baby bottle tooth decay" by
    A. Wiping the gums with a clean gauze pad
    B. Brushing with a child's soft toothbrush
    C. Using a sponge swab
    D. Brushing with a child's firm toothbrush

21. Sponge swabs are used for
    A. Persons with sore, tender mouths and for unconscious persons
    B. Cleaning dentures
    C. Oral care on children
    D. Oral care on all persons

22. You should follow Standard Precautions and the Bloodborne Pathogen Standard when giving oral hygiene because
    A. You will prevent the spread of bacteria to the person.
    B. Both will help reduce bad breath odors from the person.
    C. Both will prevent contact with bleeding gums and microbes in the mouth.
    D. You will avoid any loose teeth or rough dentures.

23. When you assist the person to perform oral hygiene in bed, arrange the items needed on the
    A. Overbed table
    B. Bedside table
    C. Sink counter
    D. Bed

24. When you are brushing the person's teeth, which of these steps would be *incorrect?*
    A. Let the person rinse the mouth with water.
    B. Use a sponge swab to clean the teeth.
    C. Brush the person's tongue gently, if needed.
    D. Floss the person's teeth.

25. Teeth are flossed to
    A. Remove plaque from the teeth.
    B. Remove tartar from the teeth.
    C. Remove food from between the teeth.
    D. All of the above are true.

26. Flossing for children should begin
    A. When the first tooth erupts
    B. When they can perform flossing by themselves
    C. When all the baby teeth have erupted (about age $2^1/_2$)
    D. When they reach school age

27. Which of these steps is incorrect to do when flossing the teeth?
    A. Start at the lower back tooth on the right side.
    B. Hold the floss between the middle fingers when flossing the upper teeth.
    C. Move the floss gently up and down between the teeth.
    D. Move to a new section of floss after every second tooth.

28. When providing mouth care for an unconscious person, position the person on one side with the head turned well to the side to
    A. Make it easier to brush the teeth.
    B. Make the person more comfortable.
    C. Prevent or reduce the risk of aspiration.
    D. Make it easier for the person to breathe.

29. A padded tongue blade is used when giving oral hygiene to an unconscious person to
    A. Keep the mouth open.
    B. Clean the teeth.
    C. Clean the tongue.
    D. Prevent aspiration.

30. Mouth care is given to an unconscious person
    A. After each meal
    B. When AM and PM care is given
    C. At least every 2 hours
    D. Once a day

31. When cleaning dentures at a sink, line the sink with a towel to
    A. Prevent infections.
    B. Prevent damage to the dentures if they are dropped.
    C. Dry the dentures.
    D. Clean the dentures.

32. If the person cannot remove the dentures, you can use ______________________ to get a good grip on the slippery dentures.
    A. Gloves
    B. Washcloth
    C. Gauze squares
    D. Bare hands

33. If dentures are not worn after cleaning, store them in
    A. Cool water or a denture-soaking solution
    B. Hot water
    C. A soft towel
    D. Soft tissues or a napkin

34. Older persons usually need a complete bath or shower two times a week because
    A. They are less active.
    B. They are often ill.
    C. They have increased perspiration.
    D. Dry skin occurs with aging.

35. If a person with dementia resists care, you should
    A. Hurry through the bath.
    B. Speak firmly in a loud voice to get the person's attention.
    C. Calm the person, and try the bath later.
    D. Use restraints so the person will not harm you.

36. The water temperature for a complete bed bath is usually between 110° F and 115° F for adults. For older persons, the temperature
    A. Should be between 110° F and 115° F
    B. May need to be lower
    C. Should be whatever you feel is comfortable
    D. May need to be warmer

37. When choosing skin care products for bathing, you should use
    A. Soap
    B. Products the person prefers
    C. Bath oils
    D. Creams and lotions

38. Before applying powder, you should
    A. Check with the nurse and care plan.
    B. Ask the person what is preferred.
    C. Check the doctor's orders.
    D. Give the person a mask to wear.

39. A complete bed bath is given to persons who are
    A. In a cast or traction
    B. Unconscious or paralyzed
    C. Weak from illness or surgery
    D. All of the above

40. When you are giving a complete bed bath, the bed linens
    A. May be changed if needed
    B. Are changed before the bath begins
    C. Are changed after the bath is completed
    D. Are changed after the person gets out of bed

41. The bedpan or urinal is
   A. Offered before the bath begins
   B. Offered after the bath ends
   C. Is left in place during the bath
   D. Not offered at all during the bath procedure

42. During the bath, the bath blanket is placed
   A. Over the top linens
   B. Under the top linens
   C. Over the top linens, and then the top linens are removed
   D. Under the person

43. Soap is not used when washing
   A. The face, ears, and neck
   B. Around the eyes
   C. The abdomen
   D. The perineal area

44. How do you avoid exposing the person when washing the chest?
   A. Keep the bath blanket over the area.
   B. Keep the top linens over the chest.
   C. Place a bath towel over the chest crosswise.
   D. Make sure the curtains are closed.

45. Bath water is changed
   A. Every 5 minutes during the bath
   B. Only if needed because it becomes cold or soapy
   C. After washing the legs and feet and after washing the back
   D. After washing the face, ears, and neck

46. A towel bath may be soothing and relaxing to a person
   A. With dementia
   B. Who has been incontinent
   C. With breaks in the skin
   D. Who needs a partial bath

47. A partial bath involves bathing
   A. Areas the person cannot reach
   B. Face, hands, axillae (underarms), back, buttocks, and perineal area
   C. Arms, legs, and feet
   D. Chest, abdomen, and underarms

48. A tub bath should not last longer than
   A. 10 minutes
   B. 15 minutes
   C. 20 minutes
   D. 30 minutes

49. When a weak or unsteady person showers, it is best to use a
   A. Shower chair
   B. Transfer belt
   C. Wheelchair
   D. Mechanical lift

50. To assist the person at home who needs to step in and out of the tub, there should be
   A. A bath mat
   B. Grab bars
   C. A shower chair
   D. A hand-held shower nozzle

51. When assisting with a tub bath or shower, which of these steps is first?
   A. Help the person undress and remove footwear.
   B. Assist or transport the person to the tub or shower room.
   C. Put the "occupied" sign on the door.
   D. Place a rubber bath mat in front of the tub or shower.

52. The best position for a back massage is
   A. Prone
   B. Supine
   C. Side-lying
   D. Semi-Fowler's

53. When giving a back massage, you should *not*
   A. Apply lotion to elbows, knees, and heels.
   B. Massage bony areas that are reddened.
   C. Wear gloves.
   D. Use lotion.

54. Back massages are dangerous for persons with all of these problems *except*
   A. Certain heart diseases
   B. Some lung disorders
   C. Arthritis
   D. Back injuries or back surgeries

55. When giving a back massage, the strokes
   A. Begin at the shoulders and end at the buttocks
   B. Should be light and gentle
   C. Begin at the buttocks and end at the shoulders
   D. Are continued for at least 10 minutes

56. When cleaning the perineal area, work from the
   A. Back to front
   B. Anal area to the urethra
   C. Urethra to the anal area
   D. Dirty to the clean area

57. When preparing water for perineal care, it should be
    A. The same temperature as water for a bed bath
    B. Warmer than bath water to clean away microorganisms
    C. Slightly cooler than bath water to prevent injury to perineal tissue
    D. Room temperature for comfort

58. When gathering equipment for perineal care, you will need
    A. One washcloth
    B. Two washcloths
    C. At least three washcloths
    D. At least four washcloths

59. When giving perineal care to a man you
    A. Retract the foreskin if he is uncircumcised.
    B. Wash from the scrotum to the tip of the penis.
    C. Use one washcloth for the entire procedure.
    D. Leave the foreskin retracted after finishing the care.

Matching

Match the skin care product with the benefits or the problem that may occur if you use the product.

60. _______	Absorbs moisture and prevents friction	A. Soaps
61. _______	Makes showers and tubs slippery	B. Bath oils
62. _______	Protects skin from the drying effect of air and evaporation	C. Creams and lotions
63. _______	Too much can cause caking and crusts that irritate the skin	D. Powders
64. _______	Masks and controls body odors	E. Deodorants and antiperspirants
65. _______	Tends to dry and irritate skin	
66. _______	Keeps skin soft and prevents drying	
67. _______	Removes dirt, dead skin, skin oil, some microbes, and perspiration	

Fill in the Blanks

68. Intact skin prevents microbes from entering the skin and causing an
    ______________________________.

69. The religion of East Indian Hindus requires at least one bath ______________________.

70. What are times when you would give oral hygiene to a person?
    ____
    ____

71. When you are delegated to give oral hygiene, what observations should you report?
    A. ______________________________
    B. ______________________________
    C. ______________________________
    D. ______________________________
    E. ______________________________
    F. ______________________________

72. If flossing is done only once a day, the best time to floss is at ________________.

73. When giving oral care to an unconscious person, explain what you are doing because you always assume ________________.

74. When following the rules for bathing in Box 16-2, you protect the skin by following these rules:

A. Rinse ________________

B. Pat ________________

C. Dry ________________

75. What two methods can be used to measure the water temperature used for a bed bath?

A. ________________

B. ________________

76. When you place a person's hand in the basin during the bed bath, have the person ________________ the hands and fingers.

77. When a person is able to bathe himself or herself, you may need to assist by washing the ________________ and ________________.

78. A tub bath can cause a person to feel ________________, especially if bedrest has been prescribed.

79. When the shower room has more than one stall or cabinet, you must protect the person's right to ________________. What are four things you can do to protect this right?

A. ________________

B. ________________

C. ________________

D. ________________

80. When giving a tub bath or shower, you use safety measures to protect the person from ________________ and ________________.

81. Lotion is applied to the elbows, knees, and heels because these bony areas are at risk for ________________.

82. When you are delegated to give a back massage, what observations should you report and record?

A. ________________

B. ________________

C. ________________

83. If a person does not understand the terms perineum and perineal, what terms might help you to explain what you need to do when giving care?

____

____

84. When assisting persons with hygiene, you should report and ________________ right away.

Labeling

85. Draw arrows on each picture to show which direction to move the toothbrush when brushing the teeth. Describe the position and motion used in each picture.

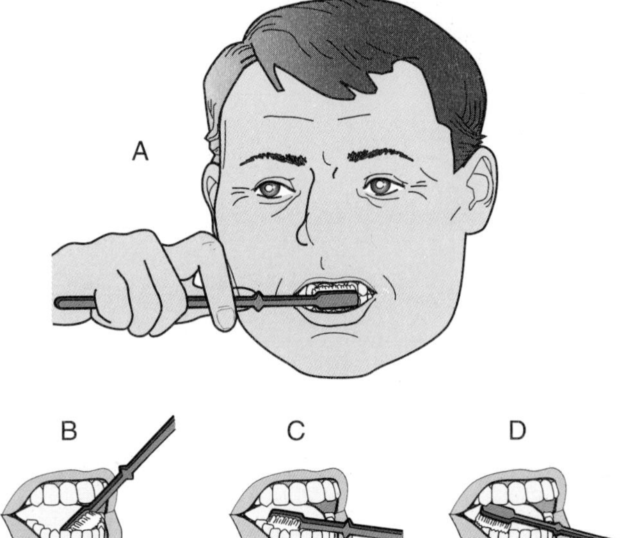

A. ______________________

B. ______________________

C. ______________________

D. ______________________

86. Look at this figure and answer these questions:

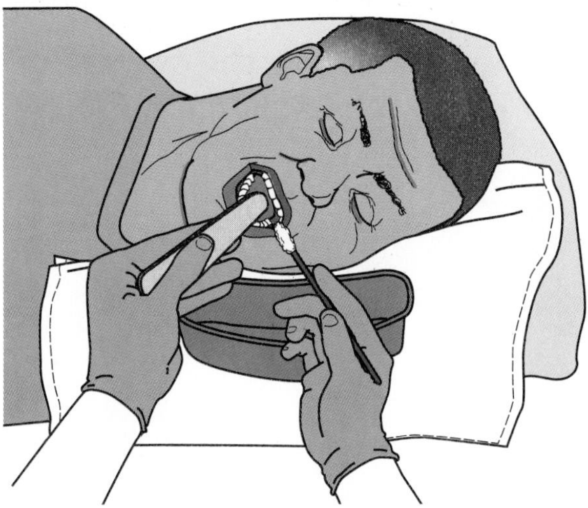

A. Why is the person positioned on his side?

____

B. What is the purpose of the padded tongue blade?

____

87. In this figure, what is the staff member using to remove the upper denture?

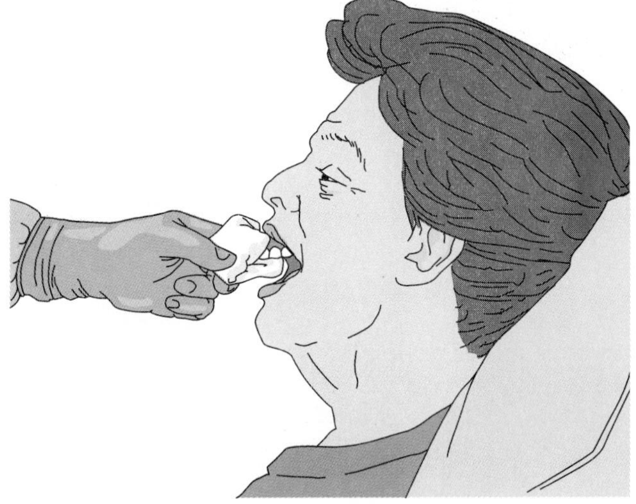

____

____

Why?

____

____

88. In this figure, explain what the staff member is doing.

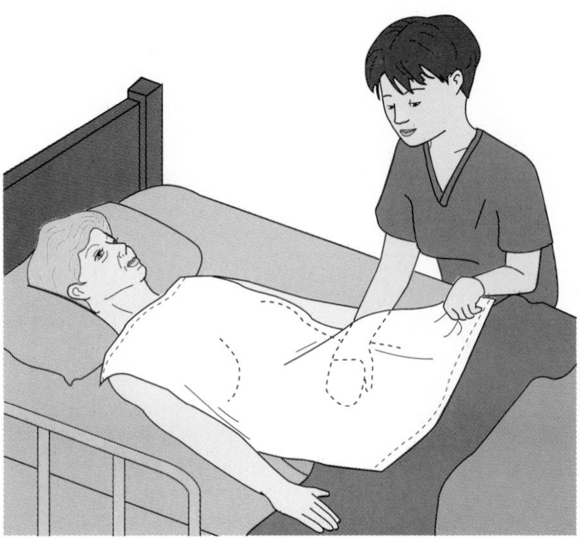

____

____

Why is the towel positioned vertically on the person?

____

____

89. Draw an arrow on the below figure to show the direction the back is washed. What rule of bathing does washing in this direction follow?

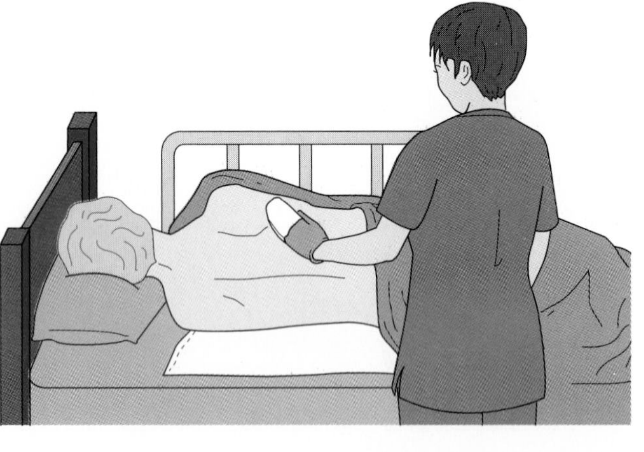

____

____

Nursing Assistant Skills Video Exercise

View the Bathing *video to answer these questions.*

90. When giving a bath, you should observe the person for

A. ____

B. ____

C. ____

D. ____

E. ____

91. If you observe any bleeding, discharge, or drainage when bathing a person, you should ____.

92. When you are giving a back massage, what should you do if you find a reddened area?

____

93. When you clean the perineal area, clean from clean to dirty areas. This means you wash from the ______________________ to the ______________________ area.

94. The water temperature should be ______________________ when you wash the perineal area.

Optional Learning Exercises

95. Hygiene promotes comfort, safety, and health. Answer these questions about hygiene:
    A. The skin is the body's first line of defense against ______________________.
    B. Intact skin prevents ______________________ from entering the body and causing an ______________________.
    C. In addition to the skin, what other areas must be clean and intact? ______________________

96. You are working the night shift and are assigned to give AM care (early morning care) to Mrs. Perez. What care is given at this time?
    A. ______________________
    B. ______________________
    C. ______________________
    D. ______________________
    E. ______________________
    F. ______________________
    G. ______________________

97. When working in long-term care, what care is given before and after afternoon naps?
    A. ______________________
    B. ______________________
    C. ______________________

98. Care given at bedtime is ______________________ and promotes ______________________.

99. What can often cause a bad taste in the mouth?
    A. ______________________
    B. ______________________
    C. ______________________

100. A dry mouth may be caused by
    A. ______________________
    B. ______________________
    C. ______________________
    D. ______________________
    E. ______________________

101. Sponge swabs are used for persons with ______________________ and for ______________________ persons.

102. Why is it important to check the foam pad on a sponge swab? ______________________

103. Why is it important to follow Standard Precautions and Bloodborne Pathogen Standard when giving oral care? ______________________

104. Flossing is done to prevent what disease? ______________________

105. Many older persons do not floss their teeth because ______________________.

106. Why is mouth care for the unconscious person especially important?
    A. ______________________
    B. ______________________
    C. ______________________

107. What do the factors listed in #106 cause?

A. ______________________________

B. ______________________________

108. To prevent aspiration when giving mouth care to an unconscious person, you should

A. ______________________________

B. ______________________________

109. What should you do if dentures are lost or damaged?

____

If you lose or damage a person's dentures, this is

______________________________ conduct.

110. List all of the benefits of bathing.

A. ______________________________

B. ______________________________

C. ______________________________

D. ______________________________

E. ______________________________

F. ______________________________

G. ______________________________

H. ______________________________

111. When you are bathing a person with dementia, what measures are important to help the person understand that you are trying to help them?

A. ______________________________

B. ______________________________

C. ______________________________

D. ______________________________

E. ______________________________

F. ______________________________

G. ______________________________

112. You are delegated to give Mrs. Johnson a bath. Before beginning, what information do you need?

A. ______________________________

B. ______________________________

C. ______________________________

D. ______________________________

E. ______________________________

F. ______________________________

113. As you are bathing Mrs. Johnson, what observations should you report and record?

A. ______________________________

B. ______________________________

C. ______________________________

D. ______________________________

E. ______________________________

F. ______________________________

G. ______________________________

H. ______________________________

I. ______________________________

J. ______________________________

K. ______________________________

114. A back massage lasts about ______________.

115. When you are preparing to give perineal care to Mrs. Johnson, why do you gather at least four washcloths?

____

____

116. What water temperature is generally used for each of these?

A. Complete bed bath __________ ° F

B. Partial bed bath __________ ° F

C. Tub bath or shower __________ ° F

D. Perineal care __________ ° F

117. What two age groups may need slightly cooler water temperatures?

____

Why?

____

Independent Learning Activities

- To understand how other persons feel when receiving personal care, answer these questions about yourself. Your answers may be kept private, or you may choose to use these questions as a discussion with several classmates. A discussion may help you understand different personal practices related to personal hygiene.
  - Do you prefer a shower or tub bath?
  - What time of day do you usually bathe?
  - What skin care products do you use to keep your skin healthy?
  - What special measures do you use when brushing your teeth? Special brush? Toothpaste? Do you floss? How often?

- As part of your preparation for caring for persons, you and your classmates may be assigned to practice back massages on each other in class. Answer these questions about how you felt when you were the person receiving the back massage.
  - How did the lotion feel on your back? Was it warm or cold?
  - Which strokes were relaxing? Which were more stimulating?
  - How long do you think the back massage lasted? Look at the clock to see the actual time.
  - What can you tell the person giving the massage that would improve his or her technique?
  - How will this practice help you when you give a back massage to another person?

- As part of your preparation for caring for persons, you and your classmates may be assigned to practice mouth care on each other in class. Answer these questions about how you felt when you were the person receiving the care.
  - What did the "nursing assistant" tell you before beginning the mouth care?
  - What choices were offered? Position? Equipment? Products?
  - How did it feel to have someone else give you mouth care? To floss your teeth?
  - How clean did your teeth feel when the mouth care was completed?
  - What can you tell the person who gave the mouth care that would help improve the procedure?
  - How will this experience help you when you give mouth care to a person you are caring for?

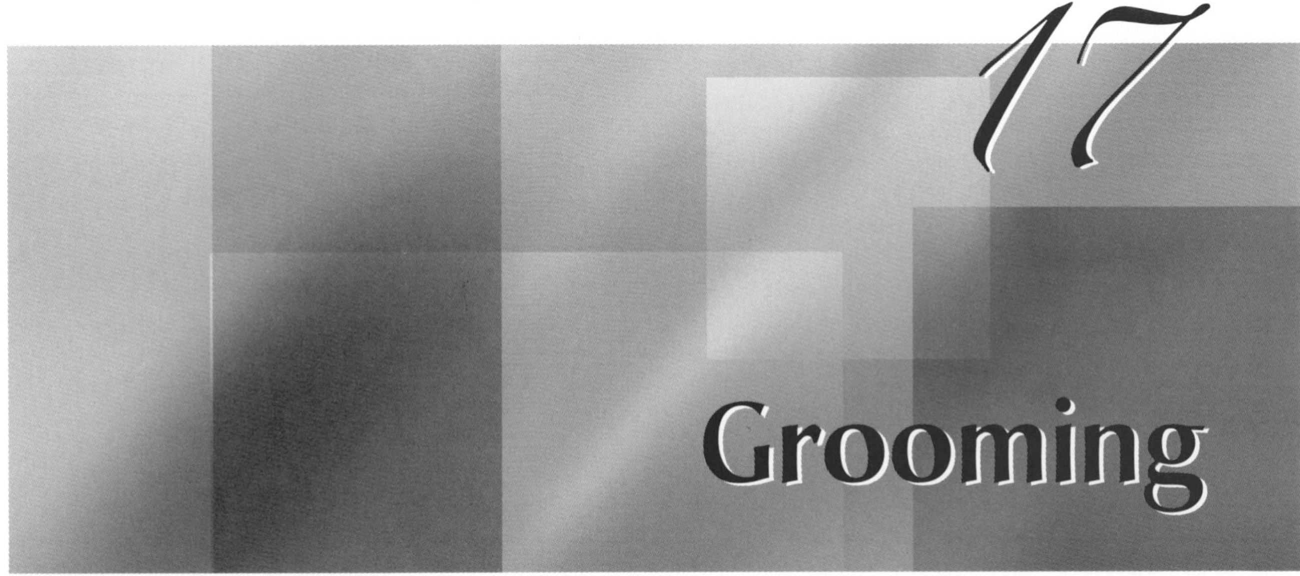

17 Grooming

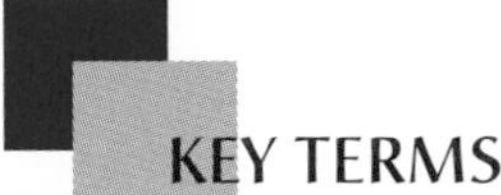

KEY TERMS

Alopecia
Dandruff
Hirsutism
Pediculosis
Pediculosis capitis
Pediculosis corporis
Pediculosis pubis

Fill in the Blanks: Key Terms

1. The infestation with lice is

   ______________________________________.

2. ______________________________ is the excessive amount of dry, white flakes from the scalp.

3. The infestation of the body with lice is

   ______________________________________.

4. Hair loss is ______________________________.

5. ______________________________________ is the infestation of lice in the pubic hair.

6. Excessive body hair in women and children is

   ______________________________________.

7. The infestation of lice in the scalp is

   ______________________________________.

Circle the BEST Answer

8. Hair care, shaving, and nail and foot care are important to people because they affect
   A. Safety and security
   B. Love and belonging and self-esteem
   C. Physical needs
   D. Self-actualization needs

9. If you see any signs of lice, you should report it to the nurse because
   A. Lice bites can cause severe infections.
   B. Lice are easily spread to other persons through clothing, furniture, bed linens, and sexual contact.
   C. Infestation can cause the person's hair to fall out.
   D. Lice will cause the hair to mat and tangle.

10. Who chooses how you will brush, comb, and style a person's hair?
    A. The person
    B. You
    C. The nurse
    D. Care plan

11. If long hair becomes matted or tangled, you should
    A. Braid the hair.
    B. Cut the hair to remove the tangles and matting.
    C. Tell the nurse, and ask for directions.
    D. Decide what is the easiest thing to do.

12. If hair is curly, coarse, and dry, which of these would *not* be done?
    A. Braid or cut the hair.
    B. Use a wide-toothed comb.
    C. Work upward, lifting and fluffing the hair outward.
    D. Apply a conditioner of petrolatum jelly to make combing easier.

13. If a person has the hair styled in small braids, when you are assisting with grooming
    A. Undo the hair, and rebraid it each day.
    B. Leave the braids intact for shampooing.
    C. Undo the braids to make lying in bed more comfortable.
    D. Ask the nurse to decide what should be done.

14. When you are caring for an older child or teenager, the hair is styled
    A. In a way that pleases the child and parents
    B. According to your standards or customs
    C. In a way to make care easier
    D. In a way the nurse directs

15. When you wash the hair
    A. It should be washed daily.
    B. Dry and style hair as quickly as possible after shampooing.
    C. Use only soap and water.
    D. Tell the person it can only be washed once a week.

16. If a woman's hair is styled in a beauty shop, you should
    A. Wash her hair only once a week.
    B. Wash her hair on the day she goes to the beauty shop.
    C. Make sure she wears a shower cap during the tub bath or shower.
    D. Wash her hair each time she gets a shower or tub bath.

17. Shampooing at the sink or on a stretcher
    A. Is not tolerated by persons with limited range-of-motion in their necks
    B. Can be used in place of shampooing in bed
    C. Is easier than shampooing in the shower or tub
    D. Is only used for persons with limited range-of-motion in the neck

18. When shampooing during the tub bath or shower, water can be kept out of the eyes by
    A. Tipping the head backward
    B. Having the person lean forward
    C. Holding a washcloth over the eyes
    D. All of the above

19. Which of these is not an observation that is made when shampooing?
    A. Scalp sores
    B. Presence of lice
    C. Amount of hair on the head
    D. Hair falling out in patches

20. Which of these statements is *not* true?
    A. You may use the agency razor for more than one person if the razor is cleaned between persons.
    B. You may use the person's own razor.
    C. It is acceptable to use disposable razors.
    D. Use safety razors to shave persons receiving anticoagulants.

21. When shaving a person, you should wear gloves
    A. When you fill the basin with water
    B. To wipe off the overbed table with paper towels
    C. To apply the shaving cream
    D. When you wash the person's face

22. You shave against the hair growth when shaving the
    A. Face
    B. Legs
    C. Underarms
    D. All of the above

23. When caring for a mustache and beard, all of these are done *except*
    A. Wash the mustache or beard daily.
    B. Comb the mustache or beard daily.
    C. Ask the person how to groom his beard or mustache.
    D. Trim or shave a beard or mustache when you feel it is needed.

24. Nursing assistants never cut or trim toenails if the person
    A. Has just taken a bath or shower
    B. Asks the nursing assistant to use nail clippers
    C. Has diabetes or poor circulation
    D. Has shoes that fit poorly

25. When caring for the fingernails or toenails, which of these is wrong?
    A. Cut the nails with small scissors.
    B. Clean under the nails with an orange stick.
    C. Clip the nails straight across with nail clippers.
    D. Shape the nails with an emery board or nail file.

26. When changing clothing, remove the clothing from
    A. The weak side first
    B. The lower limbs first
    C. The right side last
    D. The strong or "good" side first

27. When changing the gown of a person with an IV, you
    A. Turn off the IV.
    B. Lay the IV bag on the bed.
    C. Gather the sleeve of the arm with the IV, and slide it over the IV.
    D. Slide the gown over the IV and down the pole.

28. When you have finished changing the gown of a person with an IV, you should
    A. Restart the pump.
    B. Reconnect the IV.
    C. Check the flow rate, or ask the nurse to check it.
    D. Ask the person if it is running properly.

29. When you are delegated to undress a person, it is usually done
    A. In the bed
    B. With the person sitting in a chair
    C. By having the person stand at the bedside
    D. In the bathroom

30. When you are changing the person's clothes, you use good body mechanics by
    A. Have a good base of support.
    B. Hold objects close to your body.
    C. Raise the bed to a good working level.
    D. Lift with the large muscles.

31. To provide warmth and privacy when changing clothes, you should
    A. Keep the top sheets in place.
    B. Cover the person with a bath blanket.
    C. Close the curtains.
    D. Close the door.

Fill in the Blanks

32. If long hair is matted and tangled, the nurse may have you brush by taking a small section of hair near ____________________.

33. If you give hair care to a person in bed after a linen change, collect falling hair by ____________________.

34. When you brush and comb the hair, you should report and record
    A. ____________________
    B. ____________________
    C. ____________________
    D. ____________________
    E. ____________________

35. If a person cannot tip the head back as you shampoo in the shower or tub, you can protect the person's eyes by holding a ____________________.

36. When rinsing the hair, you can keep soapy water from running down the person's forehead and into the eyes by ____________________.

37. What delegation guidelines do you need when shaving a person?
    A. ____________________
    B. ____________________
    C. ____________________

38. When you are shaving the face and underarms, which direction do you shave?
    ____

39. When shaving legs, which direction do you shave?

____

40. What two actions should you take if you nick someone while shaving?

A. _______________

B. _______________

41. When you give nail and foot care, report and record

A. _______________

B. _______________

C. _______________

D. _______________

E. _______________

42. When undressing the person, if you cannot raise the person's head and shoulders you should

A. _______________

B. _______________

C. _______________

D. _______________

E. _______________

43. Before changing a person's hospital gown, what information do you need from the nurse or care plan?

A. _______________

B. _______________

C. _______________

Nursing Assistant Skills Video

View the* Personal Hygiene and Grooming *video to answer these questions.

44. What observations should be made when giving hair care?

A. _______________

B. _______________

C. _______________

D. _______________

45. When washing the hair in bed, how is the head supported in the trough?

____

46. When washing hair in bed, the water temperature should be _______________ ° F.

47. When shaving the face, keep the skin _______________ and shave at a _______________-degree angle.

48. Razors are discarded in the _______________.

49. Because injury is a risk, many centers only allow a _______________ or _______________ to trim toenails.

50. Feet and hands should be soaked for _______________ before cleaning under the nails and trimming or shaping the nails.

51. When dressing a person in bed, cover the person with a _______________.

52. To pull up the pants, have the person _______________.

Optional Learning Exercises

53. You are caring for a person who is receiving cancer treatments. What effect could this treatment have on the person's hair?

    ____

54. Dandruff not only occurs on the scalp, but it may also involve the ____________________.

55. You should immediately report any signs of lice to the nurse because infestation can easily ______________________________.

56. When brushing and combing the hair, you need to inspect the comb and brush because ______________________________.

57. Many older or disabled persons cannot tolerate having their hair shampooed at the sink because ______________________________.

58. Electric shavers are used when shaving a person who is taking anticoagulants because a ______________________________.

59. Injuries to the feet of a person with poor circulation is serious because ______________________________.

60. Why are grooming measures important? What needs does this care meet?
    - A. ______________________________
    - B. ______________________________
    - C. ______________________________
    - D. ______________________________

Independent Learning Activities

- Ask another person if you may shave him or her with a safety razor. (Some instructors may be concerned about the liability of this exercise. Make sure that the instructor approves this exercise, especially if you are using a classmate as a partner.) Ask the person you shaved to help you answer these questions.
  - What did you use for lubricating the skin? Shaving cream? Soap? Water only? How did it feel to the person? What lubricating technique worked best?
  - Which worked best, applying more pressure or applying less pressure?
  - Shave one side of the face with hair growth and one side against the hair growth. Which way is better? Why?
  - What way can the person help you shave the face better?
  - What area is the most difficult to shave? How did you deal with this area?
  - Ask the person you shaved for any tips on how to improve your shaving skills.

- Role-play this situation with a classmate. Take turns being the person and the nursing assistant. Remember to keep your left arm and leg limp when you are the person.
  Situation: Mr. Olsen is a 58-year-old man who has weakness on his left side. You are assigned to take off his sleepwear and dress him for the day. You need to remove his pajamas and dress him in a shirt, a pullover sweater, slacks, socks, and shoes.
  - How did you provide privacy?
  - How was Mr. Olsen positioned for the clothing change?
  - What difficulties did you have when you removed his pajamas?
  - Which arm did you redress first? What difficulty did you have getting his arms into the shirt?
  - How did you put on the sweater? What was the most difficult part about this?
  - What was the most difficult part of putting on the slacks?
  - How did you put on his socks and shoes?
  - What did you learn from this role-play situation? Did you follow the procedure in the chapter to assist you?
  - Discuss with each other how it felt to have someone dress you when you were "Mr. Olsen."

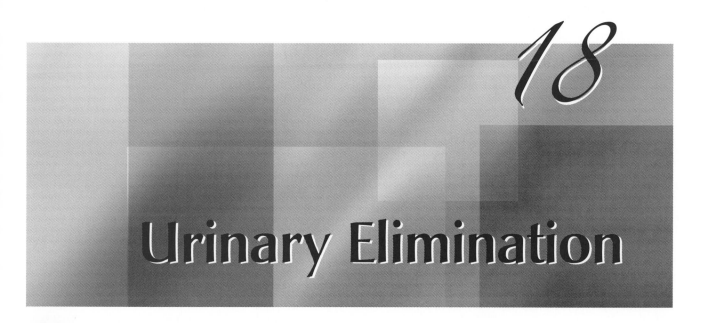

18 Urinary Elimination

KEY TERMS

Catheter
Catheterization
Dysuria
Foley catheter
Functional incontinence
Hematuria
Indwelling catheter
Micturition
Nocturia
Oliguria
Overflow incontinence
Polyuria
Reflex incontinence
Retention catheter
Straight catheter
Stress incontinence
Urge incontinence
Urinary frequency
Urinary incontinence
Urinary urgency
Urination
Voiding

Fill in the Blanks: Key Terms

1. The production of abnormally large amounts of urine is ______________________.
2. The process of inserting a catheter is ______________________.
3. ______________________ is the loss of bladder control.
4. Frequent urination at night is ______________________.
5. When the bladder is too full and urine leaks, it is ______________________.
6. Another word for urination or voiding is ______________________.
7. ______________________ occurs when the person has bladder control but cannot use the toilet in time.
8. The process of emptying urine from the bladder is micturition, voiding, or ______________________.
9. A ______________________ is also called a Foley catheter or indwelling catheter.
10. A tube used to drain or inject fluid through a body opening is a ______________________.

11. ______________________________ is the loss of urine in response to a sudden urgent need to void; the person cannot get to a toilet in time.

12. A catheter left in the bladder to enable urine to drain constantly into a drainage bag is an ______________________________ or a retention or Foley catheter.

13. ______________________________ is a scant amount of urine; less than 500 ml in 24 hours.

14. Painful or difficult urination is ______________________________.

15. Another word for urination or micturition is ______________________________.

16. A ______________________________ is also called an indwelling or retention catheter.

17. The loss of urine at predictable intervals when the bladder is full is ______________________________.

18. ______________________________ is blood in the urine.

19. Voiding at frequent intervals is ______________________________.

20. A catheter that drains the bladder and is removed is a ______________________________.

21. The need to void at once is ______________________________.

22. When urine leaks during exercise and certain movements, it is ______________________________.

Circle the BEST Answer

23. Solid wastes are removed from the body by the
    A. Digestive system
    B. Urinary system
    C. Blood
    D. Integumentary system

24. A healthy adult excretes about ____________ ml of urine a day.
    A. 200 to 300
    B. 1000
    C. 1500
    D. 2000

25. You can provide privacy when the person is voiding by doing all of these *except*
    A. Pull drapes or window shades.
    B. Stay in room.
    C. Pull the curtain around the bed.
    D. Close the room and bathroom doors.

26. If the person has difficulty starting the urine stream, you can
    A. Play music on the television.
    B. Provide perineal care.
    C. Use a stainless steel bedpan.
    D. Run water in a nearby sink.

27. The urine may be bright yellow if the person eats
    A. Asparagus
    B. Carrots and sweet potatoes
    C. Beets and blackberries
    D. Rhubarb

28. When using a steel bedpan, you should
    A. Keep the pan in the utility room.
    B. Warm the pan with water, and dry it before using.
    C. Sterilize the pan after each use.
    D. Cool the pan with water, and dry it before using.

29. When using a fracture pan, you should
    A. Warm it with water.
    B. Place the smaller end under the buttocks.
    C. Place the larger end under the buttocks.
    D. Use it only when you have a doctor's order.

30. When you are getting ready to give a person the bedpan, you should
    A. Raise the head of the bed slightly.
    B. Position the person in the Fowler's position.
    C. Wash the person's hands.
    D. Place the bed in a flat position.

31. When giving a bed pan to a person who can assist, you
    A. Turn the person onto the side away from you.
    B. Ask the person to flex the knees and raise the buttocks.
    C. Only use a fracture pan.
    D. Raise the head of the bed before offering the bedpan.

32. When a person uses the bedpan, gloves are worn
    A. When you give the bedpan
    B. When you remove the bedpan
    C. When you return the clean pan to the bedside stand
    D. All of the above

33. Urinals are placed at the bedside on
    A. Bed rails
    B. Overbed tables
    C. Bedside stands
    D. The floor

34. When using the urinal, if possible, most men prefer to
    A. Lie in bed
    B. Sit on the edge of the bed
    C. Stand at the side of the bed
    D. Sit in a chair

35. A commode chair is used when the person
    A. Is unable to walk to the bathroom
    B. Cannot sit up unsupported on the toilet
    C. Needs to be in the normal position for elimination
    D. All of the above

36. When you place a commode over the toilet
    A. Restrain the person.
    B. Stay in the room with the person.
    C. Lock the wheels.
    D. Make sure the container is in place.

37. Dribbling of urine that occurs with laughing, sneezing, coughing, lifting, or other activities mean the person has
    A. Urge incontinence
    B. Stress incontinence
    C. Overflow incontinence
    D. Functional incontinence

38. Functional incontinence occurs because
    A. The bladder is too full.
    B. The person is immobile or confused.
    C. The person has a sudden, urgent need to void.
    D. The person does not feel the need to void.

39. All of these will help the person with incontinence *except*
    A. Restricting fluid intake
    B. Dressing the person in easy-to-remove clothing
    C. Answering call bells promptly
    D. Decreasing fluid intake at bedtime

40. When providing perineal care, all of these would be correct steps *except*
    A. Provide perineal care once a day.
    B. Wash, rinse, and dry the perineal area and buttocks.
    C. Remove wet incontinent products, garments, and linens.
    D. Provide dry garments and linens.

41. A catheter that is inserted to drain the bladder and then is removed is
    A. An indwelling catheter
    B. A straight catheter
    C. A condom catheter
    D. A Foley catheter

42. An indwelling catheter is used for all of these *except*
    A. To keep the bladder empty before, during, and after surgery
    B. When a person is dying
    C. To make it easier to care for the person
    D. To protect wounds and pressure ulcers from contact with urine

43. A last resort for incontinence is
    A. Bladder training
    B. Answering signal lights promptly
    C. An indwelling catheter
    D. Adequate fluid intake

44. When cleaning a catheter, you should
    A. Wipe 4 inches up the catheter to the meatus.
    B. Disconnect the tubing from the drainage bag.
    C. Clean down the catheter from the meatus about 4 inches.
    D. Wash and rinse the catheter by washing up and down the tubing.

45. The drainage bag from a catheter should not be attached to the
    A. Bed frame
    B. Chair
    C. Wheelchair
    D. Bed rail

46. If a catheter is accidentally disconnected from the drainage bag
    A. Cover the tip of the catheter with tape.
    B. Clamp the catheter to prevent leakage.
    C. Wipe the end of the tube and the end of the catheter with separate antiseptic wipes.
    D. Discard the drainage bag, and get a new bag.

47. If a person uses a leg drainage bag, it
    A. Is switched to a drainage bag when the person is in bed
    B. Is attached to the clothing with tape or safety pins
    C. Is attached to the bed rail when the person is in bed
    D. Can be worn 24 hours a day

48. A leg bag needs to be emptied more often than a drainage bag because it
    A. Holds 1000 ml and the drainage bag holds about 2000 ml
    B. Is more likely to leak than the drainage bag
    C. Holds about 250 ml and the drainage bag holds 1000 ml
    D. Interferes with walking if it is full

49. When you empty a drainage bag, you should
    A. Disconnect the bag from the tubing.
    B. Clamp the catheter to prevent leakage.
    C. Open the clamp, and drain into a measuring container.
    D. Take the bag into the bathroom to empty it.

50. When applying a condom catheter
    A. Apply elastic tape in a spiral around the penis.
    B. Make sure the catheter tip is touching the head of the penis.
    C. Securely apply tape in a circle entirely around the penis.
    D. Remove and reapply the catheter during every shift.

51. The goal of bladder training is to
    A. Keep the person dry and clean
    B. Control urination
    C. Prevent skin breakdown
    D. Prevent infection

52. When you are assisting the person with bladder training to have normal elimination, you should
    A. Help the person to the bathroom every 15 or 20 minutes.
    B. Give the person 15 to 20 minutes to start voiding.
    C. Make sure the person drinks at least 1000 ml during each shift.
    D. Tell the person he or she can only void once during a shift.

53. When you assist with bladder training for a person with an indwelling catheter, you should
    A. Empty the drainage bag every hour.
    B. Clamp the catheter for 1 hour at first.
    C. Clamp the catheter for 3 to 4 hours at first.
    D. Give the person 15 to 20 minutes to start voiding.

Fill in the Blanks

54. What substances increase urine production?

    A. ______________________________

    B. ______________________________

    C. ______________________________

    D. ______________________________

55. A normal position for voiding for women is

    ____________________. For men, a normal

    position is ______________________.

56. Report to the nurse if an infant has not had a wet

    diaper for several hours because this is a sign of

    ______________________________.

57. What is normal for urine in the following?

    A. Color ______________________________

    B. Clarity ______________________________

    C. Odor ______________________________

    D. Particles ______________________________

58. What can you do to mask urination sounds?

    ____

    ____

59. Fracture pans are used for

A. ______________________

B. ______________________

C. ______________________

D. ______________________

E. ______________________

F. ______________________

G. Older persons with ______________________ or ______________________

60. When a person voids in a bedpan or urinal, what observations are important?

A. ______________________

B. ______________________

C. ______________________

D. ______________________

61. When you are handling bedpans, urinals, and commodes and their contents, you should follow ______________________ and ______________________.

62. If a person cannot assist in getting on the bedpan, you should

A. ______________________

B. ______________________

C. ______________________

D. ______________________

E. ______________________

63. Before assisting with urinals, what information do you need from the nurse and care plan?

A. ______________________

B. ______________________

C. ______________________

D. ______________________

E. ______________________

64. When you transfer a person to a commode from the bed, you must practice safe transfer practices and use a ______________________.

65. List four causes of urge incontinence.

A. ______________________

B. ______________________

C. ______________________

D. ______________________

66. Stress incontinence is common in women because the pelvic muscles weaken from______________________ and with ______________________.

67. Overflow incontinence may occur in men because of an enlarged ______________________.

68. Why is a person with incontinence at risk for falls?

____

____

69. When you give kindness, empathy, understanding, and patience to a person with incontinence, you protect the person's right to be free from

______________________.

70. What complications of incontinence pose serious problems for older persons?

    A. ______________________

    B. ______________________

    C. ______________________

71. When you provide perineal care after a person is incontinent, you should remember to

    A. ______________________

    B. ______________________

    C. ______________________

    D. ______________________

    E. ______________________

    F. ______________________

72. When a catheter is inserted after a person voids, it measures the amount of urine ______________________.

73. When a person has a catheter, what observations should you report and record?

    A. ______________________

    B. ______________________

    C. ______________________

    D. ______________________

    E. ______________________

74. When you give catheter care, clean the catheter about ____________ inches. Clean ____________ from the meatus with ____________ stroke.

75. What happens if a drainage bag is higher than the bladder?

    ____

    ____

76. What should you do if the drainage system is disconnected accidentally?

    A. ______________________

    B. ______________________

    C. ______________________

    D. ______________________

    E. ______________________

    F. ______________________

    G. ______________________

77. When you empty a drainage system, report and record

    A. ______________________

    B. ______________________

    C. ______________________

    D. ______________________

    E. ______________________

78. Before applying a condom catheter, you should provide ____________ and observe the penis for ______________________.

79. When bladder training is done with a person who has a catheter, the catheter is clamped

    A. At first ______________________

    B. Over time ______________________

Labeling

80. In this figure, mark two places where you would secure the catheter.

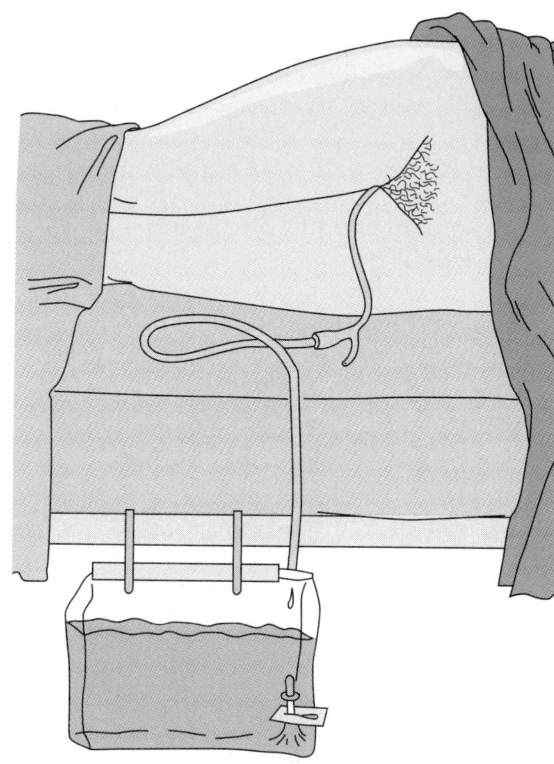

81. In this figure, mark two places where you would secure the catheter.

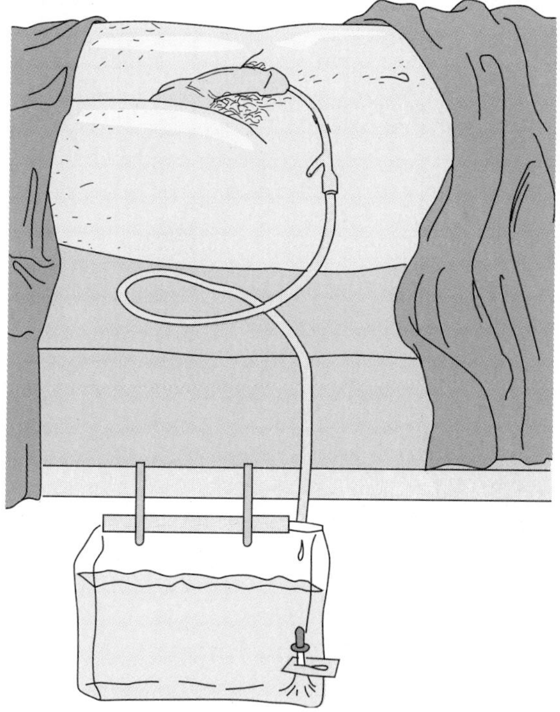

82. The following questions relate to both figures.

A. Why are the catheters secured?

Male ______________________________

____

Female ______________________________

____

B. The drainage bags are hanging from where?

Male ______________________________

____

Female ______________________________

____

C. Why are they hung there?

Male ______________________________

____

Female ______________________________

____

Crossword Puzzle

Fill in the crossword puzzle by answering the clues with words from this list.

anus
commode
dysuria
hematuria
incontinence
meatus
microbe
micturition
nocturia
oliguria
perineal
polyuria
urethra
urinal

Across

1. Chair or wheelchair with an opening for a bedpan or container
5. Another word for voiding or urination
8. Opening of urinary system to the outside of body
10. Blood in the urine
11. Abnormally large amounts of urine
12. Opening of the bowel to outside of the body
13. Tube that allows urine to leave the bladder

Down

2. Scant amount of urine, usually less than 500 ml in 24 hours
3. Container used by men to urinate at bedside
4. Painful or difficult urination
6. Temporary or permanent loss of bladder control
7. Frequent urination at night
8. Microorganism
9. Genital and anal area

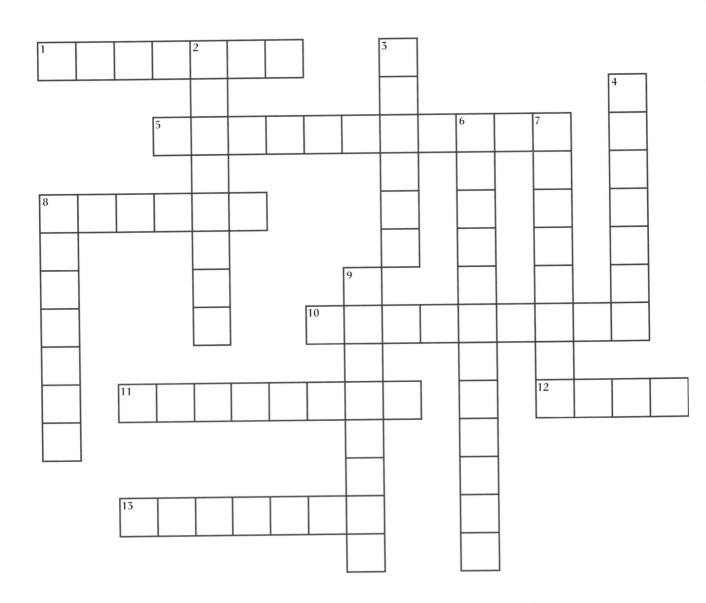

Nursing Assistant Skills Video Exercise

View the **Normal Elimination** *video to answer these questions.*

83. How much urine does a healthy adult normally produce each day?

____

84. What is the normal color of urine?

____

85. After a person has used the bedpan or urinal, you should offer _______________ and _______________.

86. Before handling a bedpan or urinal, you should put on _______________.

Optional Learning Exercises

87. How do these foods affect the urine or the body?

    A. Coffee, tea, alcohol

    ____

    B. Salt (body) _______________ (urine)

    ____

    C. Beets, blackberries, rhubarb

    ____

    D. Carrots and sweet potatoes

    ____

    E. Asparagus

    ____

88. What should be reported to the nurse after a person urinates?

    A. Ask nurse to observe

    ____

    B. Complaints of

    ____

89. Why are fracture pans used for older persons with fragile bones or painful joints?

____

90. How many pairs of gloves are needed when you assist a person with a bedpan, urinal, or commode?

____

List the activity you are preparing to do each time you put on the gloves.

A. _______________

B. _______________

C. _______________

91. How many times do you decontaminate your hands when you assist a person with a bedpan, urinal, or commode?

A. _______________

B. _______________

C. _______________

List the reason you wash your hands each time.

A. _______________

B. _______________

C. _______________

D. _______________

E. _______________

F. _______________

92. If you are caring for an incontinent person and you become short-tempered and impatient, you should _______________.

93. You know that catheters are a last resort for incontinent persons. If a person is weak, disabled, or dying, a catheter can promote

_______________________________________.

94. What are two diagnostic uses for catheters?

A. _______________________________________

B. _______________________________________

95. What can happen if microbes enter a closed drainage system?

____

____

96. What type of tape is used to apply a condom catheter?

____

Why?

____

What can happen if you use the wrong tape?

____

Independent Learning Activities

- Role-play the following situation with a classmate. Take turns playing the person using the bedpan and the nursing assistant. Answer the questions about the activity.
  Situation: Mrs. Donnelly is a 70 year old who must use the bedpan. She finds it difficult to move easily and usually does not have enough strength to raise her hips to get on the bedpan. She tells you she will try to help as much as she can.

  As Mrs. Donnelly
  - When you tried to assist, how easy was it to raise your hips? How did the nursing assistant help you get on the pan?
  - When you were rolled onto the bedpan, how did it feel? How well was the pan positioned under you?
  - How did you feel about sitting on the pan in bed? Did you feel as if this would be an easy or difficult way to void? Explain your feelings.
  - How could the nursing assistant have made this procedure better?

  As the nursing assistant
  - How did you position the bedpan to get it ready to slide under Mrs. Donnelly? Did this method work? How could you improve your method?
  - When you rolled Mrs. Donnelly onto the pan, how well was she positioned? What adjustments were necessary?
  - When you rolled her off the pan, what happened? If urine had been in the pan, what would have occurred?
  - How could you have changed some of your steps to make this procedure better?

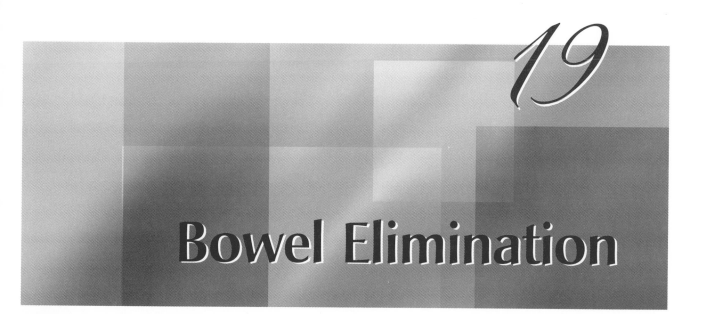

19 Bowel Elimination

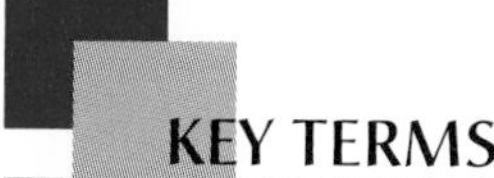

KEY TERMS

Colostomy
Constipation
Defecation
Dehydration
Diarrhea
Enema
Fecal impaction
Fecal incontinence
Feces
Flatulence
Flatus
Ileostomy
Ostomy
Peristalsis
Stoma
Stool
Suppository

Fill in the Blanks: Key Terms

1. The process of excreting feces from the rectum through the anus is a bowel movement or ______________________.
2. The excessive formation of gas in the stomach and intestines is ______________________.
3. A ______________________ is a cone-shaped solid drug that is inserted into a body opening.
4. The frequent passage of liquid stools is ______________________.
5. ______________________ is the inability to control the passage of feces and gas through the anus.
6. ______________________ is the excessive loss of water from tissues.
7. Gas or air in the stomach or intestines is ______________________.
8. The introduction of fluid into the rectum and lower colon is an ______________________.
9. Excreted feces are ______________________.

10. An artificial opening between the colon and abdominal wall is a __________________________________.

11. The prolonged retention and accumulation of feces in the rectum is __________________________________.

12. ________________________ is the alternating contraction and relaxation of intestinal muscles.

13. The passage of a hard, dry stool is __________________________________.

14. A surgically created artificial opening is a __________________________________.

15. A ________________________ is an opening such as that found in a colostomy or ileostomy.

16. The semisolid mass of waste products in the colon is ____________________________.

17. An artificial opening between the ileum and abdominal wall is an __________________________________.

Circle the BEST Answer

18. People normally have a bowel movement
    A. Every day
    B. Every 2 to 3 days
    C. 2 or 3 times a day
    D. All of the above

19. Bleeding in the stomach and small intestines causes stool to be
    A. Brown
    B. Black
    C. Red
    D. Clay colored

20. The characteristic odor of stool is caused by
    A. Poor personal hygiene
    B. Poor nutrition
    C. Bacterial action in the intestines
    D. Adequate fluid intake

21. You expect a newborn infant to have a bowel movement
    A. Once a day
    B. After every feeding
    C. Two to three times a day
    D. Every time the infant urinates

22. If you are caring for a person and observe that the stool is abnormal, you should
    A. Ask the nurse to observe the abnormal stool.
    B. Report your observation, and discard the stool.
    C. Ask the person if the stool is normal for him or her.
    D. Record your observation when you finish his or her care.

23. Which of these could interfere with normal, regular bowel elimination?
    A. Being able to relax by reading a book or newspaper
    B. Eating a diet with high-fiber foods
    C. Using a bedpan or commode in a semiprivate room
    D. Drinking six to eight glasses of water daily

24. A person who must stay in bed most of the time may have irregular elimination and constipation because of
    A. Poor diet
    B. Poor fluid intake
    C. Lack of activity
    D. Lack of privacy

25. Which of these would provide safety for the person during bowel elimination?
    A. Make sure the bedpan is warm.
    B. Place the signal light and toilet tissue within the person's reach.
    C. Provide perineal care.
    D. Allow enough time for defecation.

26. Bowel training is learned
    A. By the end of the first year of life
    B. Between ages 2 and 3 years
    C. By $1^1/_2$ years of age
    D. Between ages 4 and 5 years

27. Constipation can be relieved by
    A. Giving the person a low-fiber diet
    B. Increasing activity
    C. Decreasing fluids
    D. Ignoring the urge to defecate

28. Mr. Barton tries many times to have a bowel movement. Liquid feces seeps from the anus. He complains of abdominal discomfort, nausea, and cramping. This probably means he has
    A. Diarrhea
    B. Constipation
    C. Fecal impaction
    D. Fecal incontinence

29. If the nurse finds a fecal impaction, he or she will first try to relieve it by
    A. Changing the person's diet
    B. Telling the nursing assistant to give more fluids
    C. Removing the fecal mass with a gloved finger
    D. Increasing the activity of the person

30. A nursing assistant knows that removing a fecal impaction can be dangerous because
    A. It can stimulate the vagus nerve and slow the heart rate.
    B. It is a sterile procedure.
    C. Rectal bleeding can occur.
    D. It is uncomfortable for the person.

31. Good skin care is important when a person has diarrhea because
    A. It prevents odors.
    B. Skin breakdown and pressure ulcers are risks of diarrhea.
    C. It prevents the spread of microbes.
    D. It prevents fluid loss.

32. Which of these is *not* a sign of dehydration?
    A. Increased blood pressure
    B. Pale or flushed skin
    C. Dizziness and confusion
    D. Oliguria

33. Why are older persons at risk for dehydration?
    A. They drink more fluids.
    B. The amount of body water decreases with aging.
    C. They eat a low-fiber diet.
    D. Older persons increase their activity level.

34. As the nursing assistant, you can prevent fecal incontinence by doing all of these *except*
    A. Telling the person you will help him or her to the bathroom when you have time
    B. Answering call bells promptly
    C. Making sure a new person knows where the bathroom is located
    D. Helping with elimination after meals and every 2 to 3 hours

35. When fecal incontinence occurs, the nurse may plan all of these *except*
    A. Bowel training
    B. Assisting with elimination after meals
    C. Checking daily for a fecal impaction
    D. Providing incontinent products to keep garments and linens clean

36. If flatus is not expelled, the person may complain of
    A. Abdominal cramping or pain
    B. Diarrhea
    C. Fecal incontinence
    D. Nausea

37. When bowel training is planned, which of these is included in the care plan?
    A. Amount of stool the person expels
    B. Number of bowel movements the person has each day
    C. Usual time of day the person has a bowel movement
    D. Foods that cause flatus

38. When the nurse gives a person a suppository, you would expect the person to have a bowel movement
    A. Immediately
    B. Within about 10 minutes
    C. In about 30 minutes
    D. Between 3 and 4 hours later

39. When the nurse delegates you to prepare a soapsuds enema, you will mix
    A. 2 teaspoons of salt in 500 to 1000 ml of tap water
    B. 3 to 5 ml of castile soap in 500 to 1000 ml of tap water
    C. 5 ml of castile soap in 100 to 200 ml of tap water
    D. Mineral oil with sterile water

40. When you give a cleansing enema, it should be given to the person
    A. Within 5 minutes
    B. Over about 30 minutes
    C. In about 10 to 15 minutes
    D. Within about 15 to 20 minutes

41. The person receiving an enema is usually placed in what position?
    A. Supine
    B. Prone
    C. Semi-Fowler's
    D. Side-lying or Sims'

42. When you prepare and give an enema, you will do all of these *except*
    A. Prepare the solution at 110° F.
    B. Insert the tubing 3 to 4 inches into the rectum.
    C. Hold the solution container about 12 inches above the bed.
    D. Lubricate the enema tip before inserting it into the rectum.

43. When the doctor orders enemas until clear, you should
    A. Give one enema.
    B. Give as many enemas as necessary to return a clear fluid.
    C. Ask the nurse how many enemas to give.
    D. Give only tap water enemas.

44. If you are giving an enema and the person complains of cramping, you should
    A. Tell the person that cramping is normal and continue to give the enema.
    B. Clamp the tube until the cramping subsides.
    C. Immediately discontinue the enema, and tell the nurse.
    D. Lower the bag below the level of the bed.

45. When giving a small volume (commercial) enema, do not release pressure on the bottle because otherwise
    A. Doing so will cause cramping if pressure is released.
    B. The fluid will leak from the rectum.
    C. Solution will be drawn from the rectum back into the bottle.
    D. Do so will cause flatulence.

46. When giving a commercial enema, you should
    A. Place the person in the prone position.
    B. Insert the enema tip 2 inches into the rectum.
    C. Heat the solution to 105° F.
    D. Clamp the tubing if cramping occurs.

47. An oil-retention enema is given to
    A. Cleanse the bowel to prepare for surgery.
    B. Regulate the person who is receiving bowel training.
    C. Relieve flatulence.
    D. Soften the feces and lubricate the rectum.

48. When an oil-retention enema is given, it should be retained
    A. 5 to 10 minutes
    B. 3 to 4 hours
    C. 30 to 60 minutes or longer
    D. 15 to 20 minutes

49. The doctor may order a rectal tube
    A. To relieve flatulence and intestinal distention
    B. After rectal surgery
    C. To give cleansing enemas
    D. When the person has an impaction

50. If you feel resistance when you are inserting a rectal tube, you should
    A. Lubricate the tube more thoroughly.
    B. Push more firmly to insert the tube.
    C. Stop and call the nurse.
    D. Ask the person to take a deep breath and relax.

51. After inserting a rectal tube, you should
    A. Hold it in place until it can be removed.
    B. Have the person lie on his or her back to hold it in place.
    C. Tape the rectal tube to the buttocks.
    D. Tell the person to lie still to keep the tube in place.

52. When you are caring for a person with an ostomy, you know
    A. All of the stools are solid and formed.
    B. Stomas do not have nerve endings and are not painful.
    C. An ostomy is always temporary and is reconnected after healing.
    D. A pouch is worn to protect the stoma.

53. Which of these statements is *true* about an ileostomy?
    A. The stool is solid and formed.
    B. The stoma is an opening into the colon.
    C. The pouch is changed daily.
    D. The digestive juices in the stool can irritate the skin around the ileostomy.

54. When caring for a person with an ostomy, the pouch is
    A. Changed daily
    B. Changed every 3 to 7 days and when it leaks
    C. Only worn when the person thinks he or she will have a bowel movement
    D. Changed every time the person has a bowel movement

55. The best time to change the ostomy bag is before breakfast because
    A. The stoma is less likely to expel stool at this time.
    B. The person has more time in the morning.
    C. It should be changed before morning care.
    D. The person tolerates the procedure better before eating.

56. When cleaning the skin around the stoma, you should use
    A. Sterile water and sterile gauze squares
    B. Alcohol and sterile cotton
    C. Gauze squares or washcloths and water or soap and other cleansing agents as directed by the nurse
    D. A lubricant and sterile cotton balls

Fill in the Blanks

57. How do each of these affect the color of the stool?

    A. Bleeding in the stomach and small intestine

    ____

    B. Bleeding in lower colon

    ____

    C. Eating beets

    ____

    D. Diet high in green vegetables

    ____

    E. Diseases and infections

    ____

58. What should be observed and reported to the nurse about stools?

    A. ______________________________

    B. ______________________________

    C. ______________________________

    D. ______________________________

    E. ______________________________

    F. ______________________________

    G. ______________________________

59. Name six foods that may cause gas in the bowel.

    A. ______________________________

    B. ______________________________

    C. ______________________________

    D. ______________________________

    E. ______________________________

    F. ______________________________

60. Drinking warm fluids such as coffee, tea, cider, and warm water will increase ______________________________.

61. Constipation is a risk in older persons because the feces pass through the intestine at a ______________________________.

62. What common problem of bowel elimination can occur with each of these?

    A. Spicy foods

    ____

    B. Decreased fluid intake

    ____

    C. Drugs for pain relief

    ____

    D. Antibiotics

    ____

    E. Bed rest

    ____

    F. Milk and milk products

    ____

63. Before a nursing assistant checks for and removes impactions, he or she should make sure that

A. ______________________

B. ______________________

C. ______________________

D. ______________________

E. ______________________

64. Three serious signs of dehydration are

A. ______________________

B. ______________________

C. ______________________

65. What common problem can be caused by swallowing air while eating and drinking?

____

66. How much solution is contained in a small-volume enema?

____

67. Because it is likely you will contact stool while giving an enema, you should follow

______________________ and

______________________.

68. Only ______________ solution is used for cleansing enemas in children.

69. How much solution should be used for the following?

A. Infants

____

B. Toddlers

____

C. School-age children

____

D. 12 years and older

____

70. When you start to insert the rectal tube to give an enema, ask the person to

______________________.

71. How far is a rectal tube inserted into an adult rectum?

____

Into a child's rectum?

____

72. Which ostomy has more liquid stool—a colostomy or ileostomy?

____

Why?

____

73. What can you place in the ostomy pouch to prevent odors?

____

74. Showers and baths are delayed 1 or 2 hours after applying a new pouch to allow

______________________.

75. What observations are recorded or reported when changing an ostomy pouch?

A. ______________________

B. ______________________

C. ______________________

Labeling

Answer questions 76 through 79 using the following illustrations.

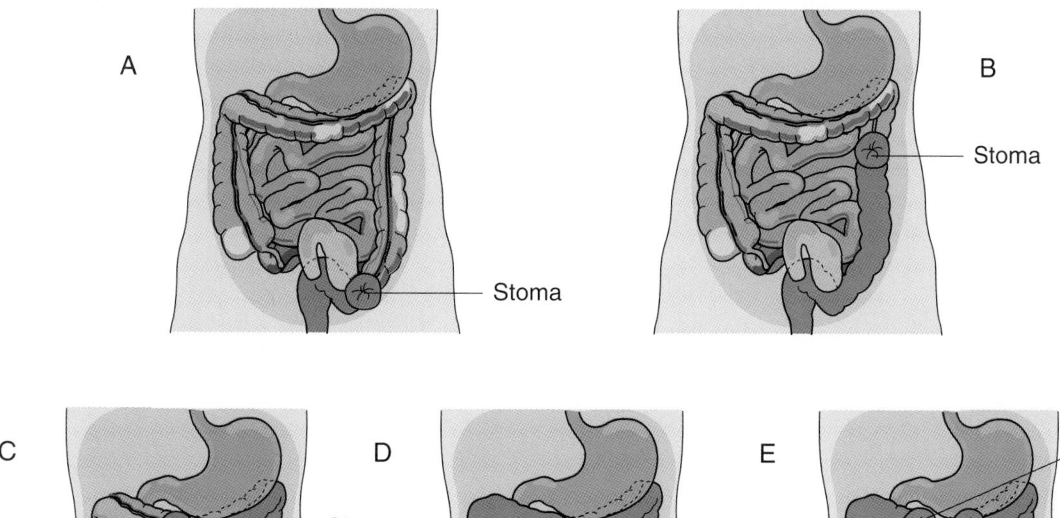

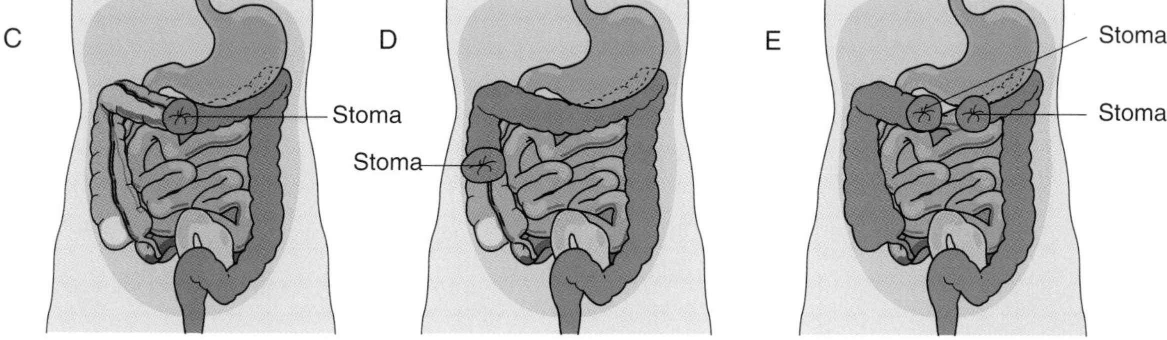

76. Name the five types of colostomies shown.

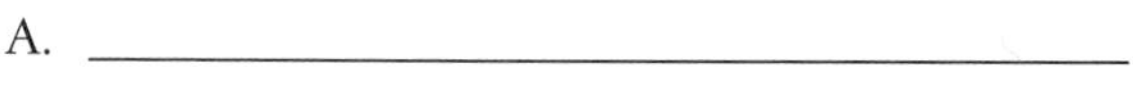

A. ______________________

B. ______________________

C. ______________________

D. ______________________

E. ______________________

77. Which colostomy will have the most solid and formed stool?

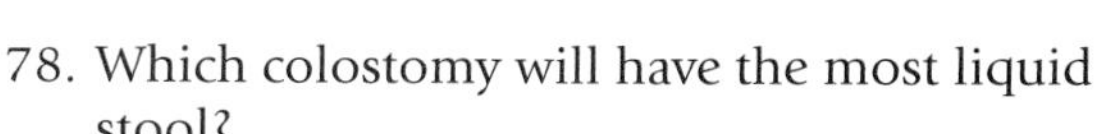

____

78. Which colostomy will have the most liquid stool?

____

79. Which colostomy is a temporary colostomy?

____

Answer questions 80 through 82 using the following illustration.

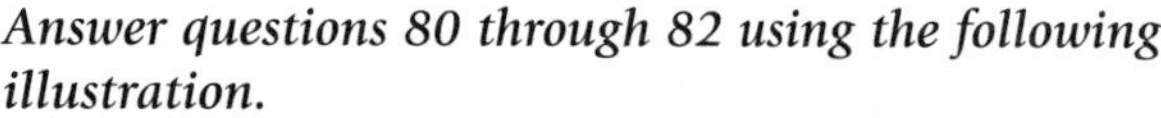

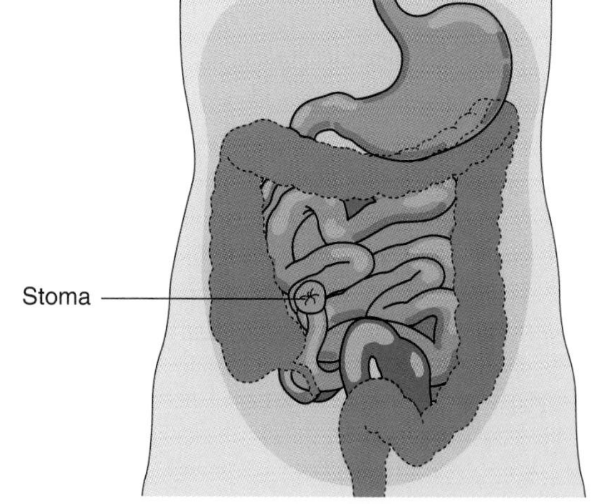

80. What type of ostomy is shown?

____

81. What part of the bowel has been removed?

____

82. Will the stool from the ostomy be liquid or formed?

____

Nursing Assistant Skills Video Exercise

View the* Normal Elimination *video (the section on Administering an enema) to answer these questions.

83. The enema tube should be ________________ in place during the enema.

84. The water temperature of an enema should be lukewarm or ________________ for an adult.

85. What is added to 1000 ml of water to prepare these enemas?

    A. Saline ________________

    B. Soap suds ________________

    C. Tap water ________________

86. After you have filled the bag and hung it from the IV, you must unclamp the tubing to ________________.

87. To relax the anal sphincter, ask the person to ________________ before inserting the tube.

88. Unless the nurse instructs you otherwise, you should lubricate the enema tube ________________ inches.

89. The enema tube is never inserted more than __________ inches.

90. Stop the enema if

    A. ________________

    B. ________________

    C. ________________

91. To prevent air from entering the rectum, you should clamp the tube and remove it before ________________.

Optional Learning Exercises

92. You are caring for Mr. Evans who is in a semi-private room. He has not had a bowel movement in 3 days, even though he has been eating well and taking medications to assist elimination. What could be a reason he has not had a bowel movement?

    ____

93. The nurse tells you to make sure Mr. Johnson eats the high fiber foods in his diet to assist in his elimination. What foods are high in fiber?

    ____

94. You offer Mr. Murphy ________________ glasses of water each day to promote normal bowel elimination.

95. Mr. Hernandez has been taking an antibiotic to treat his pneumonia and has developed diarrhea. You know he may have diarrhea because ________________.

96. You are caring for 83-year-old Mrs. Chen and helped her to the bathroom 30 minutes early; she had a bowel movement. When you enter her room to make her bed, she tells you she needs to use the bathroom for a bowel movement. You know that older people ________________.

97. The nurse delegates you to check for a fecal impaction. When you find that one is present and plan to remove it, what vital sign should be checked before you continue to remove the fecal impaction?

    ____

    Why?

    ____

98. Explain why diarrhea is more serious in infants and young children and in older persons

A. Infants and young children

____

B. Older persons

____

99. The two goals of bowel training are

A. ______________________________

B. ______________________________

100. Fill in the information about the cleansing enemas listed.

Enema	Solution and amount	Risks
Tap-water		
Soapsuds		
Saline		

Independent Learning Activities

- Think about the times when you have had a problem with bowel irregularity. Answer these questions about how you handled the problems. You do not need to share your answers with others.
  - What causes you to have irregularity? Foods? Illness? Stress? Inactivity?
  - What methods have you used to treat irregularity? Diet? Medication?
  - How does irregularity affect you physically? Your appetite? Your energy level? Sleep and rest?
  - How does irregularity affect your mood? Your daily activities?
- Interview a person who has a colostomy or an ileostomy. You may know someone who has an ostomy, or you may care for someone who has one. Your community may have an ostomy support group that you can contact. Talk with the person and ask these questions:
  - How have you had the ostomy? Is it permanent or temporary?
  - What was the hardest part of learning to live with an ostomy? What was the easiest part?
  - How has living with an ostomy affected your life? Has your work been affected? Were your leisure activities affected?
  - How has the ostomy affected your family? What changes have occurred?
  - What equipment works best for you? How expensive is the equipment? How much time is required each day to care for the ostomy?

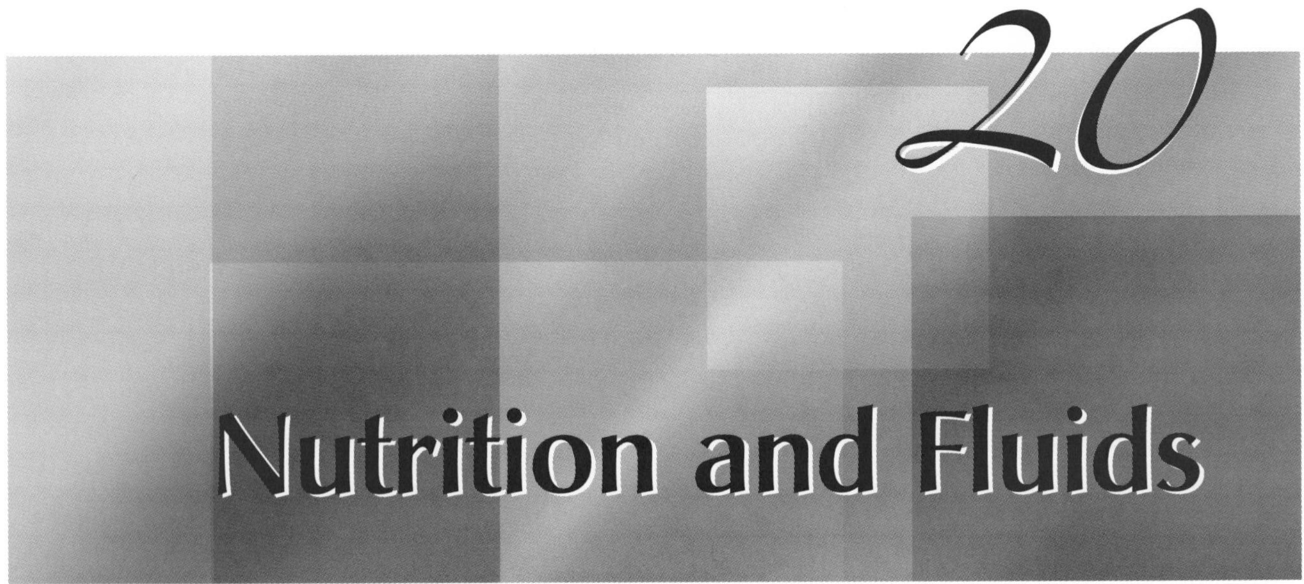

20 Nutrition and Fluids

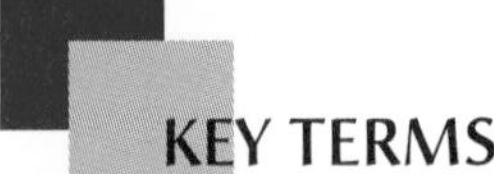

KEY TERMS

Anorexia
Aspiration
Calorie
Daily Reference Values (DRVs)
Daily Value (DV)
Dehydration
Dysphagia
Edema
Enteral nutrition
Flow rate
Gastrostomy tube
Gavage
Graduate
Intake
Intravenous therapy
Jejunostomy tube
Nasogastric tube
Nasointestinal tube
Nutrient
Nutrition
Output
Percutaneous endoscopic gastrostomy (PEG) tube
Regurgitation

Fill in the Blanks: Key Terms

1. The amount of fluid taken in is ______________________________.
2. A ______________________________ is a tube inserted through the nose into the small intestine.
3. Giving nutrition through the gastrointestinal tract is ______________________________.
4. ______________________________ is the backward flow of food from the stomach into the mouth.
5. The ______________________ is how a serving fits into the daily diet. It is expressed in a percent based on a daily diet of 2000 calories.
6. A tube inserted into the stomach through a stab or puncture wound made through the skin is a ______________________________.
7. The loss of appetite is ______________________________.
8. ______________________________ is fluid administered through a needle inserted into a vein. This is also called IV, IV therapy, and IV infusion.
9. A substance that is ingested, digested, absorbed, and used by the body is a ______________________________.

10. ______________________________ is difficulty swallowing.

11. The breathing of fluid or an object into the lungs is ______________________________.

12. The ______________________________ is the number of drops per minute (gtt/min).

13. The many processes involved in the ingestion, digestion, and absorption, as well as the use of food and fluids by the body are ______________________________.

14. A tube feeding is called ______________________.

15. The amount of energy produced when the body burns food is a ______________________.

16. A ______________________________ is a tube inserted through an opening into the middle part of the small intestine.

17. A decrease in the amount of water in body tissues is ______________________________.

18. A tube inserted into the stomach through an opening in the stomach is a ______________________________.

19. The maximum daily intake values for total fat, saturated fat, cholesterol, sodium, carbohydrate, and dietary fiber are the ______________________________.

20. A tube inserted through the nose into the stomach is a ______________________________.

21. A ______________________________ is a measuring container for fluid.

22. ______________________________ is the swelling of body tissues with water.

23. The amount of fluid lost is ______________________________.

Circle the BEST Answer

24. Which of these do *not* occur when the person has a poor diet and poor eating habits?
    A. Increased risk for infection and chronic diseases
    B. Healing problems
    C. Improved physical and mental well being
    D. Increased risk for accidents and injuries

25. Body fuel for energy is found in
    A. Vitamins
    B. Minerals
    C. Fats, proteins, and carbohydrates
    D. All of the above

26. Which of these foods are found in level 3 of the food pyramid?
    A. Rice and pasta
    B. Milk, meat, and beans
    C. Fats and sweets
    D. Vegetables and fruits

27. Which of these food groups in the food guide pyramid are low in sugar and fat?
    A. Bread, cereal, rice, and pasta
    B. Milk, yogurt, and cheese
    C. Meat, poultry, fish, and nuts
    D. Fats, oils, and sweets

28. How many servings each day are allowed from the breads, cereals, rice, and pasta group?
    A. 6 to 11
    B. 3 to 5
    C. 2 to 4
    D. 2 to 3

29. Which group in the food guide pyramid should be used sparingly?
    A. Bread, cereal, rice, and pasta
    B. Meat, poultry, fish, dry beans, eggs, and nuts
    C. Milk, yogurt, and cheese
    D. Fats, oils, and sweets

30. Which nutrient is needed for tissue growth and repair?
    A. Carbohydrates
    B. Fats
    C. Vitamins
    D. Protein

31. Food labels have all of this information *except*
    A. Serving size
    B. All vitamins and minerals
    C. Total amount of fat and saturated fats
    D. Amount of cholesterol and sodium

32. What percent of calories should come from fat?
    A. 30%
    B. 10%
    C. 50%
    D. 18%

33. A culture that eats a diet that is low in fat and high in sodium is in
    A. The Philippines
    B. China
    C. Poland
    D. Mexico

34. Persons who are Islamic are forbidden to eat
    A. All meat products
    B. Milk and meat at the same meal
    C. All pork and pork products
    D. Meat, fish, and dairy products during a fast

35. People with limited incomes often buy
    A. More protein foods
    B. Carbohydrate foods
    C. Food high in vitamins and minerals
    D. Fatty foods

36. When people buy cheaper foods, the diet may lack
    A. Fats
    B. Starchy foods
    C. Protein and certain vitamins and minerals
    D. Sugars

37. Appetite can be stimulated by
    A. Illness and medications
    B. Unpleasant sights, thoughts, and smells
    C. Aromas and thoughts of food
    D. Anxiety, pain, and depression

38. Personal choice of foods is influenced by
    A. Foods served at home
    B. Appetite
    C. Allergic reactions
    D. All of the above

39. During illness
    A. Appetite increases.
    B. Fewer nutrients are needed.
    C. Nutritional needs increase to fight infection and heal tissue.
    D. The person will prefer protein foods.

40. When you are assigned to prepare meals in home care, you need to
    A. Decide what foods you like to prepare.
    B. Plan the menu after reviewing foods allowed on the person's diet.
    C. Cook foods that you like to eat.
    D. Prepare whatever the person likes, even if it is not on the person's diet.

41. Requirements for food served in long-term care centers are made by the
    A. Food guide pyramid
    B. Omnibus Budget Reconciliation Act of 1987 (OBRA)
    C. Nursing center
    D. The Public Health Department

42. All of these are requirements for food served in long-term care centers *except*
    A. Food is prepared to meet the person's individual needs.
    B. The person's diet is well balanced and nourishing, and the food tastes good.
    C. All food is served at room temperature.
    D. Each person must receive at least three meals a day and be offered a bedtime snack.

43. A general or regular diet
    A. Is ordered for the person with difficulty swallowing
    B. Has no dietary limits or restrictions
    C. May have restricted amounts of sodium
    D. Increases the amount of sugar in the diet

44. The body needs no more sodium each day than ________________ mg.
    A. 2400
    B. 3000
    C. 5000
    D. 1000

45. When the body tissues swell with water, what organ has to work harder?
    A. Kidneys
    B. Liver
    C. Heart
    D. Lungs

46. When you are caring for a person with diabetes, you should do all of these *except*
    A. Serve the person's meals and snacks on time.
    B. Report to the nurse what the person did and did not eat.
    C. Give the person extra food and snacks whenever it is requested.
    D. Provide a between-meal nourishment if all the food was not eaten.

47. A person may be given a mechanical soft diet because
    A. Nausea and vomiting have occurred.
    B. The person has chewing difficulties.
    C. The person has been advanced from a clear-liquid diet.
    D. The person has constipation.

48. If you are serving a meal to a person on a fiber and residue-restricted diet, the meal would *not* include
    A. Raw fruits and vegetables
    B. Strained fruit juices
    C. Canned or cooked fruit without skin or seeds
    D. Plain pasta

49. A person who has serious burns would receive a ______________________ diet.
    A. Sodium-controlled
    B. Fat-controlled
    C. High-calorie
    D. High-protein

50. When a person has dysphagia, the thickness of the food served is chosen by the
    A. Person
    B. Nursing assistant
    C. Family
    D. Speech and language pathologist, dietician, and doctor or nurse

51. Which of these may be a sign of a swallowing problem (dysphagia)?
    A. Person complains that food will not go down or that food is stuck.
    B. Foods that need chewing are avoided.
    C. There is excessive drooling of saliva.
    D. All of the above are signs.

52. When assisting a person with meals, you can help to prevent aspiration while the person is eating by placing him or her in which position?
    A. Semi-Fowler's
    B. Fowler's
    C. Side-lying
    D. Supine

53. If fluid intake exceeds fluid output, the person will
    A. Have edema in the tissues
    B. Be dehydrated
    C. Have vomiting and diarrhea
    D. Have increased urinary output

54. How much fluid is needed every day for normal fluid balance?
    A. 500 ml
    B. 1000 to 1500 ml
    C. 2000 to 2500 ml
    D. 3000 to 4000 ml

55. If the person you are caring for has an order for restricted fluids, which of these should you do?
    A. Offer a variety of liquids.
    B. Thicken all fluids.
    C. Keep the water pitcher out of sight.
    D. Do not allow the person to swallow any liquids during oral hygiene.

56. When you are keeping input and output (I&O) records, you should measure all of these *except*
    A. Milk, water, coffee, and tea
    B. Mashed potatoes and creamed vegetables
    C. Soups and gelatin
    D. Ice cream, custard, and pudding

57. When you are measuring I&O, you need to know that 1 ounce equals
    A. 10 ml
    B. 500 ml
    C. 100 ml
    D. 30 ml

58. When you are using the graduate-to-measure output, you should
    A. Hold the graduate at waist level, and read the amount.
    B. Look at the graduate while it is held above eye level.
    C. Keep the container level, and read the amount at eye level.
    D. Set the graduate on the floor, and read the amount.

59. Which of the following needs to be done before the person is served a meal?
    A. Give complete personal care.
    B. Change all linens.
    C. Make sure the person is clean and dry.
    D. Make sure the person has been shaved or has makeup applied.

60. You can provide comfort during meals by
    A. Making sure unpleasant sights and sounds are removed
    B. Making sure dentures, eyeglasses, or hearing aids are in place
    C. Giving the person good oral care before and after meals
    D. All of the above

61. What should you do if a food tray has not been served within 15 minutes?
    A. Recheck the food temperatures.
    B. Serve the tray immediately.
    C. Throw the food away.
    D. Serve only the cold items on the tray.

62. How can you make sure the food tray is complete?
    A. Ask the person being served.
    B. Ask the nurse.
    C. Call the dietary department.
    D. Check items on the tray with the dietary card.

63. When you are feeding a person you should
    A. Never allow the person to assist.
    B. Give the person a fork and knife to assist with cutting the food.
    C. Feed the person in a private area to maintain confidentiality.
    D. Use a spoon because it is less likely to cause injury.

64. When feeding a person, liquids are given
    A. Only at the start of feeding
    B. Alternating with solid foods
    C. At the end of the meal when all solids have been eaten
    D. Only if the person has difficulty swallowing

65. When providing fresh water to residents, you would not
    A. Give fresh water when the pitcher is empty.
    B. Put ice in all pitchers.
    C. Practice the rules of medical sepsis.
    D. Ask the nurse about the person's fluid orders.

66. When a calorie record is kept, you should record
    A. Time the person ate
    B. Only the liquids consumed
    C. The temperature of the food
    D. What the person ate and how much

67. Enteral nutrition is used to feed a person when
    A. The person has cancer of the head, neck, or esophagus
    B. The person has trauma or surgery to the face, mouth, head, or neck
    C. The person has dementia and no longer knows how to eat
    D. When any of the above situations occur

68. Which of these is *not* a type of enteral nutrition feeding?
    A. Nasogastric tube
    B. IV therapy
    C. PEG tube
    D. Jejunostomy tube

69. A major risk with nasogastric and nasointestinal tubes is
    A. Nausea
    B. Complaints of flatulence
    C. Aspiration
    D. Elevated temperature

70. When a person has a feeding tube, it is especially important to provide
    A. Frequent sips of water
    B. Frequent oral hygiene and lubricant for the lips
    C. Linen changes every shift
    D. Snacks between meals

71. When caring for a person with a nasogastric tube, what should you do every 4 to 8 hours?
    A. Give the person sips of water.
    B. Clean the nose and nostrils.
    C. Provide oral care.
    D. Remove the tape securing the tubing.

72. When a person is seriously ill or injured, he or she may need to receive hyperalimentation, which is a highly concentrated nutritional solution given
    A. As an oral feeding
    B. Through a nasogastric tube
    C. Through an IV
    D. Through a gastrostomy tube

73. If you hear an IV pump alarm, you should
    A. Tell the nurse immediately.
    B. Reset the pump to see if it stops.
    C. Turn off the pump.
    D. Reposition the person to see if the alarm stops.

74. If you have been asked to check the flow rate of an IV, you should
    A. Count the number of drops in 1 minute.
    B. Count the number of drops in 15 seconds.
    C. Count the number of drops in 30 seconds.
    D. Look at the bag, and compare the fluid line to the time line.

75. Which of these is *not* a symptom of an IV therapy complication?
    A. Shortness of breath
    B. Confusion
    C. Normal urine output
    D. Drop in blood pressure

Fill in the Blanks

76. List seven countries in which the main meal is generally eaten at midday.

    A. ______________________

    B. ______________________

    C. ______________________

    D. ______________________

    E. ______________________

    F. ______________________

    G. ______________________

77. How many calories are in each of these?

    A. 1 g fat ______________________

    B. 1 g protein ______________________

    C. 1 g carbohydrate ______________________

78. Eating more foods from levels 1 and 2 of the food guide pyramid will help a person to eat a ______________________ diet.

79. As you move up the food guide pyramid, the amounts of ______________________ increase.

80. List the food groups in the levels of the food guide pyramid.

    A. Level 1 ______________________

    B. Level 2 ______________________ and ______________________

    C. Level 3 ______________________ and ______________________

    D. Level 4 ______________________

81. What is the size of the serving in the food guide pyramid for each of these foods?

    A. Milk or yogurt

    ____

    B. Butter or margarine

    ____

    C. Chopped, cooked, or canned fruit

    ____

    D. Cooked cereal, rice, or pasta

    ____

    E. Cooked lean meat, poultry, or fish

    ____

    F. Vegetable juice

    ____

82. How many daily servings are recommended for each level of the food guide pyramid?

    A. Breads ______________________

    B. Vegetables ______________________

    C. Fruits ______________________

    D. Milk products ______________________

    E. Meats group ______________________

    F. Fats, oils, sweets ______________________

83. How many calories are in 1 cup of whole milk?

    ____

    How many of these calories come from fat?

    ____

84. When a person eats a 12-ounce steak, how many servings of meat are used?

    ____

85. A well-balanced diet ensures an adequate intake of the essential nutrients. These nutrients are

A. ______________________________

B. ______________________________

C. ______________________________

D. ______________________________

E. ______________________________

86. Which vitamins can be stored by the body?

____

87. Which vitamins must be ingested daily?

____

88. What foods are good sources of vitamin C (ascorbic acid)?

A. ______________________________

B. ______________________________

C. ______________________________

D. ______________________________

E. ______________________________

F. ______________________________

G. ______________________________

89. Milk and milk products, liver, green leafy vegetables, eggs, breads, and cereals are good sources of which vitamin?

____

90. What mineral allows red blood cells to carry oxygen?

____

91. When the diet does not have enough

______________________________, it may affect nerve function, muscle contraction, and heart function.

92. Calcium is needed for

______________________________.

93. What information is found on food labels?

A. ______________________________

B. ______________________________

C. ______________________________

D. ______________________________

E. ______________________________

F. ______________________________

G. ______________________________

94. What religion may have groups that have restrictions about eating beef, pork, lamb, chicken, seafood, and fish?

____

95. Those who practice ______________________________ as their religion cannot eat shellfish, but they can eat fish with scales and fins.

96. List religious groups that do not allow alcohol and coffee.

A. ______________________________

B. ______________________________

C. ______________________________

D. ______________________________

E. ______________________________

97. What religious group may have members that fast from meats on Fridays, especially during Lent?

____

98. Nutritional needs increase during illness when the body must ______________________________.

99. What two OBRA requirements are related to the temperature of foods served in long-term care centers?

    A. ______________________________

    ____

    B. ______________________________

    ____

100. What foods are allowed on a clear-liquid diet?

    ____

    ____

    ____

101. When the person receives a full-liquid diet, it will include all of the foods on the clear-liquid diet, as well as these foods:

    ____

    ____

    ____

102. If a person has poorly fitted dentures and chewing difficulties, the doctor may order a ______________________________ diet.

103. A person who is constipated and has other GI disorders may receive a ______________________________ diet. The foods in this diet increase the ______________________________ to stimulate ______________________________.

104. If a person is receiving a high-calorie diet, the caloric intake is increased to about ______________________________.

105. If disease causes the body to retain extra sodium, the body retains more ______________________________.

106. When a person is receiving a diabetic diet, the same amount of ______________________________ is eaten each day.

107. If you are feeding a person a dysphagia diet, what observations should be reported to the nurse at once?

    A. ______________________________

    B. ______________________________

108. What can you do to encourage fluid intake?

    A. ______________________________

    B. ______________________________

    C. ______________________________

    D. ______________________________

109. When fluids are restricted, why is frequent oral hygiene important?

    ____

    ____

    ____

110. When you give oral hygiene to a person who is receiving nothing by mouth, the person must not ______________________________.

111. When you record I&O, what measurement system is used?

    ____

112. List the measurements for the following

A. 1 ounce equals ______________________ ml

B. 1 pint equals ______________________ ml

C. 1 quart equals ______________________ ml

113. Name the four special dining programs in nursing centers that are described.

A. Residents who need help eating are seated at horseshoe-shaped tables.

____

B. Residents eat at a dining room table with 4 to 6.

____

C. This program prevents distraction.

____

D. Food is served in bowls and on platters. Residents serve themselves.

____

114. When you are feeding a person the spoon should be filled ______________________.

115. Why should you sit facing the person while you feed him or her?

A. Shows ______________________

____

B. You can see ______________________

____

C. You can see ______________________

____

116. What should be reported after you have fed a person?

A. ______________________

B. ______________________

C. ______________________

117. Answer the following questions about tube feedings.

A. Scheduled feedings are given ______________ times a day.

B. Usually about 400 ml is given over ______________________.

C. Why is feeding tube formula given at room temperature?

____

D. Why is the person placed in semi-Fowler's position?

____

____

E. This position may be required for ______________________.

Labeling

118. Label each of the levels of the food guide pyramid in this figure, and list how many servings of each one should be eaten daily.

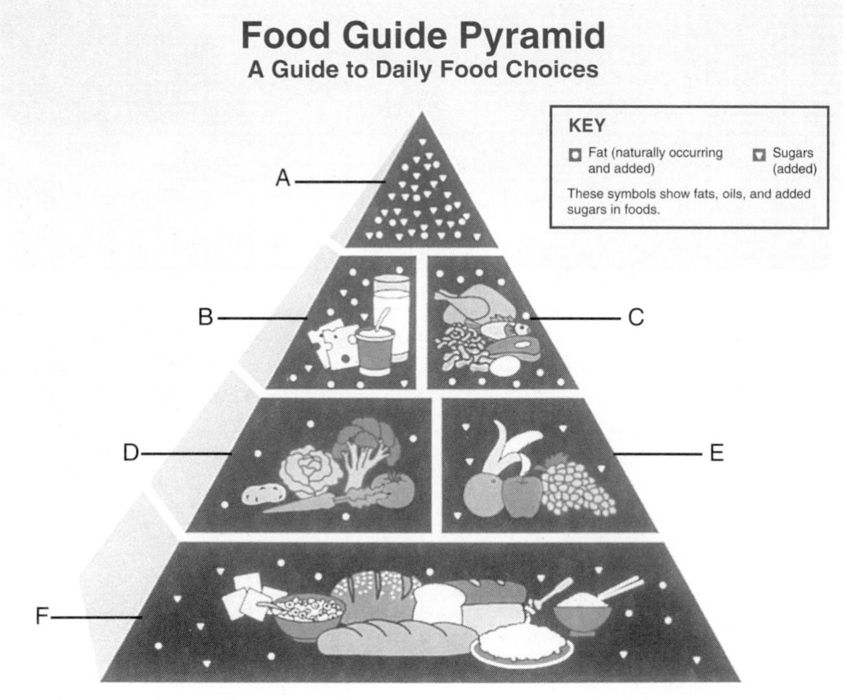

A. ______________________ ______________

B. ______________________ ______________

C. ______________________ ______________

D. ______________________ ______________

E. ______________________ ______________

F. ______________________ ______________

119. Place numbers around the plate in this figure as shown in the textbook. How would you help a visually impaired person who asks you where to find the food items on the plate?

A. Bread ______________________

B. Baked potato ______________________

C. Vegetables ______________________

D. Meat ______________________

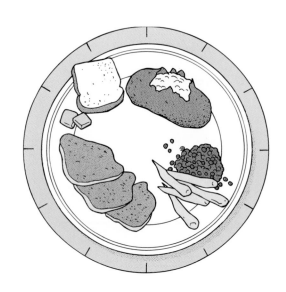

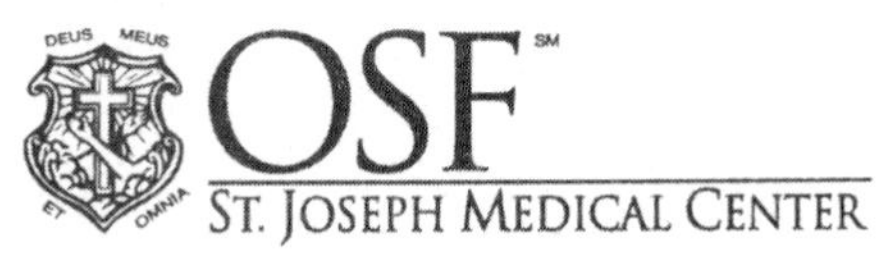

Bloomington, Illinois

DATE ______________________

FLUID BALANCE CHART

Water Glass	250cc	Ice Cream	120cc
Styrofoam Cup	180cc	Ice Chips	1/2 amt. of cc's in cup
Cup (coffee)	250cc		
Milk Carton	240cc	Pitcher (Yellow)	1000cc
Pop (1 can)	360cc		
Broth-Soup	175cc		
Juice Carton	120cc		
Juice Glass	120cc		
Jello	120cc		

INTAKE				OUTPUT					
				URINE		OTHER		CONT. IRRIGATION	
TIME	ORAL	Parenteral	Amt. cc Absbd.	Method Collected	Amt. (cc)	Method Collected	Amt. (cc)	In	Out
2400-0100		cc from previous shift							
0100-0200									
0200-0300									
0300-0400									
0400-0500									
0500-0600									
0600-0700									
0700-0800									
		8 - hour Sub-total		8-hr T		8-hr T			
0800-0900		cc from previous shift							
0900-1000									
1000-1100									
1100-1200									
1200-1300									
1300-1400									
1400-1500									
1500-1600									
		8 - hour Sub-total		8-hr T		8-hr T			
1600-1700		cc from previous shift							
1700-1800									
1800-1900									
1900-2000									
2000-2100									
2100-2200									
2200-2300									
2300-2400									
		8 - hour Sub-total		8-hr T		8-hr T			
		24 - hour Sub-total		24-hr T		24-hr T			

310' Marie Mills

Source Key:
URINE

V - Voided
C - Catheter
INC - Incontinent
U.C. - Ureteral Catheter

Source Key:
OTHER

G.I.T. - Gastric Intestinal Tube
T.T. - T. Tube
Vom. - Vomitus
Liq S. - Liquid Stool
H.V. - Hemovac

Form No. MF36722 (Rev. 5/97) MFI

120. Enter this information on the I&O record on the previous page. Total amounts for the 8-hour and 24-hour periods. (Use information at top of figure to calculate amounts in containers. Use the 8-hour shifts shown to gather information for each shift.) Amounts in parentheses indicate how much person ate or drank.

0200	Voided	300 ml
0600	Voided	500 ml
0730	**Breakfast**	
	Orange juice (whole glass)	
	Milk (1/2 carton)	
	Coffee (1 cup)	
0730	Voided	300 ml
1000	Water pitcher filled	
1130	**Lunch**	
	Soup (whole bowl)	
	Milk (1/2 carton)	
	Tea (1 Styrofoam cup)	
	Jell-O (1 serving)	
1330	Voided	450 ml
1430	Water pitcher (refilled)	500 ml
1530	Vomited	50 ml
1545	1 can of soda (whole can)	
1730	**Dinner**	
	Soup (whole bowl)	
	Tea (1 Styrofoam cup)	
	Juice (whole glass)	
	Ice cream (all)	
1730	Voided	250 ml
1830	Vomited	100 ml
1915	Voided	500 ml
2000	Milk (1 carton)	
2015	Voided	300 ml
2330	Voided	200 ml

Nursing Assistant Skills Video Exercise

View the* Nutrition and Fluids *video to answer these questions.

121. What are the signs and symptoms of dysphagia?

A. ______________________________

B. ______________________________

C. ______________________________

D. ______________________________

122. When you assist a person to eat, when should you assist them to wash the hands?

________-__________________________ and

____

123. When you assist a person to eat, when should you assist the person with oral hygiene?

______________________________ and

____

124. When you serve meal trays, what procedure guidelines should be followed?

A. ______________________________

B. ______________________________

C. ______________________________

D. ______________________________

Optional Learning Exercises

125. This is a person's food intake for 1 day. On the following page, list the foods and the servings eaten under the correct level in the food guide pyramid.

Breakfast
3/4 cup orange juice
1 cup oatmeal
2 slices toast
1/4 cup milk
2 cups black coffee

Lunch
1 cup tomato soup
Grilled cheese sandwich
1/2 cup applesauce
1 can regular soda
Candy bar

Dinner
2- to 4-ounce pork chops
Baked potato with butter
1/4 cup green beans
2 brownies
2 cups black coffee

Snacks
1 apple
1 4-ounce bag potato chips
1/3 cup nuts
1 can regular soda
1/2 cup ice cream

A. Breads ______________________________

____

Servings ______________________________

B. Vegetables ______________________________

____

Servings ______________________________

C. Fruits ______________________________

____

Servings ______________________________

D. Milk products ______________________________

____

Servings ______________________________

E. Meat ______________________________

____

Servings ______________________________

F. Fats ______________________________

____

Servings ______________________________

126. Which group or groups meet the needs for daily servings?

____

127. Which group or groups do not meet the needs for daily servings?

____

Independent Learning Activities

Now that you have learned about good nutrition, use this exercise to find out whether you eat a nutritious diet. List your intake for 1 day. Be sure to include the amount of each item—remember, the portion size is important.

- Group the foods and liquids you eat according to the parts of the food guide pyramid. Either draw a food guide pyramid and place your food items in the pyramid, or make a list of the groups of foods. Answer the following questions
  - How many servings did you eat of breads, cereals, rice, and pasta? How many of these servings were whole grain?
  - How many servings of fruit did you eat? How many were fresh fruit? Canned fruit? Fruit juice? Had added sugars?
  - How many vegetable servings did you eat? How many were raw? Cooked?
  - How many servings of milk, yogurt, and cheese did you eat? How many were low in fat or fat-free?
  - How many servings of meat, poultry, fish, dry beans, eggs, and nuts did you eat? How many were high in fat? Low in fat? High in sodium?
  - How many foods did you eat that count as fats, oils, and sweets?
  - In which food groups are you meeting your daily needs?
  - In which groups do you need to increase your intake? Decrease your intake?
  - After completing this exercise what changes in your diet will you consider?

- Role-play with a classmate, and take turns feeding each other as you would a resident. You may choose any spoon-fed foods you wish (pudding, gelatin, soup). You should also give a beverage to the person. After you have fed each other, answer these questions
  - How were your physical needs met before you were fed (toileting, handwashing, oral hygiene)?
  - Where were you fed (in a bed, in a chair, at a table)? Who made the decision about your location?
  - Which food was offered first? Who made the choice of how the food was offered? Were you offered a variety of foods?
  - When was a beverage offered? Between food items? Only at the end of feeding? How did the person feeding you decide the order of foods and beverages? What was the temperature of these items?
  - When you were being fed, how was the nursing assistant positioned? Sitting? Standing? How did the person's position make you feel?
  - What kind of conversation was carried on while you were eating? What chances were offered to rest while you were eating? Did you feel relaxed or rushed?
  - After this exercise, what would you do differently when you feed a resident?

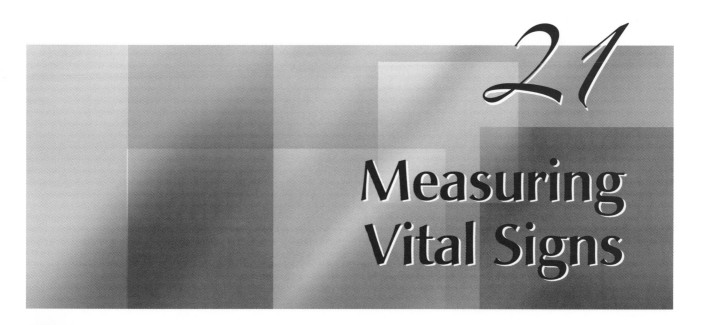

21 Measuring Vital Signs

KEY TERMS

Apical-radial pulse
Blood pressure
Body temperature
Bradycardia
Diastole
Diastolic pressure
Hypertension
Hypotension
Pulse
Pulse deficit
Pulse rate
Respiration
Sphygmomanometer
Stethoscope
Systole
Systolic pressure
Tachycardia
Vital signs

Fill in the Blanks: Key Terms

1. A rapid heart rate is ______________________. The heart rate is over 100 beats per minute.
2. The ______________________ is taking the apical and radial pulse at the same time.
3. An instrument used to listen to the sounds produced by the heart, lungs, and other body organs is a ______________________.
4. When the systolic blood pressure is below 90 mm Hg and the diastolic pressure is below 60 mm Hg, it is called ______________________.
5. The ______________________ is the number of heartbeats or pulses felt in 1 minute.
6. The amount of heat in the body that is a balance between the amount of heat produced and amount lost by the body is the ______________________.
7. ______________________ is the period of heart muscle contraction.
8. ______________________ is blood pressure measurements that remain above the normal systolic (140 mm Hg) or diastolic (90 mm Hg) pressures.
9. The cuff and measuring device used to measure blood pressure is a ______________________.

10. The beat of the heart felt at an artery as a wave of blood passes through the artery is the ______________________.

11. Temperature, pulse, respirations, and blood pressure are ______________________.

12. ______________________ is a slow heart rate; the rate is less than 60 beats per minute.

13. The amount of force it takes to pump blood out of the heart into the arterial circulation is the ______________________.

14. The period of heart muscle relaxation is ______________________.

15. The difference between the apical and radial pulse rates is the ______________________.

16. ______________________ is the amount of force exerted against the walls of an artery by the blood.

17. The act of breathing air into and out of the lungs is ______________________.

18. ______________________ is the pressure in the arteries when the heart is at rest.

Circle the BEST Answer

19. If you are unsure of your measurements of vital signs
    A. Take the vital signs several times and average the results.
    B. Promptly ask the nurse to take them again.
    C. Record the results you think you measured.
    D. Look at the person's record to compare your measurements.

20. Unless otherwise ordered, take vital signs when the person
    A. Is lying or sitting
    B. Has been walking or exercising
    C. Has just finished eating
    D. Is getting ready to take a shower or tub bath

21. Body temperature is lower in the
    A. Afternoon
    B. Morning
    C. Evening
    D. Night

22. If you take a rectal temperature, the normal range of the temperature would be
    A. 96.6° to 98.6° F (35.9° to 37.0° C)
    B. 97.6° to 99.6° F (36.5° to 37.5° C)
    C. 98.6° to 100.6° F (37.0° to 38.1° C)
    D. 98.6° F (37° C)

23. If you are taking the temperature of an older person, you would expect the temperature to be
    A. At the lower end of the normal range
    B. At the upper end of the normal range
    C. About in the middle of the normal range
    D. The same as a younger adult

24. Which of these temperature sites cannot be used for children under 6 years of age?
    A. Oral
    B. Rectal
    C. Axillary
    D. Tympanic

25. An oral temperature may be taken with a glass thermometer for a person who
    A. Is receiving oxygen
    B. Has a history of convulsive disorders
    C. Breathes through the mouth
    D. Is alert and needs a routine temperature taken

26. A rectal temperature cannot be taken if the person
    A. Breathes through the mouth
    B. Has heart disease
    C. Is unconscious
    D. Is receiving oxygen

27. A glass rectal thermometer has a
    A. Stubby tip color coded in red
    B. Long or slender tip
    C. Pear-shaped tip
    D. Slender tip color coded in blue

28. If you are caring for a child in the home setting, you should tell the nurse if
    A. A tympanic thermometer is available
    B. The parents use an electronic thermometer
    C. A mercury-glass thermometer is available
    D. The electronic thermometer is able to take rectal temperatures

29. To read a glass thermometer you should hold it at the
    A. Stem above eye level and look up to read
    B. Bulb end up and bringing to eye level
    C. Stem up and bringing to eye level
    D. Bulb at waist level and looking down to read

30. When you use a glass thermometer, which of these is *not* correct?
    A. Rinse under cool water before using.
    B. Shake down the thermometer until the substance is below the lowest number.
    C. Rinse under hot water when finished using the thermometer.
    D. Store the thermometer in a container with disinfectant.

31. If you are preparing to take an oral temperature, ask the person not to
    A. Eat, drink, or smoke for at least 15 to 20 minutes
    B. Shower or bathe right before the temperature is taken
    C. Exercise for 30 minutes before the temperature is taken
    D. Eat, drink, or smoke for at least 5 to 10 minutes.

32. A glass thermometer is inserted into the rectum
    A. 1 inch
    B. 2 inches
    C. $^1/_2$ inch
    D. 3 inches

33. When recording an axillary temperature of 97.6° F, it is written
    A. 97.6°
    B. 97.6° R
    C. 97.6° A
    D. 97.6° axillary

34. When using an electronic thermometer, you can prevent the spread of infection by
    A. Discarding the thermometer after each use
    B. Discarding the probe cover after each use
    C. Keeping a thermometer for each person at the bedside
    D. Sterilizing the thermometer after each use

35. Which pulse is most commonly used?
    A. Carotid
    B. Brachial
    C. Radial
    D. Popliteal

36. The ____________________ pulse is taken on an adult during cardiopulmonary resuscitation (CPR) and other emergencies is the
    A. Carotid
    B. Temporal
    C. Femoral
    D. Radial

37. When using a stethoscope, you can help to prevent infection by
    A. Warming the diaphragm in your hand
    B. Wiping the earpieces and diaphragm with alcohol before and after use
    C. Placing the diaphragm over the artery
    D. Placing the earpieces in your ears so the bend of the tips point forward

38. The pulse rate is the number of heartbeats or pulses felt in
    A. 30 seconds
    B. 15 seconds
    C. 1 minute
    D. 5 minutes

39. The normal adult pulse is
    A. Between 60 and 100 beats per minute
    B. Fewer than 60 beats per minute
    C. More than 100 beats per minute
    D. 72 beats per minute

40. You cannot get information about pulse ______________________ with electronic blood pressure equipment.
    A. Rhythm and force
    B. Rate
    C. Tachycardia
    D. Bradycardia

41. When taking the radial pulse, place
    A. The thumb over the pulse site
    B. Two or three fingers on the middle of the wrist
    C. Two or three fingers on the thumb side of the wrist
    D. All of the above

42. The radial pulse is counted for 1 minute if
    A. It is irregular.
    B. It is required by the center policy.
    C. It is directed by the nurse.
    D. All of the above are correct.

43. An apical pulse is taken
    A. On infants and children up to about 2 years of age
    B. On people who have heart disease
    C. When the heart rhythm is irregular
    D. All of the above

44. An apical pulse of 72 is recorded as
    A. Pulse 72
    B. 72 apical pulse
    C. 72Ap
    D. P 72

45. An apical-radial pulse is taken by
    A. Taking the radial pulse for 1 minute and then taking the apical pulse for 1 minute
    B. Subtracting the apical pulse from the radial pulse
    C. Having one staff member take the radial pulse and one staff member take the apical pulse at the same time
    D. Having two people take the apical pulse at the same time

46. When counting respirations the best way is to
    A. Stand quietly next to the person and watch the chest rise and fall.
    B. Keep your fingers or stethoscope over the pulse site so the person thinks you are still counting the pulse.
    C. Tell the person to breathe normally so you can count the respirations.
    D. Use the stethoscope to hear the respirations clearly and count for 1 minute.

47. Adult blood pressure levels are reached
    A. At birth
    B. By the time a child is 1 year of age
    C. At approximately age 12 to 13
    D. Between 14 and 18 years of age

48. The blood pressure may be higher in older people because
    A. They have orthostatic hypotension.
    B. The diet is higher in sodium.
    C. Arteries narrow and lose elasticity.
    D. They are usually overweight.

49. The blood pressure should not be taken on an arm
    A. If the person has had breast surgery on that side
    B. That has a cast
    C. That has a dialysis access site
    D. All of the above

50. You will discover the size of blood pressure cuff needed
    A. By asking the nurse
    B. By measuring the person's arm
    C. In the physician's orders
    D. By asking the person

51. When taking the blood pressure, you place the stethoscope diaphragm
    A. Over the radial artery on the thumb side of the wrist
    B. Over the brachial artery at the inner aspect of the elbow
    C. Lightly against the skin
    D. Over the apical pulse site

52. When getting ready to take the blood pressure, position the person's arm
    A. Above the level of the heart
    B. Level with the heart
    C. Below the level of the heart
    D. Abducted from the body

53. The blood pressure is inflated ________ mm Hg beyond the point at which you last felt the radial pulse.
    A. 10
    B. 20
    C. 30
    D. 40

Fill in the Blanks

54. Vital signs are taken when drugs affect the

    ________________________________ or

    ________________________________ systems.

55. When vital signs are taken report to the nurse at once if

    A. ________________________________

    B. ________________________________

    C. ________________________________

56. Sites for measuring temperature are

A. ______________________

B. ______________________

C. ______________________

D. ______________________

57. Which site has the highest baseline temperature?

____

58. Which site has the lowest baseline temperature?

____

59. If a mercury-glass thermometer breaks,

______________________ at once

because mercury ______________________.

60. When you read a thermometer, the short lines

A. On a Fahrenheit thermometer mean

____

B. On a centigrade thermometer mean

____

61. List how long the glass thermometer remains in place for the following sites:

A. Oral ______________________

or as required by center policy

B. Rectal ______________________

or as required by center policy

C. Axillary ______________________

or as required by center policy

62. When taking an oral temperature, place the tip of

the thermometer

______________________.

63. When taking an axillary temperature, the axilla

must be ______________________.

64. A tympanic membrane thermometer is useful for

children and confused individuals because of the

______________________ and

______________________ of this device.

65. If an electronic thermometer has colored probes, what does the color of the probe mean?

A. Blue ______________________

B. Red ______________________

66. When you take a rectal temperature, what is done to the tip of the thermometer or the end of the covered probe?

____

67. When taking a tympanic membrane temperature,

pull back on the ear to

______________________.

68. The pulse rate at birth is ______________________

per minute. By the time a person is an adult, the

pulse rate is ______________________ per minute.

69. List words used to describe the following

A. Forceful pulse:

____

B. Hard-to-feel pulse:

____

70. When you take a pulse, what observations should be reported and recorded?

A. ______________________

B. ______________________

C. ______________________

71. Do not use your thumb to take a pulse because

____.

72. When taking an apical pulse, each lub-dub sound counts as _________________________.

73. The apical pulse rate is never less than the

____.

74. A healthy adult has _________________________ respirations per minute.

75. What observations should be reported and recorded when counting respirations?

A. ____

B. ____

C. ____

D. ____

E. ____

F. ____

76. One respiration is counted for each

____.

77. Respirations are counted for _________________________ if they are abnormal or irregular.

78. Blood pressure is controlled by

A. ____

B. ____

C. ____

79. Blood pressure ranges for the average adult are

A. Systolic _________________________________

B. Diastolic ________________________________

80. If a person has been exercising, let the person rest for _________________________ before taking the blood pressure.

81. How is the person positioned to take the blood pressure?

A. ____

B. ____

C. The physician may order _________________ position.

82. When listening to the blood pressure

A. The first sound you hear is the _________________________ pressure.

B. The point at which the sound disappears is the _________________________ pressure.

Labeling

83. Name the types of thermometers.

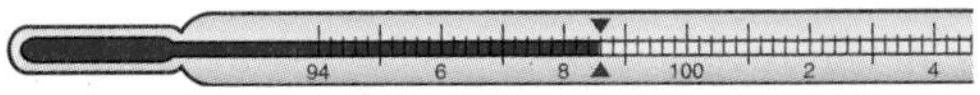

A. ____

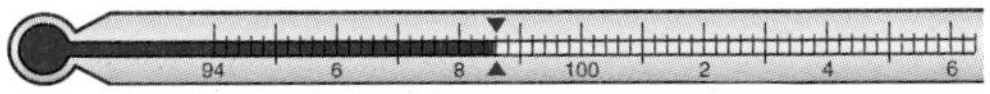

B. ____

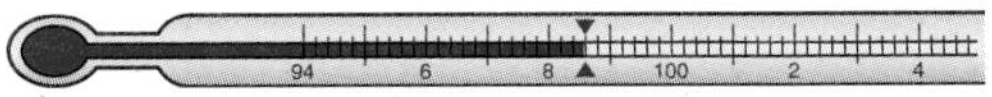

C. ____

D. Which thermometers are used for oral or axillary temperatures?

____

E. A rectal temperature is taken with the _________________________ thermometer that has a _______________ tip.

84. Name the pulse sites.

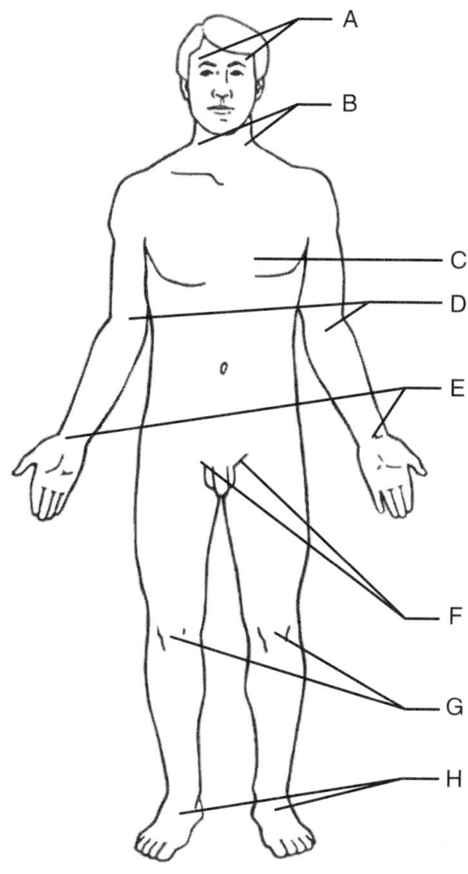

A. ______________________

B. ______________________

C. ______________________

D. ______________________

E. ______________________

F. ______________________

G. ______________________

H. ______________________

I. Which pulse is used during cardiopulmonary resuscitation on an adult?

____

J. Which pulse is most commonly taken?

____

K. Which pulse is used when taking the blood pressure?

____

L. Which pulse is found with a stethoscope?

____

85. Fill in the drawings below so that the thermometers read correctly.

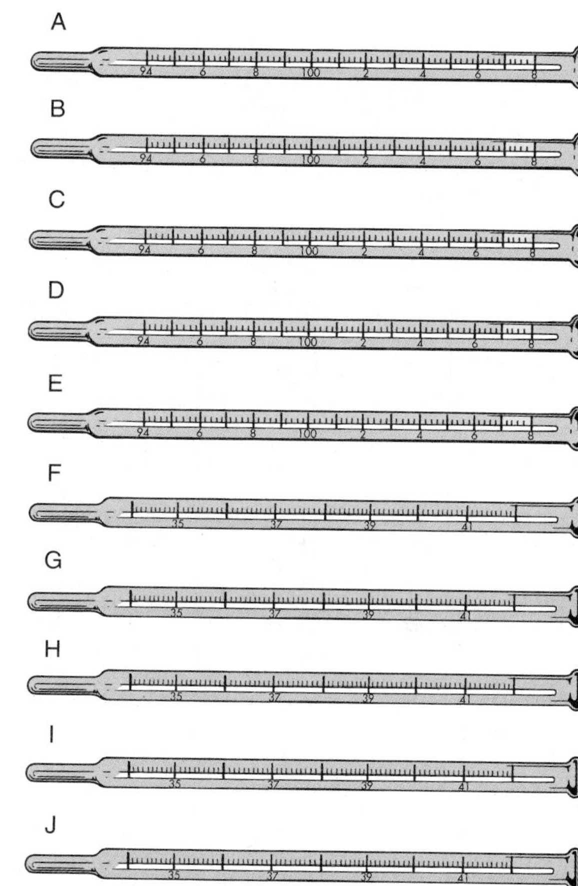

A. 95.8° F
B. 98.4° F
C. 100.2° F
D. 101° F
E. 102.6° F
F. 35.5° C
G. 36.5° C
H. 37° C
I. 38.5° C
J. 39.5° C

86. Fill in the drawings below so that the dials show the correct blood pressures.

A

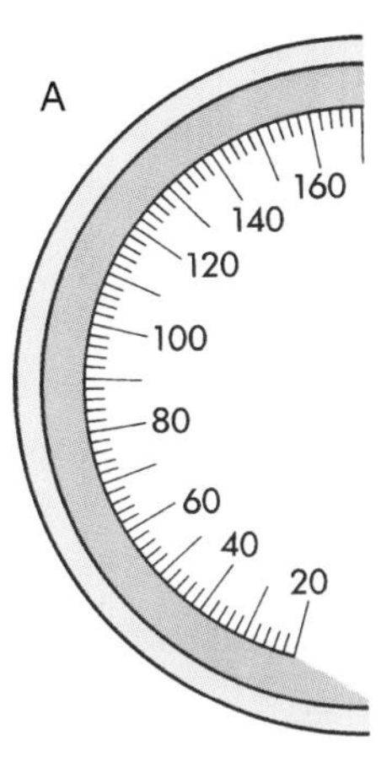

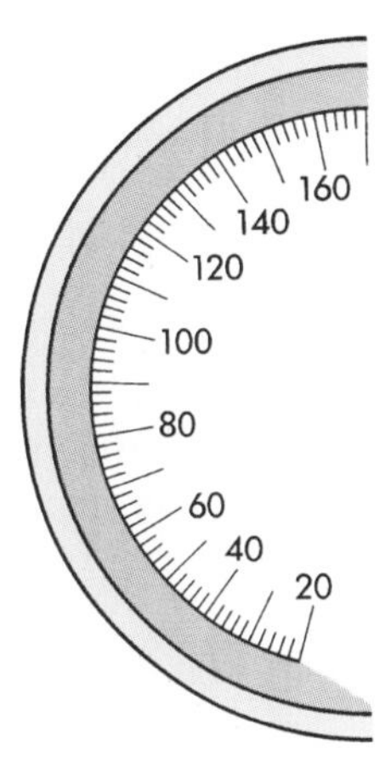

B

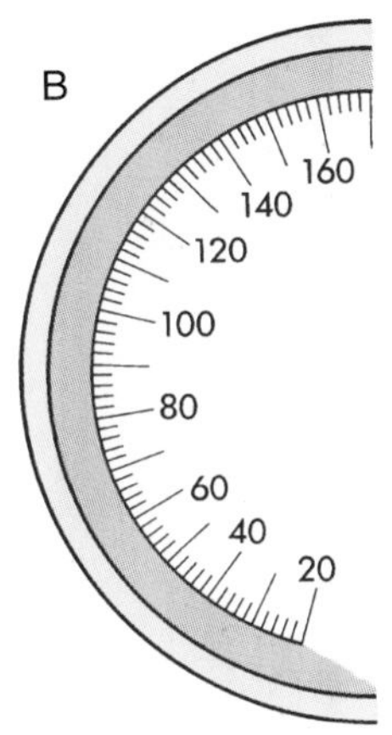

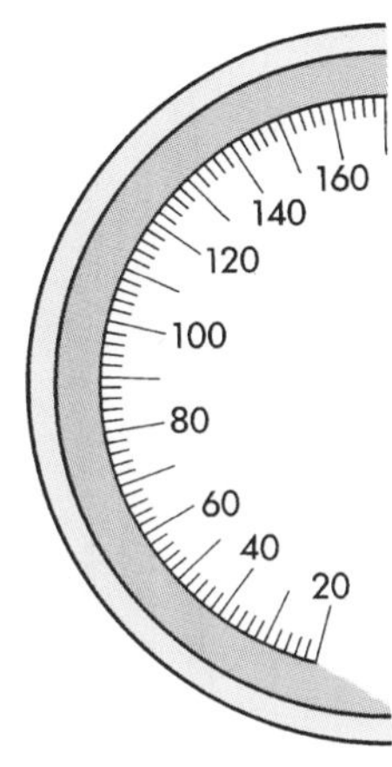

A. 168/102
B. 104/68

87. Fill in the drawings so the mercury columns show the correct blood pressures.

A

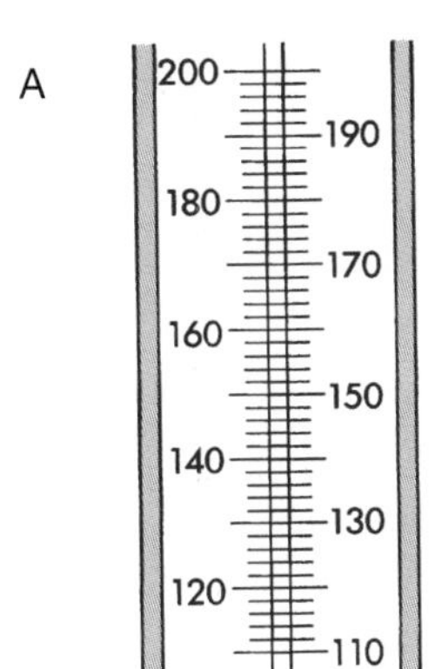

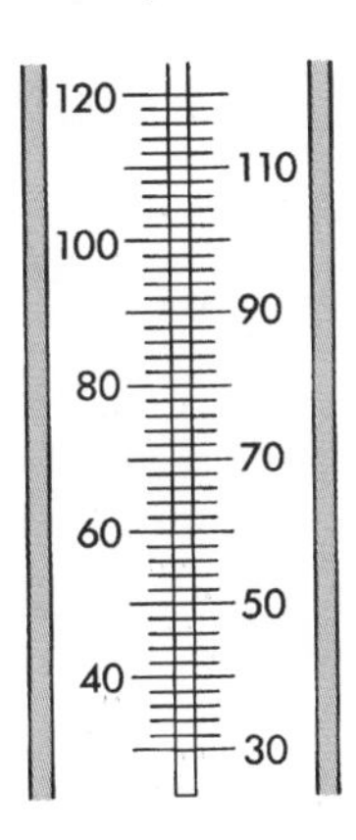

B

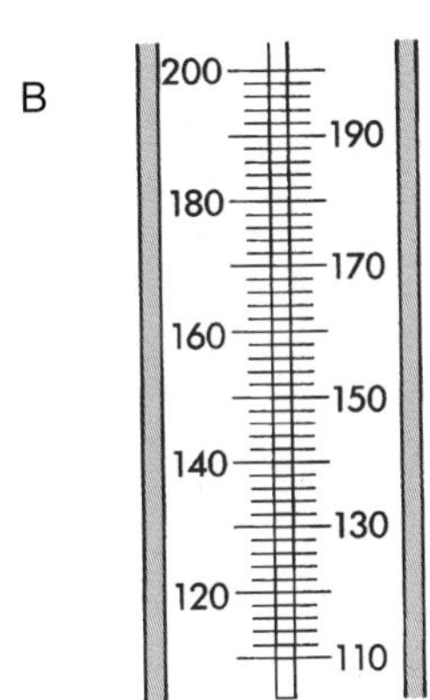

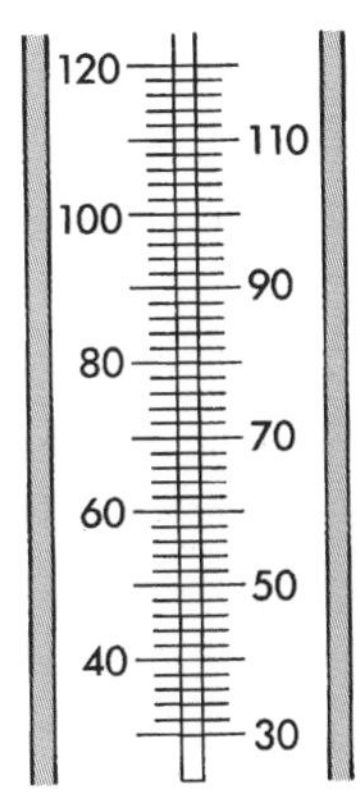

A. 152/86
B. 198/110

88. Record the readings on the thermometers pictured below.

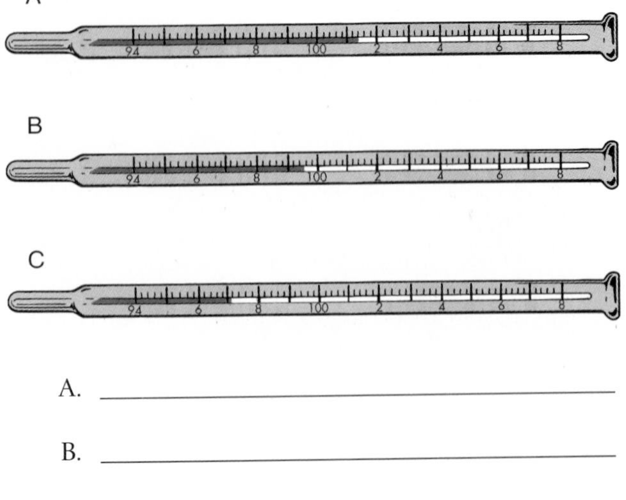

A. ______________________

B. ______________________

C. ______________________

Nursing Assistant Skills Video Exercise

View the parts of the **Measurements** *video that apply to this chapter to answer these questions.*

89. What information is needed before taking vital signs?

A. ______________________

B. ______________________

C. ______________________

D. ______________________

90. What procedure guidelines are important when taking vital signs?

A. Temperature ______________________

B. Pulse ______________________

C. Respiration ______________________

D. Blood pressure ______________________

91. Insert the rectal glass thermometer

______________________. If you meet

resistance ______________________.

92. When taking respirations in addition to counting, observe for

A. ______________________

B. ______________________

C. ______________________

93. If you use the one-step method to take the blood pressure, what do you do after inflating the blood pressure cuff until the pulse disappears?

____

____

Optional Learning Exercise

TAKING TEMPERATURES

94. You are preparing to take Mr. Harrison's temperature with a glass thermometer. When you take the thermometer from the container, it reads 97.8° F. What should you do?

____

95. If the thermometer registers between two short

lines, record the temperature to the

______________________.

96. How would you record these temperature readings?

A. An oral temperature of

97.4° F ____________ 36.5° C ____________

B. A rectal temperature of

99.8° F ____________ 38.1° C ____________

C. An axillary temperature of

96.2° F ____________ 36.1° C ____________

TAKING PULSES AND RESPIRATIONS

97. You are assigned to take Mrs. Sanchez' pulse and respirations. You note that the pulse rate and respirations are regular, so you take each one for ____________. When you complete counting the pulse, you keep your ______________________ and count ______________________. This procedure is performed so that Mrs. Sanchez will ______________________.

98. When you finish counting Mrs. Sanchez' pulse and respirations, your numbers are pulse 36 and respirations 9. What numbers should be recorded?

Pulse ____________ Respirations ____________

Why?

____

99. The nurse tells you to take an apical-radial pulse on Mrs. Hellman. Why do you ask a co-worker to help you?

____

____

100. How long is an apical-radial pulse counted?

____

After you have taken the apical-radial pulse, how do you find the pulse deficit?

____

____

TAKING BLOOD PRESSURES

101. You are assigned to take Mr. Hardaway's blood pressure. You know that he goes for dialysis three times a week. What do you need to know before you take his blood pressure?

____

Why?

____

____

102. When you inflate the cuff, you cannot feel the pulse after you pump the cuff to 130 mm Hg. How high will you inflate the cuff to take his blood pressure?

____

103. You should deflate the cuff at an even rate of

_______________________________ per seconds.

Independent Learning Activities

- Take turns measuring vital signs on three or four classmates. If possible, use glass, electronic, and tympanic thermometers for each person to determine if they give similar results. Use this table to record the results.

Person	Temperature	Pulse	Respiration	Blood Pressure
#1	Glass Electronic Tympanic	Radial Apical	Rate Rhythm Depth	
#2	Glass Electronic Tympanic	Radial Apical	Rate Rhythm Depth	
#3	Glass Electronic Tympanic	Radial Apical	Rate Rhythm Depth	
#4	Glass Electronic Tympanic	Radial Apical	Rate Rhythm Depth	

- Answer these questions about this exercise.
  - If you used different thermometers, how did the results compare?
  - What differences did you find in the radial pulses among your classmates?
  - What differences did you find in the rates and rhythms?
  - How were you able to measure respirations so that the person did not know that you were watching?
  - What differences in rhythm and depth of respirations did you find among your classmates?
  - What differences did you find in locating the brachial artery in different people?
  - How did the sounds of the blood pressure differ among your classmates?
  - What difficulties did you have with any of the measurements taken?
  - What will you change about measuring vital signs on a resident after this practice?

- Practice taking an apical-radial pulse with classmates. Take turns acting as the staff member and the person having the pulses taken. Answer these questions after the exercise is completed.
  - How was privacy maintained for the person who was having the pulse measured?
  - How did the staff member decide who would begin and end the count?
  - What problems did you have in counting for a minute?
  - How did the apical and radial counts compare?
  - What would you change about measuring the apical-radial pulses on a resident after this experience?

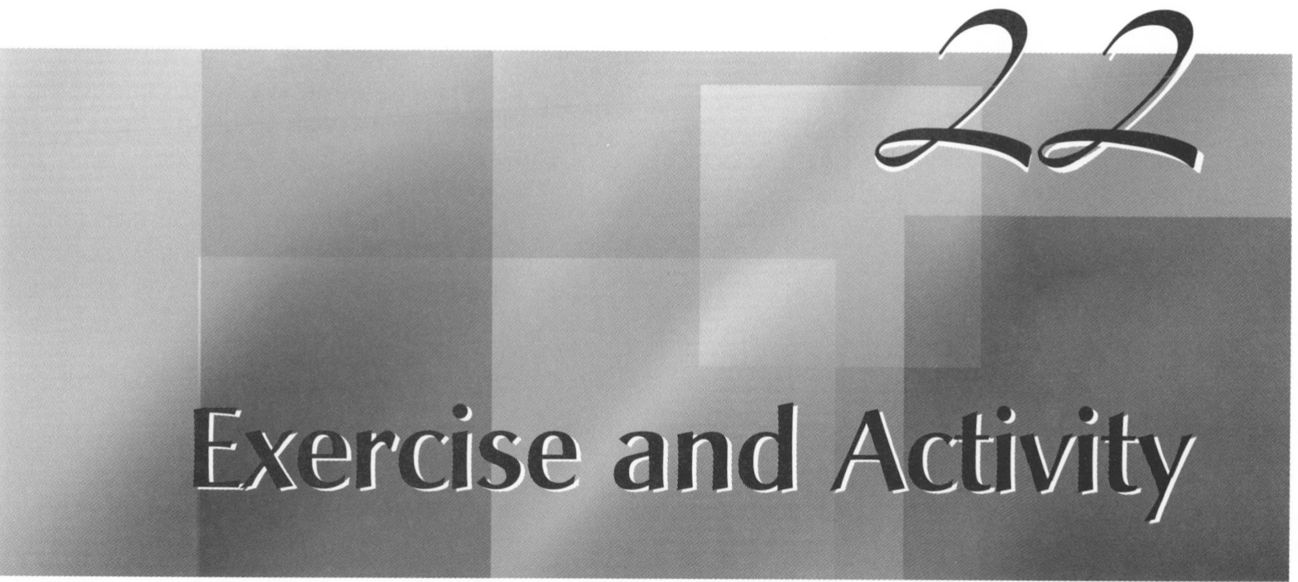

KEY TERMS

Abduction
Adduction
Ambulation
Atrophy
Contracture
Dorsiflexion
Extension
External rotation
Flexion
Footdrop
Hyperextension
Internal rotation
Orthostatic hypotension
Plantar flexion
Postural hypotension
Pronation
Range of motion (ROM)
Rotation
Supination
Syncope

Fill in the Blanks: Key Terms

1. If ______________________________ or foot drop is present, the foot is bent down at the ankle.
2. A brief loss of consciousness or fainting is ______________________________.
3. Bending a body part is ______________________________.
4. Moving a body part away from the midline of the body is ______________________________.
5. ______________________________ is the movement of a joint to the extent possible without causing pain.
6. Turning the joint outward is ______________________________.
7. A drop in blood pressure when the person stands is postural hypotension or ______________________________.
8. ______________________________ occurs when moving a body part toward the midline of the body.
9. Turning upward is called ______________________________.
10. A toe-up motion of the foot at the ankle is ______________________________.
11. Excessive straightening of a body part is ______________________________.

12. A decrease in size or a wasting away of tissue is

_______________________________________.

13. Turning the joint is ___________________________.

14. ___________________________________ is straightening of a body part.

15. ___________________________________ is another name for orthostatic hypotension.

16. ___________________________ is permanent plantar flexion; the foot falls down at the ankle.

17. The act of walking is

_______________________________________.

18. ___________________________ is turning downward.

19. ___________________________________ is turning the joint inward.

20. The lack of joint mobility caused by abnormal shortening of a muscle is a

_______________________________________.

Circle the BEST Answer

21. If a person is on bed rest, the person
    A. May be allowed to perform some activities of daily living
    B. Can use the bedside commode for elimination needs
    C. May not perform any activities of daily living
    D. Can use the bathroom for elimination needs

22. Complications of bedrest include all of the following *except*
    A. Contractures in fingers, wrists, knees and hips
    B. Urinary tract infections and renal calculi
    C. Increased appetite and improved muscle strength
    D. Orthostatic hypotension and syncope

23. If a contracture develops
    A. Extra range-of-motion exercises to correct the problem is required.
    B. You need to position the person in good body alignment.
    C. The person is permanently deformed and disabled.
    D. The problem will be relieved as soon as the person is able to walk and exercise.

24. When you are assisting a person who has orthostatic hypotension out of bed
    A. Raise the head of the bed such that the person is in Fowler's position.
    B. Have the person get out of bed quickly to prevent weakness.
    C. Keep the bed flat when helping the person get out of bed.
    D. Have the person walk around immediately to decrease weakness and dizziness.

25. You can prevent complications from bed rest with good nursing care, such as
    A. Positioning in good body alignment
    B. Range-of-motion exercises
    C. Frequent position changes
    D. All of the above

26. If a person who is sitting on the edge of the bed complains of weakness, dizziness, or spots before the eyes, you should
    A. Assist the person to stand.
    B. Help the person to sit in a chair or walk around.
    C. Place the person to Fowler's position.
    D. Tell the person that this is a normal response, and continue to get the person out of bed.

27. Bed boards are used to
    A. Keep the person in alignment by preventing the mattress from sagging.
    B. Prevent plantar flexion that can lead to footdrop.
    C. Keep the hips abducted.
    D. Keep the weight to top linens off the feet.

28. Plantar flexion must be prevented to
    A. Keep the feet from bending down at the ankle.
    B. Keep the hips from rotating outward.
    C. Keep the wrist, thumb, and fingers in their normal position.
    D. Maintain good body alignment.

29. To prevent the hips and legs from turning outward, you can use
    A. Bed cradles
    B. Hip abduction wedges
    C. Trochanter rolls
    D. Splints

30. Exercise occurs when
    A. ADLs are done.
    B. The person turns and moves in bed without help.
    C. The person uses a trapeze to lift the trunk off the bed.
    D. All of the above are correct.

31. When another person moves the joints through their range of motion, it is called
    A. Active range of motion
    B. Activities of daily living
    C. Active-assistive range of motion
    D. Passive range of motion

32. Range-of-motion exercises are performed on the ______________________ only if it is allowed by center policy.
    A. Shoulder
    B. Neck
    C. Hip
    D. Knee

33. Active range-of-motion exercises for children are done by
    A. Showing the child each movement and making sure the child exercises
    B. Performing active-assistive range of motion
    C. Encouraging play activities within the child's activities limits
    D. Scheduling play activities that will exercise every joint completely

34. In long-term care activities
    A. Must be attended by all residents
    B. Are planned only if all residents are interested in the activity
    C. Must allow the person the right to personal choice
    D. Are designed to meet only physical needs

35. When exercising the wrist, you will perform all of these motion *except*
    A. Abduction
    B. Hyperextension
    C. Flexion
    D. Extension

36. Which joint is adducted and abducted?
    A. Neck
    B. Hip
    C. Forearm
    D. Knee

37. When you help a person who is weak and unsteady to walk, you should
    A. Use a gait belt.
    B. Encourage the person to use the hand rails along the wall.
    C. Check the person for orthostatic hypotension.
    D. All of the above are correct.

38. If you are walking a person, and he or she starts to fall, you should
    A. Support the person and prevent the fall.
    B. Call for help while you hold the person upright.
    C. Ease the person to the floor.
    D. Let the person fall so you do not injure him or her by stopping the fall.

39. When the person is walking with crutches, the person should wear
    A. Soft slippers on the feet
    B. Clothes that fit well
    C. Clothes that are loose
    D. A gait belt

40. When walking with a cane, it is held
    A. On the strong side of the body
    B. On the weak side of the body
    C. In the right hand
    D. On the left side of the body

41. When a person is using a walker, it is
    A. Picked up and moved 3 to 4 inches in front of the person
    B. Moved forward with a rocking motion
    C. Moved first on the left side and then on the right
    D. Picked up and moved 6 to 8 inches in front of the person

42. When you are caring for a person who wears a brace, it is important to report immediately
    A. How far the person walks
    B. What care the person can do alone
    C. The amount of mobility in joints when doing range-of-motion exercises
    D. Any redness or signs of skin breakdown when you remove a brace

Fill in the Blanks

43. You will find information about the person's activity level and needed exercises in the

_______________.

44. Bedrest is ordered to

A. _______________

B. _______________

C. _______________

D. _______________

E. _______________

45. The nurse tells you that the person is on bedrest, but the bathroom can be used for elimination. This information means that the person is ordered to _______________.

46. What joints can develop permanent contractures?

A. _______________

B. _______________

C. _______________

D. _______________

E. _______________

F. _______________

G. _______________

H. _______________

I. _______________

47. When a person is moved from a lying or sitting to a standing position, the blood pressure may _______________. This patient status is called _______________.

48. Bed boards prevent the mattress from sagging, which keeps the person in good

_______________.

49. When you use a foot board, the soles of the feet are _______________ against it to prevent _______________.

50. A trochanter roll is placed along the body to prevent the hips and legs from

_______________.

51. Hand rolls or grips prevent _______________ of the thumb, fingers, and wrists.

52. A device that is used to keep the wrist, thumb, and fingers in the normal position is a

_______________.

53. Bed cradles are used because the weight of top linens can cause _______________ and _______________.

54. A _______________ allows the person to lift the trunk off the bed. It also allows the person to _______________ and _______________ in bed.

55. When range-of-motion exercises are done, what should be reported or recorded?

A. _______________

B. _______________

C. _______________

D. _______________

E. _______________

56. When performing range-of-motion exercises, each movement should be repeated ______________________ times or the ______________________.

57. List the rules to follow when performing range-of-motion exercises.

A. ______________________

B. ______________________

C. ______________________

D. ______________________

E. ______________________

F. ______________________

G. ______________________

58. When you help a person walk, where do you walk?

____

59. What are two ways you provide support when you help a person walk?

A. ______________________

B. ______________________

60. If a person falls, do not allow him or her to move or get up before the ______________________.

61. If a person falls, what is reported to the nurse?

A. ______________________

B. ______________________

C. ______________________

D. ______________________

E. ______________________

Labeling

62. The drawings below show the exercises for the ______________________.

Name the movements shown in each drawing.

A B C

A. (1) ______________________

(2) ______________________

(3) ______________________

B. (1) ______________________

(2) ______________________

C. (1) ______________________

(2) ______________________

63. What joint is being exercised in the drawings shown below?

____

Name the movements shown in each drawing.

A. ______________________

B. ______________________

A B

64. What joint is being exercised in the following drawing?

____

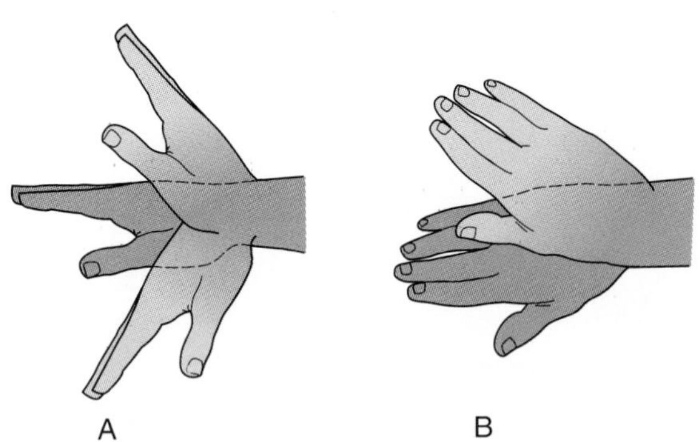

Name the movements in each drawing.

A. (1) _______________

(2) _______________

(3) _______________

B. (1) _______________

(2) _______________

65. The _______________ is being exercised in the drawings shown below.

Name the movements in each drawing.

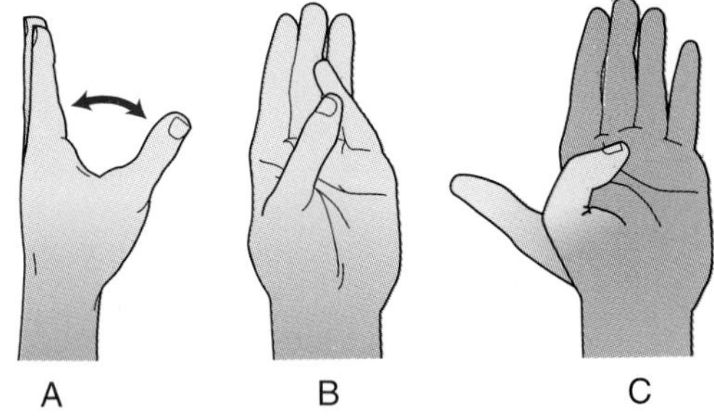

A. (1) _______________

(2) _______________

B. _______________

C. (1) _______________

(2) _______________

66. What joint is being exercised in the drawing shown below?

____

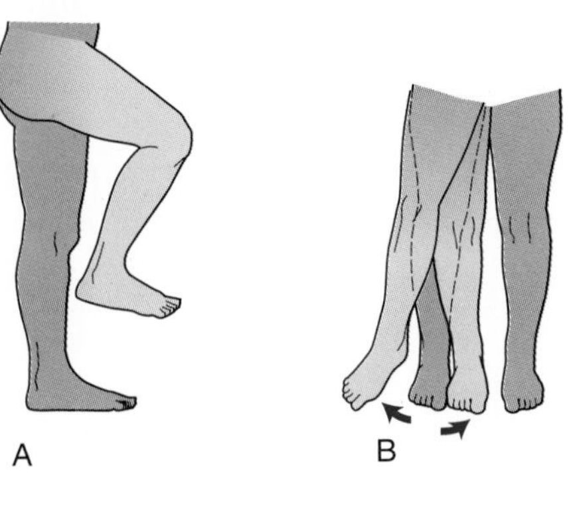

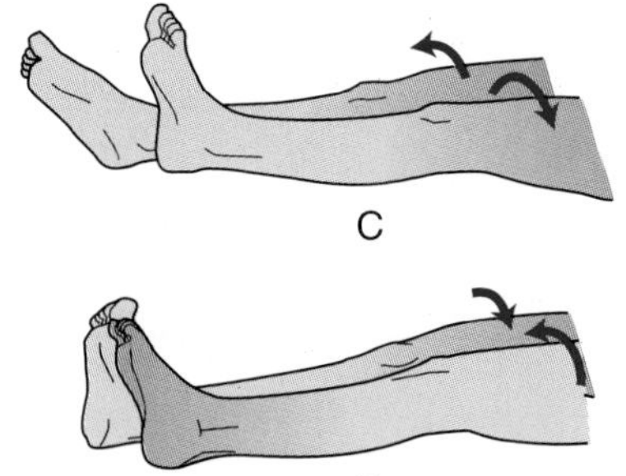

Name the movements shown in each drawing.

A. (1) _______________

(2) _______________

B. (1) _______________

(2) _______________

C. _______________

D. _______________

Crossword Puzzle

Fill in the crossword puzzle by answering clues with words from the following list.

abduction
adduction
dorsiflexion
extension
external rotation
flexion
hyperextension
internal rotation
key
plantar flexion
pronation
ROM
rotation
supination

Across

1. Turning the joint upward
5. Turning the joint outward (rotation)
6. Moving a body part toward the midline of the body
7. Straightening a body part
8. Turning the joint
9. Bending a body part
10. Bending the toes and foot up at the ankle
11. Moving a body part away from the midline of the body
12. Excessive straightening of a body part

Down

2. Bending the foot down at the ankle (two words run together)
3. Turning the joint downward
4. Turning the joint inward (rotation)
8. Range-of-motion

Nursing Assistant Skills Video

View the related portions of the* Body Mechanics and Exercise *video to answer these questions.

67. When doing range-of-motion exercises, you should support the ______________________________.

68. When exercising the knee, your hands should be under the ______________________________ and the ______________________________.

69. The person should wear ______________________ footwear when being ambulated.

70. When using a gait belt, you should grasp the belt ______________________________ when helping the person to stand.

71. When ambulating the person, grasp the gait belt at the ______________________________ and the ______________________________.

72. What observations should be reported after ambulating a person?

    A. ______________________________

    B. ______________________________

Optional Learning Exercises

73. What kind of range-of-motion exercises would be used with each of the following individuals?

    A. The person needs complete care for bathing, grooming, and feeding.

    ____

    B. The person takes part in many activities in the center. She walks to most activities independently.

    ____

    C. The person has weakness on his left side. He is able to feed himself or herself, but needs help with bathing and dressing.

    ____

74. As you plan to help a person out of bed, you are concerned about orthostatic hypotension. To make sure that the person is able to stand and get up safely, you plan to take the blood pressure, pulse, and respirations several times. When would you take the blood pressure?

    A. ______________________________

    B. ______________________________

    C. ______________________________

    D. ______________________________

    E. ______________________________

Independent Learning Activities

- Role-play with a classmate, and take turns acting as the nursing assistant and a person with left-sided weakness. Perform range-of-motion exercises on the person. Answer these questions about how you felt after this activity.
    - What did the nursing assistant explain to you before performing the exercises?
    - How were you positioned for exercising? What did the nursing assistant ask about your comfort and personal wishes in the position used?
    - How was your privacy maintained? Did anything make you feel exposed or embarrassed?
    - How were your joints supported during the exercises? Did you feel any discomfort or pain during the exercises?
    - What exercises were you encouraged to carry out independently? With some assistance?
    - Which exercises were down first? Were the exercises carried out in an organized pattern? How did you know what exercise would be done next?
    - After this activity, what will you do differently when giving range-of-motion exercises to a person?

- With a classmate, role-play assisting a weak, older person to ambulate. Take turns acting as the person and as the nursing assistant. Answer these questions about how you felt and what you learned.
  - What did the nursing assistant tell you before preparing to walk with you? What choices were offered about the time you were to ambulate, what clothing to wear, and where you were going to walk?
  - What safety devices were used? What did the nursing assistant tell you about the devices or equipment that were to be used?
  - What assessments were made before you sat up? When you dangled? After walking?
  - Did the nursing assistant make you feel secure during ambulation? How did the nursing assistant hold you?
  - What did you learn from this activity that will help you when you ambulate a person?

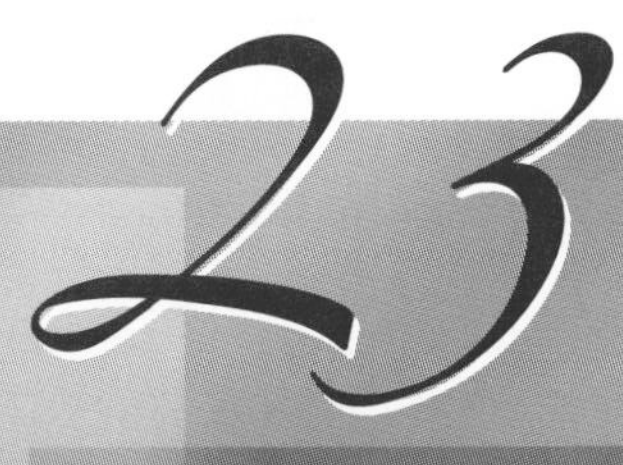

Comfort, Rest, and Sleep

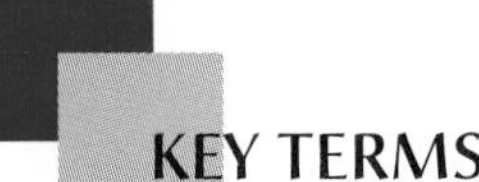

KEY TERMS

Acute pain
Chronic pain
Circadian rhythm
Comfort
Discomfort
Distraction
Enuresis
Guided imagery
Insomnia
NREM sleep
Pain
Phantom pain
Radiating pain
Relaxation
REM sleep
Rest
Sleep

Fill in the Blanks: Key Terms

1. To ache, hurt, or be sore is ______________________ or discomfort.
2. ______________________ is pain that is felt suddenly from injury, disease, trauma, or surgery; it generally lasts less than 6 months.
3. ______________________ is a way to change a person's center of attraction.
4. A state of unconsciousness, reduced voluntary muscle activity, and lowered metabolism is ______________________.
5. Pain lasting longer than 6 months is ______________________; it is constant or occurs off and on.
6. ______________________ is to be free from mental or physical stress.
7. ______________________ is a state of well-being. The person has no physical or emotional pain and is calm and at peace.
8. To be calm, at ease, and relaxed is to ______________________. The person is free of anxiety and stress.
9. Creating and focusing on an image is ______________________.
10. The stage of sleep when there is rapid eye movement is ______________________.

11. ________________________ is a chronic condition in which the person cannot sleep or stay asleep throughout the night.

12. The day-night cycle or body rhythm is also called ________________________. This daily rhythm is based on a 24-hour cycle.

13. ________________________ is pain felt at the site of tissue damage and in nearby areas.

14. The stage of sleep when there is no rapid eye movement is ________________________.

15. ________________________ is also called pain.

16. Pain felt in a body part that is no longer there is called ________________________.

17. Urinary incontinence in bed at night is ________________________.

Circle the BEST Answer

18. Comfort, rest, and sleep are needed for
    A. Well-being and energy
    B. To decrease function and quality of life
    C. Increasing muscle strength
    D. All of the above

19. OBRA requirements related to comfort, rest, and sleep include
    A. Only two people in a room
    B. Bright lighting in all areas
    C. Room temperature between 65° and 71° F
    D. Adequate ventilation and room humidity

20. When a person complains of pain
    A. The person has pain.
    B. It must be carefully measured to see if the person really has pain.
    C. You can easily measure to find out how much pain is present.
    D. You can tell if the person really has pain by the way he or she acts.

21. When a person complains of pain that is nearby areas of tissue damage, this is ____________ pain.
    A. Acute
    B. Chronic
    C. Radiating
    D. Phantom

22. Which of the following will *not* be likely to affect how a person handles pain?
    A. Knowing what to expect after surgery or an illness
    B. Being served meals on a special diet
    C. Personal and family support
    D. Having support from family and friends

23. When a person has anxiety, the person
    A. Will usually feel increased pain
    B. Will usually feel less pain
    C. May deny having pain
    D. May be stoic and show no reaction to pain

24. If pain is ignored or denied, it may be because the person thinks that pain is a sign of weakness. Which factor that affects pain would this be?
    A. Attention
    B. Past experience
    C. Value or meaning of pain
    D. Support from others

25. Pain may seem worse at night because
    A. Lying in bed makes pain more intense.
    B. The person is hungry.
    C. The person has more time to think about the pain.
    D. The circadian rhythm causes more pain at night.

26. A person from ________________________ may refuse pain relief the first time it is offered.
    A. Vietnam
    B. China
    C. Mexico
    D. Philippines

27. How can you know if a young child or infant is having pain?
    A. The child will support the area of pain.
    B. The child or infant may cry, fuss, and be restless.
    C. Children are able to point to the area of pain.
    D. Children do not have as much pain as adults.

28. An older person may not tell you that they have pain because the person may
    A. Have decreased pain sensations
    B. Think it relates to a known health problem
    C. Deny or ignore pain because of what it may mean
    D. All of the above

29. When you ask a person "Where is the pain?" you are asking the person to
    A. Describe the pain.
    B. Explain the intensity of the pain.
    C. Tell you the onset and duration of the pain.
    D. Tell you the location of the pain.

30. When a person tells you that he or she has pain when coughing or deep breathing, this is
    A. A factor causing pain
    B. A measurement of the onset of pain
    C. Words used to describe the pain
    D. The location of the pain

31. A distraction measure to promote comfort and relieve pain may be
    A. Asking the person to focus on an image
    B. Learning to breathe deeply and slowly
    C. Listening to music or playing games
    D. Contracting and relaxing muscle groups

32. If the nurse has given a person pain medication, you should
    A. Give the person a bath.
    B. Walk the person according to the care plan.
    C. Wait 30 minutes before giving care.
    D. Give care before the medication makes the person sleepy.

33. You may help to promote comfort and relieve pain by doing all of these *except*
    A. Allow family members and friends at the bedside as requested by the person.
    B. Keep the room brightly lit and play loud music.
    C. Provide blankets for warmth and to prevent chilling.
    D. Handle the person gently.

34. Which of the following is an example of guided imagery?
    A. Having the person take a deep breath and breathe out slowly
    B. Helping the person imagine a pleasant scene and focus on the scene
    C. Concentrating on relaxing muscle groups throughout the body
    D. Encouraging the person to watch television or listen to music

35. You can help to promote rest by
    A. Meeting physical needs such as thirst, hunger, and elimination needs
    B. Making sure the person feels safe
    C. Allowing the person to practice rituals or routines before resting
    D. All of the above

36. When caring for an ill or injured person, you know that the person may need more rest. You can help the person to get rest by making sure you
    A. Provide plenty of exercise to prevent weakness.
    B. Provide rest periods during or after a procedure.
    C. Give complete hygiene and grooming measures quickly.
    D. Spend time talking with the person to distract him or her.

37. Which of the following does *not* occur during sleep?
    A. The person is unaware of the environment.
    B. Metabolism is reduced during sleep.
    C. Blood pressure, temperature, pulse, and respirations are higher during sleep.
    D. No voluntary arm or leg movements are present.

38. Some people function better in the morning because of
    A. The circadian rhythm
    B. Getting enough sleep
    C. Interference with the body rhythm
    D. Changes in the work schedule

39. During REM sleep, the person
    A. Is hard to arouse
    B. Has a gradual fall in vital signs
    C. Is easily aroused
    D. Will relax all muscles completely

40. Which stage of sleep is usually not repeated during the cycles of sleep?
    A. REM
    B. Stage 1 NREM
    C. Stage 2 NREM
    D. Stage 3 NREM

41. Which age-group requires the least amount of sleep?
    A. Toddlers
    B. Young adults
    C. Adolescents
    D. Older adults

42. Which of the following factors increases the need for sleep?
   A. Illness
   B. Weight loss
   C. A diet high in L-tryptophan
   D. Drugs and other substances

43. When a person takes sleeping pills, sleep may not restore the person mentally because
   A. Caffeine prevents sleep.
   B. Some people have difficulty falling asleep.
   C. The length of REM sleep is reduced.
   D. Sleep aids upset the usual sleep routines.

44. Exercise should be avoided for 2 hours before sleep because
   A. Energy is required.
   B. People usually feel good after exercise.
   C. Exercise causes the release of substances in the bloodstream that stimulate the body.
   D. The person tires after exercise.

45. People who are ill or in intensive care units are at great risk for
   A. Sleep deprivation
   B. Sleepwalking
   C. Insomnia
   D. Increased sleep times

46. If a person has decreased reasoning, red, puffy eyes, and coordination problems, report these signs to the nurse because the person
   A. Is having a reaction to sleeping medications
   B. Has signs and symptoms of sleep disorders
   C. Needs more exercise before bedtime
   D. May need an increase in sleeping pills

47. Which of the following measures would *not* help to promote sleep?
   A. Providing blankets or socks for those who tend to be cold
   B. Having the person void or make sure incontinent persons are clean and dry
   C. Following bedtime rituals
   D. Offering the person a cup of coffee or tea at bedtime

Fill in the Blanks

48. OBRA has requirements about the person's room. List the requirements that relate to each of the following:
   A. Suspended curtain
   ____
   B. Linens
   ____
   C. Bed
   ____
   D. Room temperature
   ____
   E. People in room
   ____

49. Name the type of pain described in the following
   A. A person with an amputated leg may still sense leg pain.
   ____
   B. Tissue damage is present. The pain decreases with healing.
   ____
   C. Pain from a heart attack is often felt in the left chest, left jaw, left shoulder, and left arm.
   ____
   D. The pain remains long after healing. Common causes are arthritis and cancer.
   ____

50. What is the reason that people from the Phillipines may appear stoic in reaction to pain?
   ____

51. Older people may ignore or deny pain because

A. ______________________________

B. ______________________________

52. When the person uses words to describe pain such as aching, knifelike, or sore, what do you report to the nurse?

____

53. When gathering information about a person in pain, you can use a scale of 1 to 10. Which end of the scale is the most severe pain?

____

54. What happens to vital signs when the person has acute pain?

____

55. What body responses may be signs that the person has pain?

A. ______________________________

B. ______________________________

C. ______________________________

D. ______________________________

E. ______________________________

56. What changes in the following behaviors may be symptoms of pain?

A. Speech

____

B. Affected body part

____

C. Body position

____

57. List nursing measures to promote comfort and relieve pain related to these clues.

A. Position of the person

____

B. Linens

____

C. Blankets

____

D. Pain medications

____

E. Family members

____

58. If a person is receiving strong pain medication or sedatives, what safety measures are important?

A. ______________________________

B. ______________________________

C. ______________________________

D. ______________________________

59. What can you give an infant or young child that will provide comfort when the child has pain?

A. ______________________________

B. ______________________________

C. ______________________________

60. When you explain the procedure before it is performed, you may help a person rest better because you met the need for

______________________________.

61. A clean, neat, and uncluttered room can promote rest by meeting ____________________ needs.

62. When the mind and body rest, the body saves energy, and body functions slow during

______________________________.

63. Mental restoration occurs during a phase of sleep called ______________________________.

64. The deepest stage of sleep occurs during

______________________________.

65. If work hours are during the evening or night, the body must adjust to changes in the

______________-______________ cycle and the ______________________ rhythm.

66. How does weight gain and weight loss affect sleep needs?

A. Weight gain

____

B. Weight loss

____

67. Alcohol tends to cause drowsiness and sleep, but it interferes with

______________________________.

68. Insomnia may be caused by

A. Fear of

____

B. Afraid of not

____

C. Fear of not being able to

____

D. Physical and emotional

____

Optional Learning Exercises

69. You are caring for two residents who both have arthritis. Mr. Forman tells you that this is the first time that he has had any health problems. Mrs. Wegman tells you that she has had several surgeries and has had three children. Which of these two people is likely to be more anxious about the pain and would be unable to handle the pain well?

____

Why?

____

____

70. Mr. Forman tells you that his pain seems much worse at night. What might be the reason for this reaction?

____

____

____

71. You are caring for Mrs. Reynolds. She tells you that she misses her children who have moved to another state. Today, Mrs. Reynolds is complaining of pain in her abdomen. In spite of nursing comfort measures, she still rates her pain at a level of 7. What is a possible reason that Mrs. Reynolds is not getting relief of her pain?

____

____

72. When a person is ill, how is sleep affected?

A. Treatments and medications

____

B. Traction or a cast

____

C. Emotions that affect sleep include

____

73. Certain foods affect sleep. Explain how these foods affect sleep, and list foods that contain the substances.

    A. Caffeine ______________________ sleep.

       It is found in ______________________.

    B. L-Trytophan ______________________ sleep.

       It is found in ______________________.

Independent Learning Activities

- Form a group with several classmates and share your personal experiences with pain. Discuss these questions to understand the different ways you respond to and treat the pain.
  - What experiences have you had with pain? Accidents? Illnesses? Childbirth? Surgery?
  - What type of pain have you had? Acute? Chronic? Other types?
  - How would you rate your pain on a scale of 1 to 10? How long did the pain last?
  - How did your family and friends respond to your pain? How much support did you receive from them? How did the support (or lack of it) affect the pain?
  - What measures were used to treat the pain? Which measures were the most effective? The least effective?
  - What did you learn from this discussion with others about their pain? How will this information help you as you care for others with pain?

- Form a group with several classmates to talk about differences in sleep habits. Answer the following questions to understand differences in personal practices concerning rest and sleep.
  - How many hours do you sleep each day? How many hours of sleep do you think you should get each day?
  - If you did not have to follow a schedule (work, school, and so forth) when would you go to bed and wake up?
  - What rituals do you perform before going to bed? How is your sleep affected if you cannot perform these rituals?
  - What factors interfere with your sleep? What do you do to avoid these factors?
  - When do you feel most alert? Morning? Afternoon? Night?
  - How do you feel when you wake up? Alert? Pleasant? Grouchy? Tired?
  - How often do you take naps? What time of day do you like to nap? How do you feel when you wake from a nap?
  - How will this discussion help you understand differences in sleep patterns when you are caring for others? How will sleep affect the way you help people in your care get the rest and sleep they need?

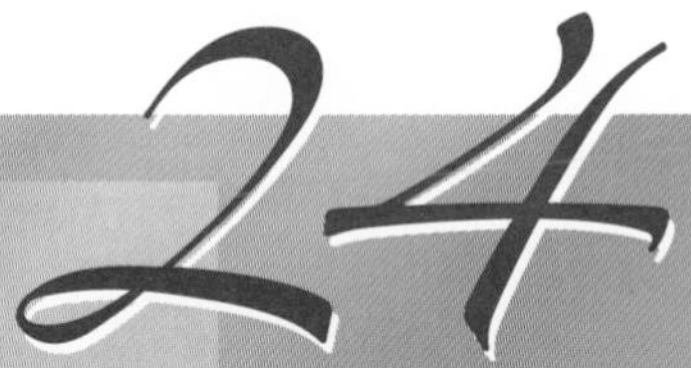

Admitting, Transferring, and Discharging Persons

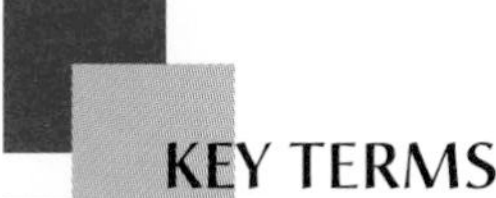

KEY TERMS

Admission
Discharge
Transfer

Fill in the Blanks: Key Terms

1. ______________________ is moving a person from one room or nursing unit to another.
2. The official entry of a person into a nursing center or nursing unit is ______________________.
3. ______________________ occurs with the official departure of a person from a nursing center or nursing unit.

Circle the BEST Answer

4. Usually, ______________________ is a happy time.
   A. Admission
   B. Discharge
   C. Transfer
   D. Home care
5. If a person develops pain or distress during admission, transfer, or discharge, you should
   A. Complete what you are doing and then go get the nurse.
   B. Call for the nurse at once.
   C. Ask the person to take several deep breaths to relax.
   D. Offer the person something to drink.
6. Where does the admissions process start?
   A. In the admitting office
   B. When the nurse greets the person
   C. When you take the person to the assigned room
   D. When the physician arrives to give the person a physical
7. When a person with dementia is admitted to a nursing center, the person
   A. Is usually depressed
   B. May have an increase in confusion
   C. May have a decrease in confusion
   D. Usually feels safer in the new setting

8. If a person being admitted arrives by stretcher, you should
   A. Raise the bed to its highest level.
   B. Leave the bed closed.
   C. Raise the head of the bed to the Fowler's position.
   D. Lower the bed to its lowest level.

9. Introduce yourself by telling the person
   A. Only your first name
   B. Details about your life
   C. Your name and title
   D. Only your title

10. During admission in long-term care, you can help the person feel more comfortable by
   A. Offering the person and the family beverages to drink
   B. Writing down names of roommates and other nearby residents
   C. Assisting the person to hang pictures or display photos
   D. All of the above

11. When you are delegated to admit a person, you will do all of these *except*
   A. Give the person a complete bath.
   B. Weigh and measure the person.
   C. Obtain a urine specimen.
   D. Orient the person to the room, nursing unit, and the agency.

12. When weighing a resident, have the person
   A. Wear socks and shoes and bathrobe.
   B. Remove regular clothes, and wear a gown or pajamas.
   C. Wear regular street clothes.
   D. Remove clothing after weighing and then weigh the clothes.

13. Chair and lift scales are used for people who
   A. Can transfer from a wheelchair to the chair scale
   B. Cannot stand
   C. Can stand and walk independently
   D. Are in the supine position

14. When measuring the length of a child under 2 years of age
   A. Have the child stand still against the wall.
   B. Ask the parent the length of the child.
   C. Lay the child down and have two people hold the child still.
   D. Measure the child with a tape measure while the child is sleeping.

15. Before measuring the weight, ask the person to
   A. Void
   B. Remove all clothing
   C. Tell you how much he or she weighs
   D. Wear a robe to avoid chilling

16. When a person cannot stand on the scale to have the height measured
   A. Ask the person or the family the height of the person.
   B. Have the person sit in a chair and use a measuring tape from head to toe.
   C. Position the person in supine position, and use a measuring tape.
   D. Estimate the height of the person by observing him or her.

17. Who is notified when a person is transferred?
   A. The physician
   B. The social worker
   C. The family and business office
   D. The person's roommate

18. When you are transferring a person, you should do all of these *except*
   A. Identify the person by checking the identification bracelet with the transfer slip.
   B. Explain the reasons for the transfer.
   C. Collect the person's personal belongings and bedside equipment.
   D. Introduce the person to the receiving nurse.

19. If a person wishes to leave the center without the physician's permission, you should
   A. Tell the person that leaving is not allowed.
   B. Prevent the person from leaving.
   C. Tell the nurse at once.
   D. Try to convince the person to stay.

20. When you assisting a person who is being discharged, you should
   A. Check all drawers and closet.
   B. Check off the clothing list.
   C. Help the person dress as needed.
   D. All of the above are correct.

Fill in the Blanks

21. When you are delegated to assist with admissions, transfers, or discharges, what information should you have from the nurse?

    A. ______________________

    B. ______________________

    C. ______________________

    D. ______________________

    E. ______________________

22. What supplies and equipment are collected and placed in the room before a person arrives?

    A. ______________________

    B. ______________________

    C. ______________________

    D. ______________________

    E. ______________________

    F. ______________________

    G. ______________________

    H. ______________________

    I. ______________________

    J. ______________________

    K. ______________________

23. Why is having a person urinate before being weighed important?

    ____

    When you ask the person to void, you may collect a ______________________.

24. How is the balance scale prepared before using it to weigh a person?

    A. ______________________

    B. ______________________

    C. ______________________

25. When using a lift scale, the person should be raised approximately ____________ off the bed.

26. When measuring a person in the supine position, the ruler is placed

    ______________________.

27. If you transfer a person to a new unit, you can help the person by introducing him or her to the ____________ and ____________.

28. When you assist the discharge of a person, you should report and record

    A. ______________________

    B. ______________________

    C. ______________________

    D. ______________________

    E. ______________________

Nursing Assistant Skills Video Exercise

View the portions of the Measurements *video that apply to this chapter and answer these questions.*

29. Before weighing a person, you should empty any

    ______________________.

30. You can provide balance for the person standing on a scale by keeping your

    ______________________.

Optional Learning Exercises

Answer the questions about the following person and situation. Rosa Romirez, age 65, is being admitted to the hospital where you work.

31. Because you know that Mrs. R. is arriving by wheelchair, you leave the bed ____________, and position it in the ____________ level.

32. The nurse asks you to greet and admit Mrs. R.

after the nurse makes sure Mrs. R. has no

______________________ or

______________________.

33. You greet Mrs. R. by name and ask her if she

prefers a certain ______________________.

34. When you orient Mrs. R. to the area, what information is given?

A. ______________________

B. ______________________

C. ______________________

D. ______________________

E. ______________________

F. ______________________

G. ______________________

H. ______________________

I. ______________________

J. ______________________

35. Mrs. R. has some weakness on her left side. She can safely transfer from the wheelchair to a chair or the bed but cannot stand. The nurse tells you to weigh Mrs. R. with the what kind of scale?

____

When you arrive at work one day, you are told Mrs. Romirez is being transferred to another unit and you are asked to assist. Answer these questions about transferring her.

36. When you transport Mrs. R. in a wheelchair, she

is covered with a ______________________.

37. What items are taken with Mrs. R. to the new unit?

____

38. What information is recorded and reported about the transfer?

A. ______________________

B. ______________________

C. ______________________

D. ______________________

E. ______________________

f. ______________________

Several weeks later, you are assigned to assist Mrs. R. when she is discharged. Answer these questions about her discharge.

39. Before a person is discharged, the physician must

______________________.

40. What should you do with Mrs. R. before you tell the nurse that the patient is ready for the final visit?

A. ______________________

B. ______________________

C. ______________________

Independent Learning Activities

Have a discussion with three or four classmates to share experiences you have had with admissions to health care agencies. You may have had personal experience or you may have observed a friend or family member being admitted. If you have not had this experience, perhaps you can relate the feelings you have had when visiting a physician's office. Use these questions during the discussion.

- Who was the first person you met when you arrived to be admitted? How were you greeted? Did you feel welcome?
- How did you arrive at your room? Were you escorted, or did you have to find your own way?
- How long did you wait in the room before a staff member came to admit you? How did this wait affect your feelings about the place?
- How were you addressed? First name? Last name? Did anyone ask you what you preferred?
- What information were you given to make you feel more comfortable? What printed information was provided?
- Overall, how did the admission procedure affect your feelings about the facility? Negative? Positive?
- How will your personal experience and the experiences of others in this group affect your approach to new people in a care facility?

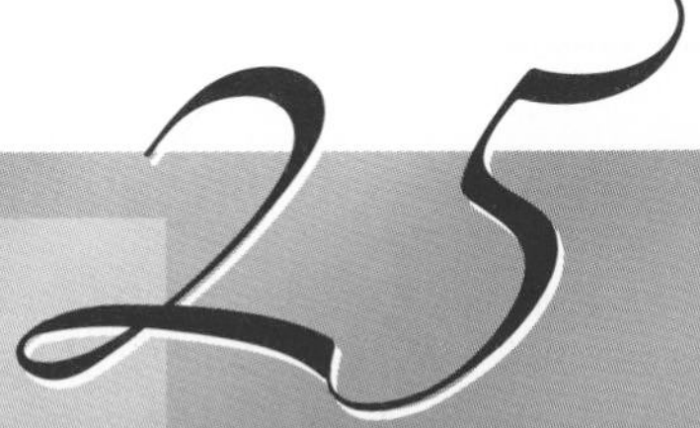

Assisting With the Physical Examination

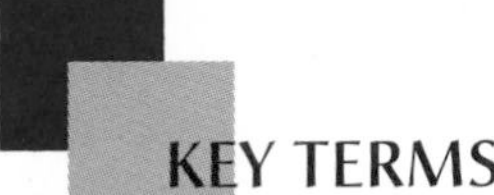

KEY TERMS

Dorsal-recumbent position
Horizontal-recumbent position
Knee-chest position
Laryngeal mirror
Lithotomy position
Nasal speculum
Ophthalmoscope
Otoscope
Percussion hammer
Tuning fork
Vaginal speculum

Fill in the Blanks: Key Terms

1. An instrument used to test hearing is a ________________________.
2. When a person is in the ________________________, the hips are brought down to the edge of the examination table, the knees are flexed, the hips are externally rotated, and the feet are supported in stirrups.
3. The supine or back-lying examination position in which the legs are together is called the ________________________.
4. An ________________________ is a lighted instrument used to examine the external ear and the eardrum (tympanic membrane).
5. A ________________________ is an instrument used to open the vagina so that it and the cervix can be examined.
6. When a person kneels and rests the body on the knees and chest, and the head is turned to one side, the arms are above the head or flexed at the elbows, the back is straight, and the body is flexed approximately 90 degrees at the hip, the person is in the ________________________.
7. A ________________________ is an instrument used to tap body parts to test reflexes.
8. An instrument used to examine the mouth, teeth, and throat is called a ________________________.

9. An instrument used to examine the inside the nose is a ______________________________.

10. The dorsal recumbent position is also called the ______________________________.

11. An ______________________________ is a lighted instrument used to examine the internal structures of the eye.

Circle the BEST Answer

12. Examinations are done to
    A. Promote health
    B. Determine fitness for work
    C. Diagnose disease
    D. All of the above

13. If a person is having a physical examination, you may be asked to do all of the following *except*
    A. Measure vital signs, height, and weight.
    B. Assist the doctor or nurse with an examination.
    C. Explain why the examination is being done and what to expect.
    D. Position and drape the person.

14. When the doctor is examining the person's mouth, teeth, and throat, you may be asked to hand him or her the
    A. Ophthalmoscope
    B. Percussion hammer
    C. Tuning fork
    D. Laryngeal mirror

15. Which of the following would *not* protect the right to personal choice for a person having a physical examination?
    A. The person is told to urinate before the examination begins.
    B. The person is told who will do the examination and when it will be done.
    C. The doctor or nurse explains the procedure.
    D. A family member is allowed to be present if the person requests.

16. The right to privacy is protected by
    A. Removing all clothes for a complete examination.
    B. Explaining the reasons for the examination.
    C. Exposing only the body part being examined.
    D. Explaining the examination results with a family member who is present.

17. Having a person empty the bladder is important before an examination because
    A. An empty bladder allows the examiner to feel the abdominal organs.
    B. A full bladder can change the normal position and shape of organs.
    C. A full bladder can cause discomfort when the abdominal organs are felt.
    D. All of the above are correct.

18. Which of the following will *not* provide warmth during the physical examination?
    A. Exposing only the body part being examined
    B. Having an extra bath blanket nearby
    C. Preventing drafts to protect the person from chilling
    D. Not leaving the person unattended

19. After you have taken the person to the examination room and placed the person in position, you should
    A. Put the signal light on for the nurse or examiner.
    B. Leave the room.
    C. Go to the nurse or examiner to report that the person is ready.
    D. Open the door, so the nurse or examiner knows you are ready.

20. When the abdomen, chest, and breasts are to be examined, you will place the person in the
    A. Lithotomy position
    B. Sims position
    C. Dorsal recumbent (horizontal recumbent) position
    D. Knee-chest position

21. Which position is rarely used for older people?
    A. Lithotomy
    B. Knee-chest
    C. Dorsal recumbent
    D. Sims

22. If a person is asked to stand on the floor during an examination, you should
    A. Help the person put on his or her shoes or slippers.
    B. Place paper or paper towels on the floor.
    C. Place a sheet on the floor.
    D. Wipe the floor carefully with an antiseptic cleaner before the person stands on it.

23. When a child or infant is examined, the parent is asked to
    A. Hold the child still during some parts of the procedure.
    B. Wait outside to avoid upsetting the child.
    C. Firmly tell the child to be cooperative.
    D. Sit quietly, and avoid touching the child.

24. If an older person is confused and resists an examination
    A. Several staff members may be needed to help with the examination.
    B. The examination is attempted at another time.
    C. The nurse explains the reason for the examination.
    D. A family member holds the person still during the examination.

25. If you are cross-trained to draw blood for laboratory study, you are
    A. An EKG technician
    B. A phlebotomist
    C. An ECG technician
    D. An x-ray technician

Fill in the Blanks

You are collecting equipment for a physical examination. What equipment is used for the examinations listed in #26 through #28?

26. Ear examinations
    A. ______________________
    B. ______________________

27. Eye examinations
    A. ______________________
    B. ______________________

28. Nose, mouth, and throat examinations
    A. ______________________
    B. ______________________
    C. ______________________
    D. ______________________

29. How is privacy protected during the physical examination?
    A. A patient gown reduces the ______________________.
    B. The person is covered with ______________________.
    C. The door is ______________________.
    D. The only body part that is exposed is the part ______________________.

30. When preparing children for an examination, how are they dressed?
    A. Babies ______________________
    B. Baby boys ______________________
    C. Toddlers, preschool children, and school-age children ______________________

31. What should you tell the person about the examination position?
    A. ______________________
    B. ______________________
    C. ______________________
    D. ______________________

32. After the examination is completed, you may need to wipe or clean the person's ______________________ or ______________________ because ______________________ is used during the examination.

33. If you are cross-trained, you can receive your training

A. ___

B. ___

C. ___

D. ___

Labeling

Answer #34 through #38 using the following illustration.

34. Name the instruments.

A. ___

B. ___

C. ___

D. ___

E. ___

F. ___

G. ___

35. Which instrument is used to examine the nose?

___

36. When the eye is examined, the examiner uses the

___.

37. If a person has a sore throat, the examiner will look at the throat with the

___.

38. The reflexes are examined by using the

___.

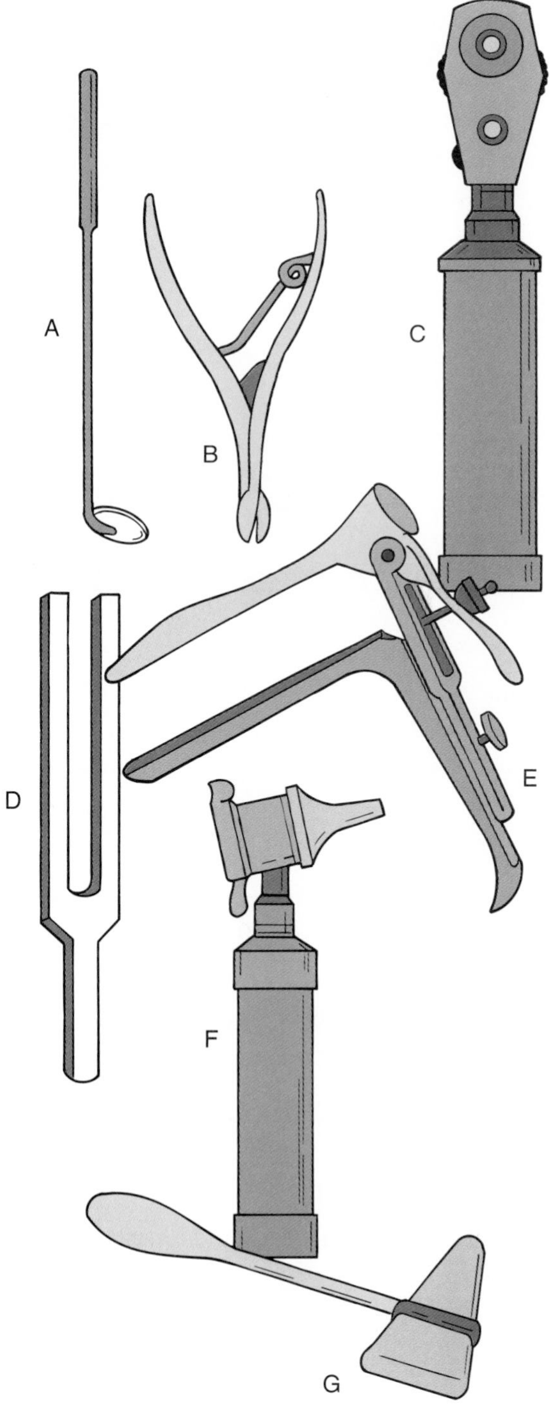

Answer #39 through #42 using the following illustration.

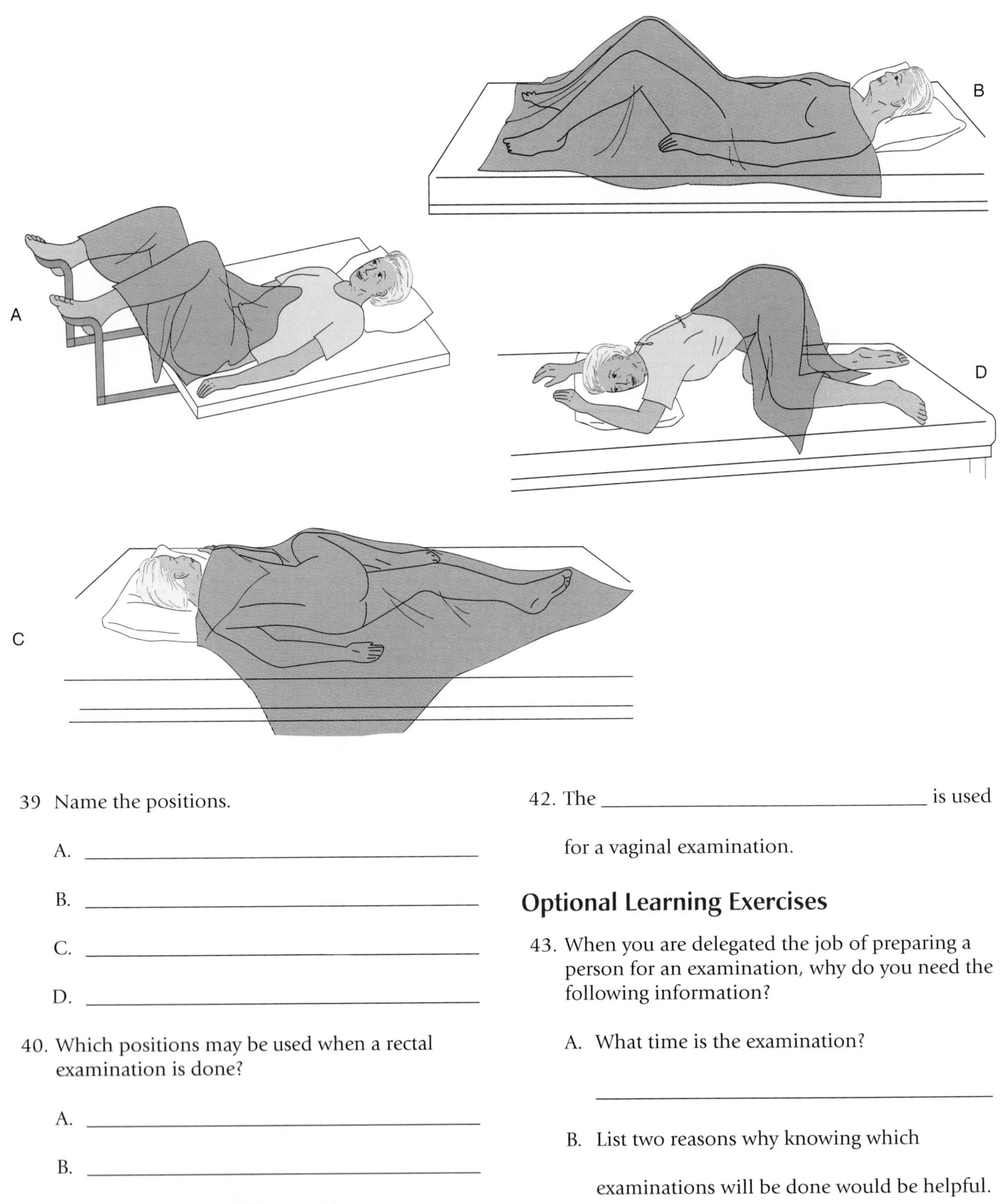

39 Name the positions.

A. ______________________

B. ______________________

C. ______________________

D. ______________________

40. Which positions may be used when a rectal examination is done?

A. ______________________

B. ______________________

41. When the abdomen, chest, and breasts are examined, the person is placed in ______________________.

42. The ______________________ is used for a vaginal examination.

Optional Learning Exercises

43. When you are delegated the job of preparing a person for an examination, why do you need the following information?

A. What time is the examination?

____

B. List two reasons why knowing which examinations will be done would be helpful.

____

____

C. What equipment will you need if you are assigned to take vital signs?

____

____

44. You are a female nursing assistant who is assisting a male examiner with an examination of a female person. The nurse tells you to stay in the examination room during the entire procedure. Why is this precaution important to the examiner and to the woman?

____

____

Independent Learning Activities

- You probably have had a physical examination at some time. Perhaps you needed one to be a student in this class. Answer these questions about your experience when you had the physical done to you.
  - Who explained what to expect during the examination? What were you told about any discomfort?
  - What steps were taken to give you privacy? While you changed clothes? During the examination?
  - Who was present during the examination? Were you given a choice of having another person in the room with you and the examiner? How did you feel about having (or not having) another person in the room?
  - How did you know what was being done? How much information were you given about procedures? Positions? Tests?
  - What positions were used during the examination? Which positions shown in this chapter were used?

- How comfortable did you feel? How did the examiner and assistant help to make you more comfortable with the positions?
  - What questions did you have during the examination? Who was able to answer these questions? How well were they answered to make you understand what was being done?
  - How comfortable did you feel about the examination? What might have been done to make you more comfortable physically and psychologically?
  - How did this experience help you understand the feelings of people you may assist during an examination?

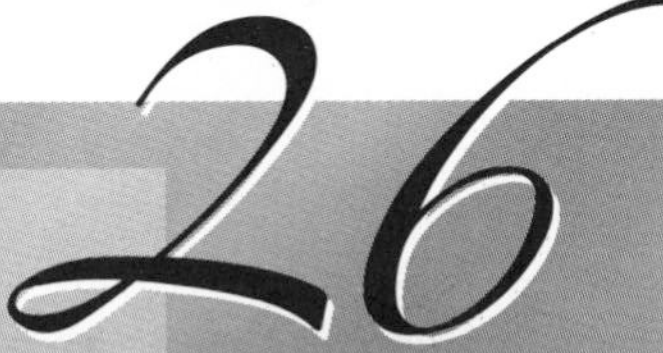

Collecting and Testing Specimens

KEY TERMS

Acetone
Glucosuria
Glycosuria
Hematuria
Hemoptysis
Ketone
Ketone body
Melena
Sputum

Fill in the Blanks: Key Terms

1. Bloody sputum is ______________________.
2. A ketone or acetone is also called ______________________.
3. A black, tarry stool is ______________________.
4. ______________________ is glucosuria or sugar in the urine.
5. ______________________ is mucus from the respiratory system that is expectorated through the mouth.
6. Acetone is called ______________________ or ketone body.
7. A substance that appears in urine from the rapid breakdown of fat for energy is ______________________.
8. Sugar in the urine is called glycosuria or ______________________.
9. ______________________ is blood in the urine.

Circle the BEST Answer

10. Specimens are collected and tested for all of these reasons *except* to
    A. Measure the specimen
    B. Prevent diseases
    C. Detect diseases
    D. Treat diseases

11. When you are collecting a specimen, which of the following is *incorrect?*
    A. Use a clean container for each specimen.
    B. Gloves are not needed.
    C. Do not touch the inside of the container or lid.
    D. Place the specimen container in a plastic bag.

12. When collecting a urine specimen from a toddler or young child, it is useful to use a
    A. Collection bag applied to the genital area
    B. Potty chair
    C. Catheter
    D. Paper bag to cover the specimen container

13. A random urine specimen is collected
    A. First thing in the morning
    B. After meals
    C. At any time
    D. At bedtime

14. When a person is collecting a random urine specimen, ask the person to put the toilet tissue in
    A. The wastebasket or toilet
    B. In the specimen container
    C. In the specimen pan
    D. Any of the above

15. When obtaining a midstream specimen, the perineal area is cleaned to
    A. Remove all microbes from the area.
    B. Reduce the number of microbes in the urethral area.
    C. Follow Standard Precautions and Bloodborne Pathogen Standards.
    D. Reduce infection during the specimen collection.

16. When collecting a midstream specimen, which of the following is correct?
    A. Collect the entire amount of urine voided.
    B. Collect approximately 4 oz (120 ml) of urine.
    C. Have the person void and then pass the receptacle into the stream of urine.
    D. Collect several specimens and mix them together.

17. When collecting a 24-hour urine specimen, the urine is kept
    A. On ice or refrigerated during the time
    B. At room temperature
    C. In a sterile container at the nurses' station
    D. In a drainage collection bag at the bedside

18. A 24-hour urine specimen collection is started
    A. At the beginning of a shift
    B. After a meal
    C. At night
    D. After the person voids and that urine is discarded

19. The last step in a 24-hour specimen collection is
    A. Collecting a urine specimen at the end of the 24-hour period
    B. Writing down any missed or spilled urine
    C. Recording the amount of urine collected
    D. All of the above

20. When collecting a double-voided specimen, the first specimen is
    A. Discarded without testing
    B. Mixed with the second specimen collected
    C. Tested in case you cannot obtain a second specimen
    D. Sent to the laboratory

21. When a collection bag is used to collect a urine specimen from a child, you should
    A. Restrain the child so the the child cannot remove the bag.
    B. Cut a slit in a diaper and pull the bag through the slit.
    C. Connect the bag to a collection bag at the bedside.
    D. Ask the parents to hold the bag in place until the child voids.

22. When testing urine, which of the following tests are best if done with a double-voided specimen?
    A. Test for pH
    B. Test for blood
    C. Test for melena
    D. Test for glucose and ketones

23. When you test urine with a reagent strips, it is important that you
    A. Follow the directions on the bottle carefully.
    B. Use a sterile urine specimen.
    C. Wear sterile gloves.
    D. Make sure the urine is cold.

24. When you are assigned to strain a person's urine, you
    A. Have the person void directly into the strainer.
    B. Send all specimens to the laboratory.
    C. Have the person void into the bedpan and then pour the urine through the strainer.
    D. Discard the strainer after it is used to strain any crystals, stones, or particles from the urine.

25. If a warm stool specimen is required, it is
    A. Placed it in an insulated container
    B. Taken to the laboratory at once
    C. Tested at once on the nursing unit
    D. Placed in a special heated area on the nursing unit

26. When collecting a stool specimen, ask the person to
    A. Void and have a bowel movement in a bedpan.
    B. Use only a bedpan or commode to collect the specimen.
    C. Void first, then place the specimen container at the back of the toilet to collect the stool specimen.
    D. Place the toilet tissue in the bedpan, commode, or specimen pan with the stool.

27. When collecting the stool specimen
    A. Pour it into the specimen container.
    B. Use your gloved hand to obtain a specimen to place in the container.
    C. Use a tongue blade to take about 2 tablespoons of stool from the middle of the formed stool.
    D. Use a tongue blade to place the entire stool specimen in the container.

28. When you test a stool specimen for blood
    A. It must be sent to the laboratory.
    B. The specimen must be sterile.
    C. You will need to test the entire stool specimen.
    D. Use a tongue blade to obtain a small of amount of stool.

29. A sputum specimen is more easily collected
    A. On awakening
    B. After eating
    C. At bedtime
    D. After activity

30. Before obtaining a sputum specimen, ask the person to
    A. Rinse the mouth with water.
    B. Brush the teeth and use mouthwash.
    C. Cough and discard the first sputum expectorated.
    D. Sit in an upright position to loosen secretions.

31. Postural drainage is used when collecting a sputum specimen to
    A. Collect specimens from children.
    B. Make the sputum specimen more liquid.
    C. Stimulate coughing.
    D. Help secretions drains by gravity.

Fill in the Blanks

32. When collecting urine specimens what observations are reported and recorded?

    A. ______________________________

    B. ______________________________

    C. ______________________________

    D. ______________________________

33. How much urine is collected for a random urine specimen?

    ____

34. When collecting a midstream urine specimen, the person starts to void and then stops ______________________________. After the specimen container is positioned, the person ______________________________.

35. When you are obtaining a midstream specimen from a woman, spread the labia with your thumb and index finger with your ______________________________ hand.

36. When cleaning the female perineum for a midstream specimen, clean from ______________________________.

37. When cleaning the male perineum for a midstream specimen, clean the penis starting ______________________________.

38. When you make labels for a 24-hour urine collection to place in the room and bathroom, what information is marked?

    ____

    ____

39. Another name for a double-voided specimen is a

______________________.

40. When collecting a double-voided specimen, the second voiding is collected __________ minutes after the first voiding.

41. Make sure that you do not cover the ______________________ when applying the a urine collection bag to a child.

42. Urine pH measures if the urine is ______________ or ______________.

43. When you use reagent strips, you read the strip by comparing it to the ______________.

44. When you strain urine, you are looking for stones that can develop in the

______________________.

45. The strainer or gauze are placed in the specimen container if any ______________ appear.

46. Stool specimens are studied and checked for

A. ______________________

B. ______________________

C. ______________________

D. ______________________

E. ______________________

47. When collecting a stool specimen from a child who is wearing diapers, you can

______________________.

48. After collecting a stool specimen, place the container in a ______________________.

49. When stools are black and tarry, bleeding is present in the ______________________.

50. Blood in the stool that is hidden is called

______________________.

51. Mouthwash is not used before a sputum specimen is collected because it

______________________.

52. To collect a sputum specimen from infants and small children, the RN or respiratory therapist gives a ______________________. The nurse then ______________________ for the specimen.

53. When you are delegated to collect a sputum specimen, report and record

A. ______________________

B. ______________________

C. ______________________

D. ______________________

E. ______________________

F. ______________________

G. ______________________

H. ______________________

54. When you are assisting a person to collect a sputum specimen, ask the person to take two or three ______________________ and ______________________ the sputum.

Crossword Puzzle

Fill in the crossword puzzle by answering the clues with words from the following list.

calculi
dysuria
expectorated
labia
midstream
occult
postural
random
specimens
suctioning

1 2 3 4 5 6 7 8 9 10

Across

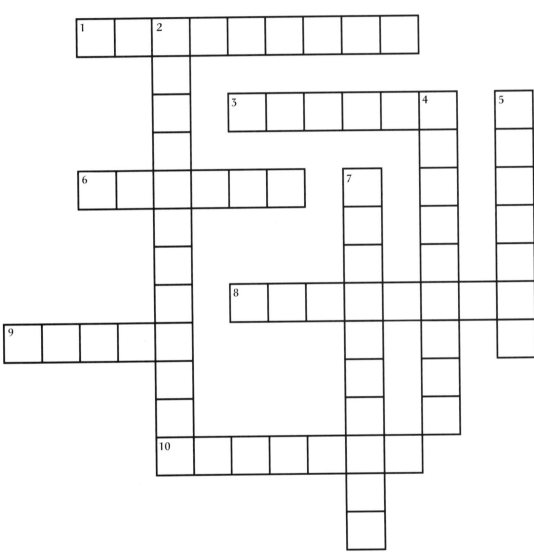

1. Samples
3. A urine specimen that can be collected at any time
6. Hidden, as in blood in the stool
8. Position with head lower than body used to cause fluid to flow down
9. Folds of tissue on each side of the vagina
10. Pain when urinating

Down

2. Expelled, as in sputum through the mouth
4. A urine specimen that is collected after the person starts to void
5. Stones that develop in kidneys, ureters, or bladder
7. Removal of sputum from the trachea with a machine

Optional Learning Exercises

55. You are assigned to collect a urine specimen from a young child. How will you explain to the child what you need?

____

56. Why would you place a urine specimen container in a paper bag when you ask an adolescent for a urine specimen?

____

57. If you are collecting a midstream specimen, what should you do if the person had difficulty stopping the stream of urine?

____

58. You are caring for a person who is having a 24-hour urine specimen test. He tells you that he forgot to save a specimen an hour ago. What should you do and why?

____

59. When collecting a double-voided specimen, why do you test the first specimen?

____

60. When collecting a double-voided specimen, what can you do to help the person void 30 minutes after the first voiding?

____

61. What is normal pH for urine?

____

What can cause changes in the normal pH?

____

62. When the body cannot use sugar for energy, it uses fat. When this happens, ____________________ appear in the urine.

61. What food is *not* eaten for 3 days before a stool test for occult blood?

____

What else can affect test results?

____

____

62. Why is privacy important when collecting a sputum specimen?

____

____

Independent Learning Activities

Answer the following questions about collecting specimens

- What specimens may be collected by nursing assistants in your state?
- What special training is given to make sure nursing assistants understand how to collect specimens?
- Ask permission to look at specimen containers used in your clinical site.
- Are any directions included with the containers?
- Where is information about collecting specimen kept at the clinical site?

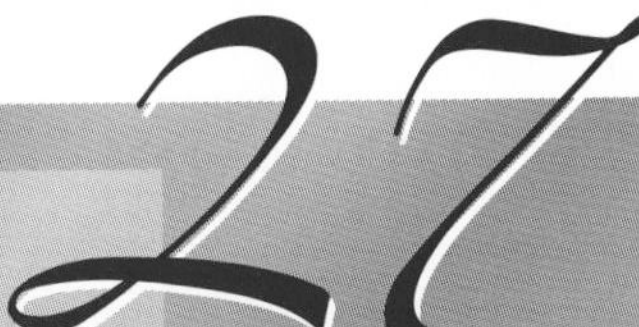

27 The Person Having Surgery

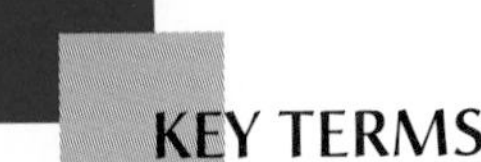

KEY TERMS

Anesthesia
Douche
Elective surgery
Embolus
Emergency surgery
General anesthesia
Local anesthesia
Preoperative
Postoperative
Regional anesthesia
Thrombus
Urgent surgery

Fill in the Blanks: Key Terms

1. The loss of consciousness and all feeling or sensation is ______________________.
2. ______________________ is surgery done by choice to improve the person's life or well-being.
3. A blood clot is called a ______________________.
4. ______________________ is the loss of feeling or sensation produced by a drug.
5. An ______________________ is a blood clot that travels through the vascular system until it lodges in a distant blood vessel.
6. ______________________ is before surgery.
7. ______________________ is surgery needed for the person's health. Surgery is done soon to prevent further damage or disease.
8. The introduction of a fluid into the vagina and the immediate return of the fluid is a ______________________.
9. ______________________ is after surgery.
10. The loss of feeling or sensation in a large area of the body is ______________________.
11. Surgery done immediately to save life or function is ______________________.
12. ______________________ is the loss of feeling or sensation in a small area.

Circle the BEST Answer

13. Surgery is done to
    A. Remove a diseased body part.
    B. Make a diagnosis.
    C. Restore function.
    D. All of the above are correct.

14. A surgery that is done soon to prevent further damage or disease is
    A. Emergency
    B. Elective
    C. Urgent
    D. General

15. When an accident occurs, the person often requires
    A. Elective surgery
    B. Emergency surgery
    C. General anesthesia
    D. Urgent surgery

16. When a person tells you about fears and concerns before surgery, you should
    A. Explain that the surgeon is highly skilled.
    B. Tell the person not to worry.
    C. Respect the person's fears and concerns.
    D. Change the subject and talk about something else.

17. When a patient ask you about test results or the diagnosis
    A. Answer the questions honestly.
    B. Refer the questions to the nurse.
    C. Tell the person that information is not available.
    D. Explain that you do not know but will find out.

18. Which of the following is not part of your role when caring for a surgical patient?
    A. Explain the care you will give.
    B. Perform procedures and tasks with skill and ease.
    C. Tell the person about your own experience with the same surgery.
    D. Report a request to see a member of the clergy to the nurse.

19. The nurse will tell the patient that deep-breathing and coughing exercises will be done after surgery
    A. Once a shift
    B. Every 1 or 2 hours when the person is awake
    C. Every 4 hours
    D. Every 2 hours for the first 48 hours after surgery

20. How is a child prepared for surgery?
    A. The parents are responsible for explaining the surgery to the child.
    B. A doll may be used to show the site of the surgery.
    C. Children are not told about the surgery as it may frighten them.
    D. A child does not need an explanation because the idea of surgery is too difficult for the child to understand.

21. If blood loss is expected during surgery, what test is done preoperatively?
    A. Type and crossmatch
    B. Complete blood count
    C. Urinalysis
    D. Electrocardiogram

22. A person is NPO 6 to 8 hours before surgery to reduce
    A. Breathing problems after surgery
    B. Pain postoperatively
    C. Diarrhea
    D. Vomiting and aspiration during and after surgery

23. Cleansing enemas may be ordered before surgery to
    A. Clear the colon of feces.
    B. Prevent incontinence after surgery.
    C. Prevent diarrhea after surgery.
    D. Prevent pain.

24. The person being prepared for surgery needs to void
    A. Right before leaving the room
    B. The morning of surgery
    C. Before the nurse gives the preoperative drugs
    D. Before an enema is given

25. Makeup, nail polish, and artificial nails are removed before surgery because
    A. This reduces wound infection.
    B. It reduces the number of microbes on the body.
    C. The skin, lips, and nail beds are observed for color during and after surgery.
    D. It makes the person more comfortable after surgery.

26. When preparing a child for surgery, it is important to report
    A. A dry mouth
    B. Any loose teeth
    C. Any missing teeth
    D. That you removed hair clips from the hair

27. If a person is allowed to wear a wedding ring during surgery, you should
    A. Record this information on the chart.
    B. Secure the ring in place with gauze and tape.
    C. Make sure the ring fits well and will not come off.
    D. Put a clean glove on the person's hand.

28. If you are assigned to do a skin preparation preoperatively, you should be careful
    A. Not to cut, scratch, or nick the skin
    B. To shave against the direction of hair growth
    C. To shave the entire body
    D. Not to shave too closely to the skin

29. To protect yourself from being accused of sexual abuse when giving a vaginal douche
    A. Explain the procedure to the person.
    B. Get her consent to proceed.
    C. Protect her right to privacy.
    D. All of the above are correct.

30. The surgery consent
    A. Is signed by the person and the nearest relative
    B. Is signed by the person's attorney
    C. May be obtained by nursing assistant
    D. Is obtained by the doctor or nurse

31. Preoperative medications are given
    A. To prevent pain
    B. Approximately 45 minutes to I hour before surgery
    C. Immediately before surgery
    D. In the operating room

32. When a child is transported to the operating room, the parents
    A. Must stay in the child's room
    B. May be with the child while anesthesia is given
    C. Are allowed to go with the child as far as the operating room entrance
    D. May stay with the child during surgery

33. A person stays in a recovery room for 1 to 2 hours after surgery or until
    A. Vital signs are stable
    B. Respiratory function is good
    C. The person can respond and call for needed help
    D. All of the above

34. When you prepare a room for a person to return from surgery
    A. You make a closed bed.
    B. The bed is in the lowest position.
    C. The bed is in the highest position.
    D. You make an open bed.

35. You may be assigned to take the vital signs after surgery. They are usually measured
    A. Once a shift
    B. Every 15 minutes for the first hour
    C. Every 2 hours
    D. Every 5 minutes for the first hour

36. When positioning a person postoperatively, the head may be turned to the side to
    A. Prevent aspiration if vomiting occurs.
    B. Make breathing easier.
    C. Make the person more comfortable.
    D. All of the above are correct.

37. Coughing and deep breathing exercises are done after surgery to
    A. Make the person more comfortable.
    B. Prevent pneumonia and atelectasis.
    C. Decrease pain and discomfort.
    D. Prevent nausea and vomiting.

38. Leg exercises are important to prevent
    A. Pneumonia and atelectasis
    B. Thrombus and embolus from forming
    C. Pain at the surgical site
    D. Low blood pressure

39. Elastic stockings help to
    A. Prevent swelling in the legs
    B. Prevent orthostatic hypotension
    C. Prevent thrombi
    D. Increase blood pressure

40. When applying elastic stockings, you should have the person
    A. Lie in a supine position.
    B. Sit in a chair.
    C. In a Fowler's position.
    D. First walk around the room for few minutes.

41. When applying elastic bandages
    A. Start at the proximal part of the extremity.
    B. Completely cover the fingers or toes.
    C. Apply the bandages very loosely.
    D. Expose the fingers and toes.

42. When you assist a person to walk after surgery, you should first measure the
    A. Person's temperature
    B. Blood pressure and pulse
    C. Distance from the bed to the door
    D. Person's weight

43. If a person is NPO after surgery, it is important for you to
   A. Offer frequent oral hygiene.
   B. Give ice chips frequently.
   C. Offer sips of cool water.
   D. Avoid mentioning anything about food or liquids.

44. Reporting the time and amount of the first voiding after surgery is important because the person must void
   A. Within 2 hours after surgery
   B. During the first 24 hours after surgery
   C. Within 8 hours after surgery
   D. At least 1000 ml within the first 4 hours after surgery

45. You can help the person be comfortable post-operatively by
   A. Offering frequent oral care
   B. Changing the gown whenever it is wet or soiled
   C. Telling the nurse promptly when the person complains of pain
   D. All of the above

Fill in the Blanks

46. If a person has outpatient, 1-day, or ambulatory surgery, the person is admitted in the morning and ____________________.

47. Why is the following personal care given before surgery?

   A. Baths ____________________

   ____

   B. Removing makeup ____________________

   ____

   C. Hair care ____________________

   ____

   D. Oral hygiene ____________________

   ____

48. Some people do not like being seen without their dentures. How can you promote dignity and self-esteem when dentures must be removed before surgery?

   ____

   ____

49. When you are delegated a skin preparation, what is reported and recorded?

   A. ____________________

   B. ____________________

   C. ____________________

50. If you are delegated to give a douche what is the temperature of the solution?

   ____

   ____

51. What vital signs are recorded on the preoperative checklist?

   ____

   ____

52. After the preoperative drugs are given, the person is not allowed ____________________.

53. When a person returns to the room after surgery how often are vital signs usually measured?

   A. ____________________

   B. ____________________

   C. ____________________

   D. ____________________

54. You may be able to turn a person who has had surgery by yourself when the person's condition ____________________.

55. Why are older people at risk for respiratory complications?

A. ______________________________

B. ______________________________

C. ______________________________

56. Leg exercises are done at least every

______________________________.

These exercises are done ____________ times.

57. Leg exercises are

A. ______________________________

B. ______________________________

C. ______________________________

D. ______________________________

58. When you apply elastic stockings you avoid twist because they can ______________________________.

Creases and wrinkles can cause

______________________________.

59. When you apply elastic bandages, what observations are reported and recorded?

A. ______________________________

B. ______________________________

C. ______________________________

D. ______________________________

E. ______________________________

F. ______________________________

G. ______________________________

60. Early ambulation prevents

A. ______________________________

B. ______________________________

C. ______________________________

D. ______________________________

E. ______________________________

Labeling

61. Color in the area on the figure that needs a skin preparation for the surgery listed.

A. Breast surgery

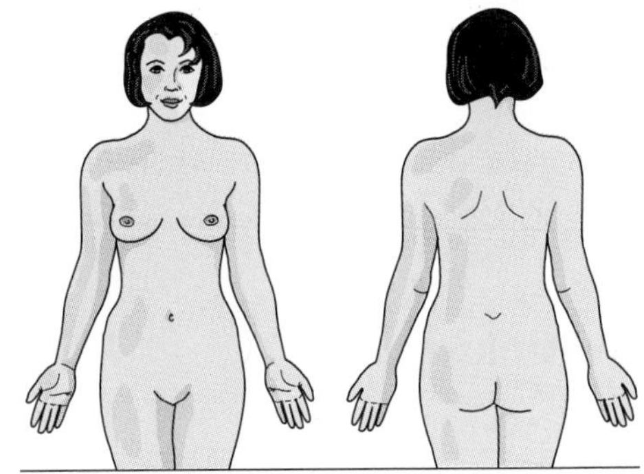

B. Cervical spine surgery

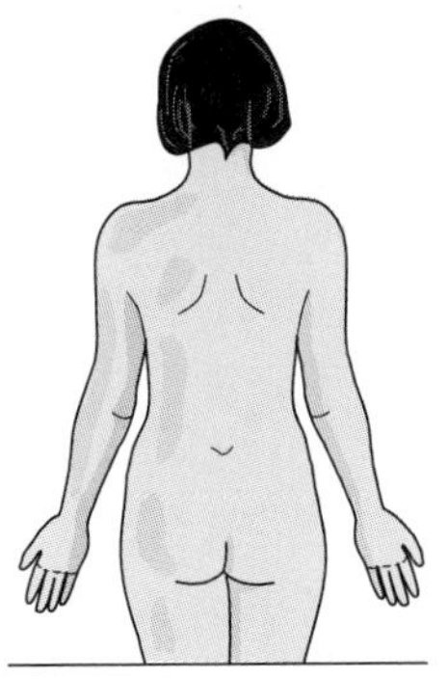

C. Knee surgery

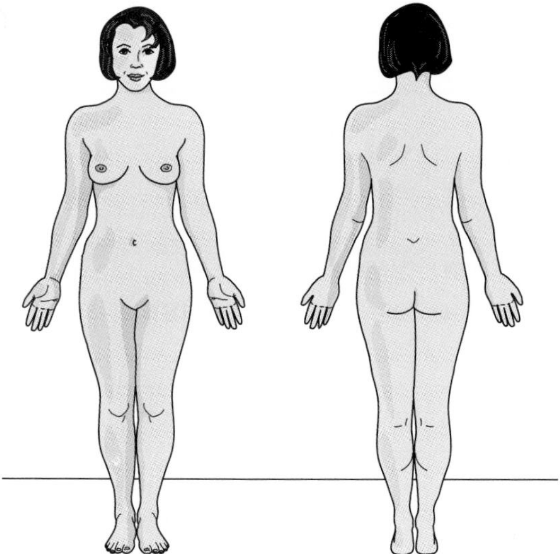

D. Abdominal and leg surgery

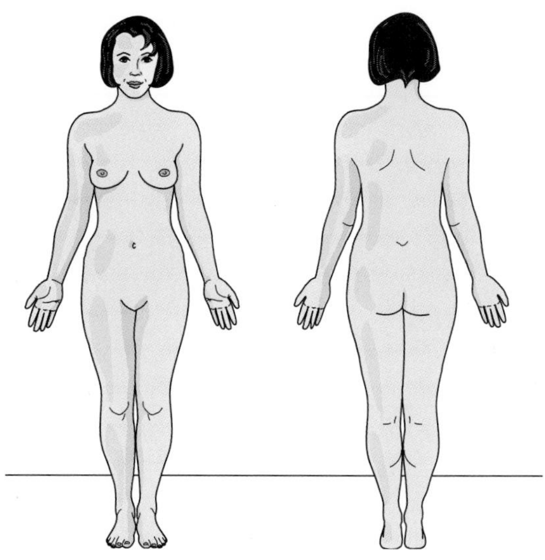

62. A preoperative checklist is completed before a person is sent to surgery. Mark the steps that a nursing assistant can do and report to the nurse.

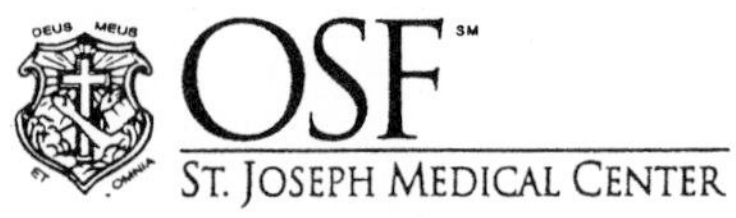

2200 E. Washington Street, Bloomington, Illinois 61701
Phone (309) 662-3311

PRE-OPERATIVE CHECKLIST

DATE OF SURGERY: ______________________

CHART PREPARATION	ADEQUATE INITIAL HERE	NOT ADEQUATE INITIAL HERE AND EXPLAIN
1. HISTORY AND PHYSICAL ON CHART HT. ______ WT. ______		
2. SURGICAL CONSENT ON CHART, SIGNED		
3. CONSENT FOR ADM BLOOD/BLOOD PROD.		
4. PREGNANCY TEST OBTAINED WHEN INDICATED		
5. URINALYSIS REPORT ON CHART		
6. BLOOD WORK TYPE ______		
7. TYPE AND CROSSMATCH		
8. CHEST X-RAY REPORT ON CHART		
9. EKG REPORT ON CHART READ ______		
10. KNOWN ALLERGIES AND SENSITIVITIES NOTED ON CHART		
11. KNOWN EXPOSURE AND/OR ALLERGY TO **LATEX** NOTED ON CHART		

PATIENT PREPARATION	ADEQUATE INITIAL HERE	NOT ADEQUATE INITIAL HERE AND EXPLAIN
12. FAMILY NOTIFIED OF SURGERY NAME ______ DATE/TIME ______		
13. PATIENT IDENTIFICATION ON WRIST		
14. ALL PROSTHESIS REMOVED (INCLUDING DENTURES, WIGS, HAIRPINS, CONTACT LENSES, COSMETICS, NAIL POLISH, ARTIFICIAL EYES, LIMBS, ETC.)		
15. ALL JEWELRY REMOVED		
16. CLOTHING REMOVED EXCEPT HOSPITAL GOWN WITH TIES		
17. SURGICAL PREP DONE		
18. TIME OF LAST MEAL OR FLUIDS ______ TIME		
19. PRE-OP TPR AND BP: T______ P______ R______ BP______		
20. VOIDED TIME ______ OR FOLEY		
21. PRE-OP IV AND/OR ANTIBIOTIC: TIME:		

	DRUG	DOSAGE	ROUTE
PREOPERATIVE MEDICATION GIVEN,			

TIME ______ GIVEN BY ______

☐ SIDE RAILS UP

READY FOR O.R. DATE ______ TIME ______ SIGNATURE ______

PATIENT IDENTIFIED BY TRANSPORTER AND STAFF NURSE TIME ______

FLOOR NURSE SIGNATURE ______ OR TRANSPORTER SIGNATURE ______ OR NURSE SIGNATURE ______

IDENTIFICATION OF INITIALS

INITIALS	SIGNATURE	INITIALS	SIGNATURE

Crossword Puzzle

Fill in the crossword puzzle by answering the clues with words from this list.

anesthetist
atelectasis
CBC
cyanosis
distal
electrocardiogram
hypoxia
PACU
PAR
prostheses
proximal
urinalysis

Across

1. Test done to detect cardiac problems
5. Lack of oxygen
8. Lower part of an extremity
9. Complete blood count
10. Post anesthesia room
11. Laboratory test of the urine
12. RN with advances study to give anesthesia

Down

2. Collapse of a portion of the lung
3. Bluish color of lips or nails
4. Upper part of an extremity
6. Artificial body parts such as eyeglasses, artificial eyes, hearing aids, and artificial limbs
7. Postanesthesia care unit

Optional Learning Exercises

Mr. Shafer is an 82-year-old man who was admitted for knee replacement surgery. Answer the questions about Mr. Shafer and his preoperative care.

63. This surgery is done by choice and is an

    ________________ surgery.

64. When you are in the room, you listen quietly while Mr. Shafer talks about his fears and concerns. By sitting quietly, and showing concern for his feelings, you can assist in Mr. Shafer's

    ________________ care.

65. The nurse comes to Mr. Shafer's room. What kind of preoperative teaching will be given to him?

    A. ________________

    B. ________________

    C. ________________

    D. ________________

    E. ________________

    F. ________________

    G. ________________

    H. ________________

    I. ________________

    J. ________________

66. The nurse tells you she will give Mr. Shafer his preoperative drugs in 10 minutes. What should you do?

    ____

Mrs. Johnson is a 70-year-old woman who is scheduled for abdominal surgery. Answer the questions about her care.

67. The nurse delegates a female nursing assistant to give Mrs. Johnson a vaginal douche. What information does the nursing assistant need?

    A. ________________

    B. ________________

    C. ________________

    D. ________________

    E. ________________

68. After the douche is completed, what information should be reported and recorded?

    A. ________________

    B. ________________

    C. ________________

    D. ________________

    E. ________________

69. The nurse tells you that she is busy and asks you to have Mrs. Johnson sign the operative permit. What should you do?

    ____

    ____

70. Mrs. Johnson returns to her room 2 hours after the surgery is completed. You know she is returned to her room when

    A. ________________

    B. ________________

    C. ________________

71. How is the room prepared for Mrs. Johnson's return?

    A. ________________

    B. ________________

    C. ________________

    D. ________________

    E. ________________

72. When Mrs. Johnson returns to her room, she has sequential compression devices (SCD) on her legs. What is the purpose of SCD?

____

____

73. You are caring for Mrs. Johnson 3 days after her surgery, and she tells you that she has not had a bowel movement since before surgery. You know that one reason for constipation can be drugs given for _____________________.

Independent Learning Activities

- Answer the following questions about a person's experience with surgery. If you have had surgery, use your own experience. If you have not had surgery, ask a family member or friend who has surgery to answer the questions.
  - What type of surgery did you have—elective, urgent, or emergency?
  - What information were you given before surgery? Who gave you the information? If you did not understand the information, how well were your questions answered?
  - What preparations were needed before surgery—skin prep, enemas, and so forth? Who explained the procedures needed? How did you feel about having these done?
  - What fears did you have about the surgery? How did you express these feelings to others? How did the person respond to your concerns?
  - How much pain did you have after surgery? How was it treated? Did you get relief from the medications and care?

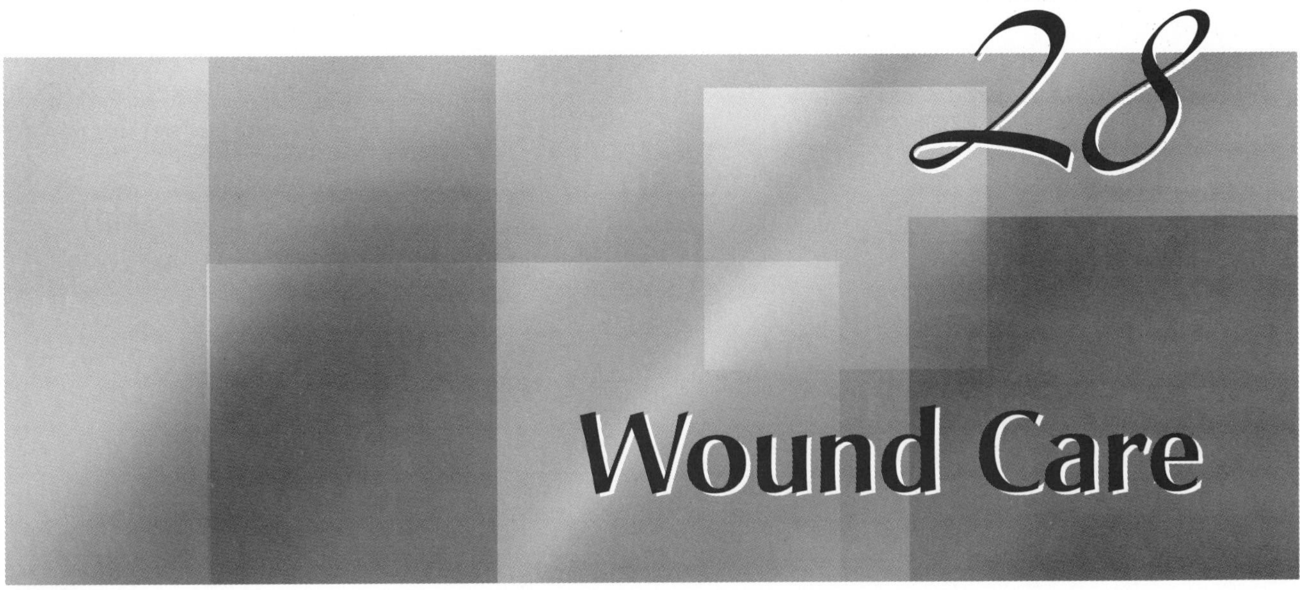

28 Wound Care

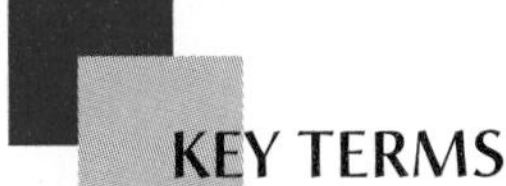

KEY TERMS

Abrasion
Arterial ulcer
Bedsore
Chronic wound
Circulatory ulcer
Clean wound
Clean-contaminated wound
Closed wound
Contaminated wound
Contusion
Decubitus ulcer
Dehiscence
Dirty wound
Epidermal stripping
Evisceration
Full-thickness wound
Gangrene
Hematoma
Hemorrhage
Incision
Infected wound
Intentional wound
Laceration
Open wound
Partial-thickness wound
Penetrating wound
Pressure sore
Pressure ulcer
Puncture wound
Purulent drainage
Sanguineous drainage
Serosanguineous drainage
Serous drainage
Shock
Skin tear
Stasis ulcer
Trauma
Unintentional wound
Vascular ulcer
Venous ulcer
Wound

Fill in the Blanks: Key Terms

1. A ______________________________ is a break or rip in the skin that separates the epidermis from underlying tissue.
2. An open wound with clean, straight edges, usually made intentionally with a sharp instrument is an ______________________________.
3. ______________________ is another name for a pressure ulcer, pressure sore, or decubitus ulcer.
4. A wound in which tissues are injured but the skin is not broken is a ______________________________.
5. ______________________________ is thick green, yellow, or brown drainage.
6. A wound in which the dermis and epidermis of the skin are broken is called a ______________________________.

7. A ______________________________ is a break in the skin or mucous membrane.

8. A wound that is not infected and microbes have not entered the wound is a ______________________________.

9. An ______________________________ is a partial-thickness wound caused by the scraping away or rubbing of the skin.

10. Another name for a pressure ulcer, pressure sore, or bedsore is a ______________________________.

11. Thin, watery drainage that is tinged with blood is called ______________________________.

12. An ______________________________ is a wound that contains large amounts of bacteria and shows signs of infection. This type of wound is also called a dirty wound.

13. A vascular wound or a ______________________________ is an open wound on the lower legs and feet caused by a decrease in blood flow through arteries and veins.

14. Removing the epidermis as tape is removed from the skin is called ______________________________.

15. A ______________________________ is a collection of blood under the skin and tissues.

16. A wound with a high risk of infection is a ______________________________.

17. A condition in which there is death of tissue is ______________________________.

18. Any injury caused by unrelieved pressure is a ______________________________ or a decubitus ulcer, bedsore, or pressure sore.

19. A ______________________________ is an open wound with torn tissues and jagged edges.

20. A wound resulting from trauma is an ______________________________.

21. An ______________________________ is an open wound on the lower legs and feet caused by poor arterial blood flow.

22. Clear, watery fluid is ______________________________.

23. The excessive loss of blood in a short time is ______________________________.

24. A ______________________________ is also called a bedsore, decubitus ulcer, or a pressure ulcer.

25 An infected wound is a ______________________________.

26. A wound occurring from the surgical entry of the urinary, reproductive, respiratory, gastrointestinal system is a ______________________________.

27. A ______________________________ is a wound that does not heal easily.

28. A stasis ulcer is also called a ______________________________.

29. An open wound made by a sharp object is a ______________________________. The entry of the skin and underlying tissues may be intentional or unintentional.

30. A wound created for therapy is an

______________________________.

31. A ______________________________ is an open wound in which the skin and underlying tissues are pierced.

32. ______________________________ is the separation of wound layers.

33. A circulatory ulcer is also called a

______________________________.

34. ______________________________ is a condition that results when blood supply to organs and tissues is insufficient.

35. A ______________________________ occurs when the dermis, epidermis, and subcutaneous tissue are penetrated. Muscle and bone may be involved.

36. An accident or violent act that injuries the skin, mucous membranes, bones, and internal organs is called ______________________________.

37. The separation of the wound along with the protrusion of abdominal organs is

______________________________.

38. A ______________________________ is an open wound on the lower legs and feet caused by poor blood return through the veins. It is also called a venous ulcer.

39. Bloody drainage is called

______________________________.

40. A closed wound caused by a blow to the body is a ______________________________.

41. An ______________________________ occurs when the skin or mucous membrane is broken.

Circle the BEST Answer

42. Wounds are
    A. Any break in the skin or mucous membranes
    B. Only made as the result of trauma
    C. Only caused by surgical incisions
    D. Always open breaks in the skin

43. Mrs. Seymour complains that her elbow hurts from pushing herself up in bed. When you inspect her elbow, you find some of the skin is rubbed away. You would report this to the nurse as a(an)
    A. Laceration
    B. Abrasion
    C. Contusion
    D. Incision

44. Mr. Telford catches his arm on a chair. When you look at his arm, the tissue is torn with jagged edges. You report this injury to the nurse and tell her Mr. Telford has a
    A. Puncture wound
    B. Abrasion
    C. Penetrating wound
    D. Laceration

45. Which of these would *not* place a person at risk for skin tears?
    A. The person is older.
    B. The person requires complete help in moving.
    C. A lift sheet is not used to move the person.
    D. The person is alert and oriented.

46. A person is at great risk for pressure ulcers because of
    A. Chronic disease
    B. Dry skin
    C. Good fluid balance
    D. Being obese or very thin

47. A pressure ulcer occurs because
    A. The person is restless and moves about in the bed or chair.
    B. Too much fluid in taken in the diet.
    C. Unrelieved pressure occurs between hard surfaces.
    D. The person is repositioned too frequently.

48. Epidermal stripping can cause occur in newborns especially because
    A. Babies at this age are immobile.
    B. The skin is very fragile.
    C. They have circulatory problems.
    D. They have problems sensing pain or pressure.

49. The first sign of a pressure ulcer in an area would be
    A. Reddened skin
    B. Swelling in the area
    C. A break in the skin
    D. Exposed tissue and some drainage from the area

50. Mrs. Greene keeps sliding down in bed. The nurse tells you raise the head of the bed no more than 30 degrees. This position will help prevent tissue damage caused by
    A. Pressure over hard surfaces
    B. Shearing
    C. Poor body mechanics
    D. Poor fluid balance

51. Pressure ulcers can occur
    A. Over bony areas such as the hips
    B. Underneath the breasts
    C. Between abdominal folds
    D. All of the above

52. When following a repositioning schedule, the person should be repositioned
    A. According to the schedule in the person's care plan
    B. Every 2 hours
    C. Every 15 minutes
    D. As often as you have time

53. One way to prevent friction in the bed is to
    A. Use soap when cleansing the skin.
    B. Rub or massage reddened areas.
    C. Use pillows and blankets to prevent skin from being in contact with skin.
    D. Apply a thin layer of cornstarch to the bottom sheet.

54. Bed cradles are used to
    A. Position the person in good body alignment.
    B. Prevent pressure on the legs and feet.
    C. Keep the heels off the bed.
    D. Distribute body weight evenly.

55. When the person is using an eggcrate-like mattress, it is covered with a special cover and
    A. Only a bottom sheet
    B. A bottom sheet and a waterproof pad
    C. A bottom sheet and a draw sheet
    D. Several layers of waterproof materials, a lift pad, and a bottom sheet

56. Circulatory ulcers of the feet and legs are caused by
    A. Poorly fitted shoes
    B. Decreased blood flow to and from the legs and feet
    C. Increased activity
    D. Increased fluid intake

57. A measure to prevent stasis ulcers is
    A. Use elastic or rubber band type garters to hold the person's socks in place.
    B. Keep the person's legs crossed while sitting in a chair.
    C. Apply elastic stockings or elastic bandages to legs according to the care plan.
    D. Rub the feet and legs thoroughly when bathing drying.

58. When caring for a person at risk for arterial ulcers, you should do all of the following *except*
    A. Remind the person to sit with the legs uncrossed.
    B. Assist the person to apply garters to hold up socks or hose.
    C. Make sure the shoes fit well.
    D. Encourage the person to stop smoking.

59. When a person is at risk for arterial ulcers the nursing assistant may be delegated to all of the following *except*
    A. Make sure shoes fit well.
    B. Clean and dry between the toes.
    C. Use elastic or rubber type of garters to hold socks in place.
    D. Keep pressure off heels and other bony areas with pillows.

60. During wound healing, what phase is happening when the wound is approximately 1 year of age?
    A. Initial phase
    B. Inflammatory phase
    C. Maturation phase
    D. Proliferative phase

61. A wound that is closed by bringing the wound edges together with sutures, staples, or adhesive strips is a type of wound healing called
 A. Primary-intention healing
 B. Secondary-intention healing
 C. Tertiary-intention healing
 D. Delayed-intention healing

62. Good nutrition will help wound healing because
 A. It prevents infection.
 B. Protein is needed for tissue growth and repair.
 C. It increases circulation.
 D. Pathogens will grow and multiply.

63. A sign of internal bleeding would be
 A. Bloody drainage
 B. Pooling of blood under a body part
 C. A hematoma
 D. Dressings soaked with blood

64. Which of the following symptoms is *not* a sign of shock?
 A. Pulse that is rapid and weak
 B. Skin that is warm and dry to touch
 C. Blood pressure that falls
 D. Respirations that are rapid

65. If a person tells you a wound is painful and tender, it may mean the person has
 A. Internal bleeding
 B. Shock
 C. An infection
 D. Dehiscence

66. The nurse tells you to make sure Mrs. Reynolds supports her abdominal wound when she coughs. The nurse wants this done to protect against
 A. Secondary intention healing
 B. Infection
 C. Scarring
 D. Dehiscence

67. When you are caring for Mrs. Reynolds, you notice thin, watery drainage from her wound that is blood-tinged. When you report your observations, you would tell the nurse that the wound has ______________________ drainage.
 A. Purulent
 B. Serosanguineous
 C. Serous
 D. Sanguineous

68. Which of the following methods used in wound care will prevent microbes from entering a draining wound?
 A. Wet-to-dry dressings
 B. Hemovac suction
 C. A Penrose drain
 D. Nonadherent gauze

69. Wound dressings are used to for all of the following *except*
 A. Prevent drainage
 B. Remove dead tissue
 C. Cover unsightly wounds
 D. Provide a moist environment for wound healing

70. When wet-to-dry dressings are used, they
 A. Are removed when dry
 B. Are kept moist
 C. Allow air to reach the wound, but fluids and bacteria cannot
 D. Do not stick to the wound

71. Plastic and paper tape may be used to secure a dressing
 A. Because they allow movement of the body part
 B. When the dressing must be changed frequently
 C. If the person is allergic to adhesive tape
 D. Because they stick well to the skin

72. If you are changing a dressing and the person has Montgomery ties, you should
 A. Replace the cloth ties each time to change the dressing.
 B. Replace the adhesive strips only when they are soiled.
 C. Replace the adhesive strips each time you change the dressing.
 D. Apply tape to hold the dressing in place.

73. If you are delegated to apply a dressing, make sure that you know
 A. What kind of medication the person receives
 B. The person's diagnosis
 C. When pain medication was given and how long until it takes effect
 D. What activity the person is allowed

74. You can make the person more comfortable when changing a dressing by doing all of the following *except*
 A. Control your nonverbal communication when looking at the wound.
 B. Remove the tape and dressing gently.
 C. Encourage the person to look at the wound.
 D. Make sure the person does not see the soiled side of the dressing when it is removed.

75. When you are assigned to change dressings, you should
    A. Follow Standard Precautions and the Bloodborne Pathogen Standard.
    B. Use sterile technique.
    C. Wear gloves only to remove old dressings.
    D. Use one pair of gloves throughout the dressing change.

76. A binder may be used when the person has a dressing to
    A. Prevent infection
    B. Prevent drainage
    C. Promote circulation
    D. Prevent bleeding

77. Which of these measures will *not* help to meet the person's basic needs?
    A. Tell the person that the wound looks fine and that he or she should not be upset.
    B. Encourage the person to eat well so that the body can heal better.
    C. Remove any soiled dressings from the room as soon as possible.
    D. Allow pain medications to take effect before giving wound care.

Matching

Match the type of wound with the description

78. ______ A wound created for therapy

79. ______ The dermis and epidermis of the skin are broken

80. ______ Unintentional wound or the result of break in surgical asepsis

81. ______ Caused by a bruise, twist, or sprain

82. ______ Wound that does not heal easily such as a pressure sore

83. ______ Surgical entry into body systems that are not sterile and contain normal flora

84. ______ Contains large amounts of bacteria and shows signs of infection

85. ______ Microbes have not entered the wound

86. ______ Involves muscle and bone as well as the dermis, epidermis and subcutaneous tissue

A. Chronic
B. Clean
C. Clean-contaminated
D. Closed
E. Contaminated
F. Full thickness
G. Infected (dirty)
H. Intentional
I. Partial-thickness

Fill in the Blanks

87. You can cause a skin tear when moving, repositioning, and transferring by holding on to a person's arm or leg ______________________.

88. Friction can cause a skin tear and it becomes a portal of entry for ______________________.

89. Name the stage of pressure ulcer described in each of the following

    A. The skin is gone, and underlying tissues are exposed.

    ____

    B. The skin is red. The color does not return to normal when the skin is relieved of pressure.

    ____

    C. Muscle and bone are exposed and damaged. Drainage is likely.

    ____

    D. The skin cracks, blisters, or peels.

    ____

90. You can help to prevent shearing by raising the head of the bed only ______________________.

91. Remind the person sitting in a chair to shift position every ______________________ to decrease pressure on ______________________.

92. Explain how these protective devices help to prevent pressure ulcers.

    A. Bed cradle prevents pressure on

    ______________________.

    B. Elbow protectors prevent ______________ between ______________________.

    C. Heel elevators raise

    ______________________.

    D. Eggcrate-like mattress distributes

    ______________________.

    E. Special beds allow person to ______________________ on the mattress so body weight is ______________________. Little pressure occurs on

    ______________________.

93. If you are caring for a person with poor circulation. When you check the person's legs and feet, you should report ______________________

    ______________________.

94. What two diseases are common causes of arterial ulcers?

    A. ______________________

    B. ______________________

95. The inflammatory phase of wound healing last about ______________________.

    A. During this phase, the blood brings

    ______________________.

    B. Signs and symptoms of

    ______________________ appear.

96. The proliferative phase lasts

    ______________________.

    The tissue cells multiply to

    ______________________.

97. The maturation phase can last up to

_______________ years.

During this phase, the scar gains

_______________ and becomes

_______________.

98. With primary intention healing the wound edges are held together with

_______________.

99. Secondary intention healing is used for

____

wounds. Because healing takes longer the threat of _______________ is great.

100. When you check a person for external bleeding check under a body part for

_______________.

101. If a person shows signs of hemorrhage or shock you should _______________.

102. Surgical emergencies that can occur are

A. _______________

B. _______________

C. If these occur, you must

_______________.

103. When you observe a wound, what would you report about the appearance?

A. _______________

B. _______________

C. _______________

D. _______________

104. Name the type of wound drainage described.

A. Thick green, yellow, or brown

____

B. Bright or darker bloody drainage

____

C. Clear, watery fluid

____

D. Thin, watery drainage that is blood-tinged

____

105. Wound drainage is measured by

A. Noting _______________

B. Weighing _______________

C. Measuring _______________

106. A transparent adhesive film dressing allows

_______________ to reach wound.

107. When wet-to-dry dressings are removed, what else is removed?

____

108. When taping a dressing in place, the tape should not encircle the entire body part because

_______________.

109. When delegated to apply dressings, list what observations should be reported and recorded.

A. ______________________

B. ______________________

C. ______________________

D. ______________________

E. ______________________

F. ______________________

G. ______________________

H. ______________________

I. ______________________

Labeling

Answer questions 110 and 111 using the following illustration.

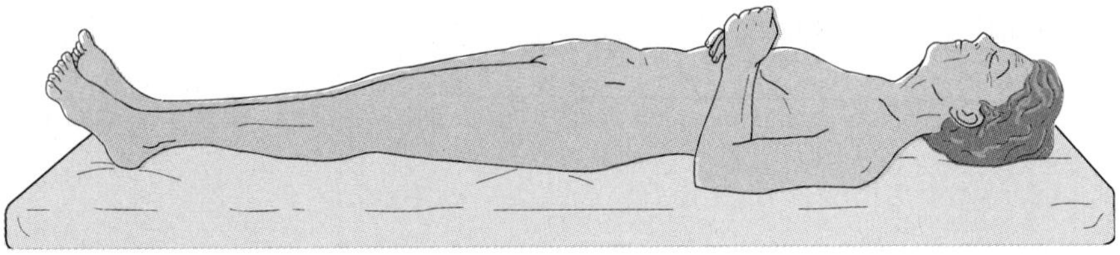

110. Name this position ______________________

111. Place an "X" on each of the five pressure points. Name the bony point for each one.

A. ______________________

B. ______________________

C. ______________________

D. ______________________

E. ______________________

Answer questions 112 and 113 using the following illustration.

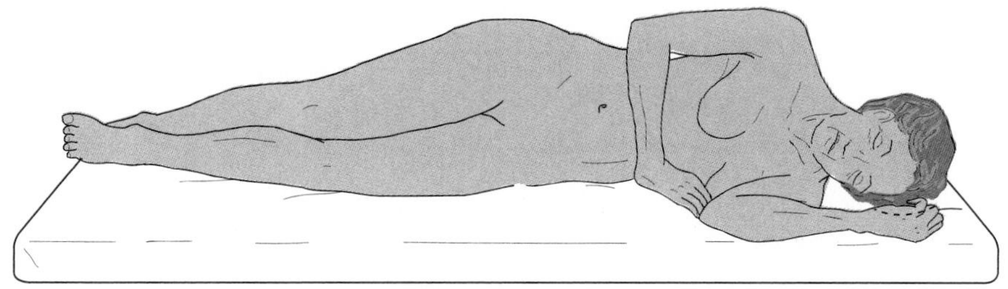

112. Name this position ______________________________

113. Place an "X" on the seven pressure points. Name the bony point(s) for each one.

A. ______________________________

B. ______________________________

C. ______________________________

D. ______________________________

E. ______________________________

F. ______________________________

G. ______________________________

Answer questions 114 and 115 using the following illustration.

114. Name this position ______________________________

115. Place an "X" on the six pressure points. Name the bony point for each one.

A. ______________________________

B. ______________________________

C. ______________________________

D. ______________________________

E. ______________________________

F. ______________________________

Answer questions 116 and 117 using the following illustration.

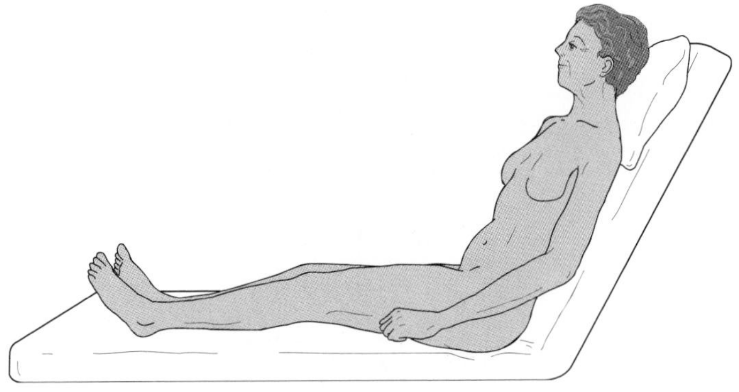

116. Name this position ______________________________

117. Place an "X" on the three pressure points. Name the bony point for each one.

   A. ______________________________

   B. ______________________________

   C. ______________________________

Answer questions 118 and 119 using the following illustration.

118. Name the position ______________________________

119. Place an "X" on the five pressure points. Name the bony point for each one.

   A. ______________________________

   B. ______________________________

   C. ______________________________

   D. ______________________________

   E. ______________________________

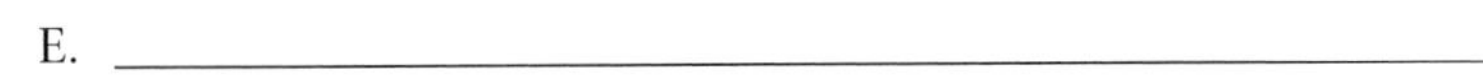

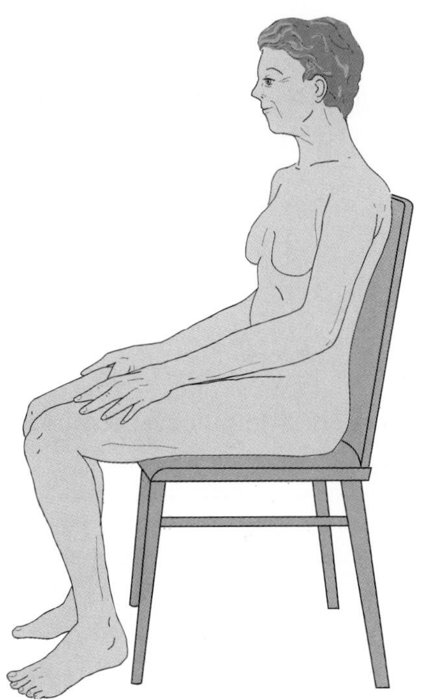

Crossword Puzzle

Fill in the crossword puzzle by answering the clues with words from this list.

adhesive	hemovac	proliferate
eggcrate	incontinence	serum
epidermis	infection	shearing
gauze	montgomery	sutures
hemoglobin	penrose	

Across

2. Tape that sticks well, but can irritate skin
7. Closed drainage system that removes drainage from a wound with suction
8. Rubber tube that drains onto a dressing from a wound
10. Top layer of skin
12. Disease state resulting from the invasion and growth of microorganisms in the body
13. Multiply rapidly
14. Stitches used to close a wound

Down

1. Consists of adhesive strips and cloth ties; designed to hold dressing in place (ties)
3. Substance in red blood cells that carries oxygen to body tissues
4. Clear, thin, fluid portion of the blood
5. Loss of control of bladder or bowels
6. Type of dressing absorbs moisture; comes in rolls, squares, rectangles, and pads
9. Mattress made with peaks of foam in mattress to distribute person's weight
11. Occurs when skin sticks to a surface and deeper tissues move downward

Nursing Assistant Skills Video Exercise

View the **Preventing and Treating Pressure Ulcers** *video to answer the following questions.*

120. What are the basic principles of preventing and treating pressure ulcers?

A. ______________________________

B. ______________________________

C. ______________________________

D. ______________________________

121. What stage of a pressure ulcer is the most serious? ______________________________.

Describe this stage.

______________________________.

122. When tissue is squeezed between two hard surfaces, oxygen and nutrients cannot get to the tissue and so the tissue ____________________.

123. Name four pressure sites in obese individuals.

____

____

____

____

124. If skin is dry you may apply ______________________________ but do not ______________________________.

Optional Learning Exercises

You are assigned to care for Mrs. Stevens. She is 87 years of age and has diabetes and high blood pressure. She walks with difficulty, and spends most of her day sitting in her chair. She is somewhat overweight and tells you that she had a knee replacement 5 years ago and had phlebitis after surgery. The nurse tells you to watch carefully for signs of circulatory ulcers.

125. What risk factors does Mrs. Stevens have that place her at risk for circulatory ulcers?

A. ______________________________

B. ______________________________

C. ______________________________

D. ______________________________

E. ______________________________

F. ______________________________

G. ______________________________

126. What signs and symptoms may be present if Mrs. Stevens has stasis ulcers?

____

____

127. If arterial ulcers develop, they are usually found

______________________________.

Mr. Hawkins, age 74, was in an automobile accident and has a wound on his leg that is large and open. The wound has become infected, and he is being treated with antibiotics. When you are talking with him, he tells you he has smoked for 55 years and has poor circulation in his legs. He lives alone and generally eats takeout foods or eats cereal when he is at home.

128. Why is he receiving antibiotics?

____

____

129. What factors would increase Mr. Hawkins risk for complications?

A. ______________________

B. ______________________

C. ______________________

D. ______________________

130. What is missing in Mr. Hawkins diet that is needed to help in healing the wound?

____

____

You are assisting the nurse with wound care. She is changing dressings for two different persons. Mrs. Henderson has a wound that has a large of amount of drainage. Mr. Wendel has a drain in his wound that is attached to suction.

131. Why does the nurse weigh Mrs. Henderson's new dressings before applying them to the wound and the old dressings when they are removed?

____

____

132. How does she find out the amount of drainage from Mr. Wendel's wound?

____

____

133. What other ways can be used to measure drainage?

A. ______________________

B. ______________________

C. ______________________

D. ______________________

E. ______________________

F. ______________________

134. When you are changing a nonsterile dressing, why do you need two pairs of gloves?

____

____

135. When a wound is infected and has poor circulation, the wound may be left open at first and then closed later. This type of wound healing is called healing through ______________. This type of healing combines ______________________ and ______________ intention healing.

Independent Learning Activities

- Take turns with a classmate and carry out the following exercises. These exercises will help you understand how a person who cannot move without help feels when pressure is unrelieved. NOTE: These exercises work best if the person wears thin clothes so the discomfort is more noticeable.
- Place a pencil or similar hard object on the seat of a chair and have a classmate sit on the object for 10 minutes. Keep time and remind the person not to move in order to make it more uncomfortable. Remember, people who are at risk for pressure ulcers are often unable to change position without assistance.
- Position a classmate in bed, making sure the bedclothes are wrinkled to form lumps under bony pressure points. (For example, place a wrinkle under the sacrum in the supine position, or under the hip or shoulders in the lateral position.)
- Answer these questions about the exercises done.
  - How long did it *seem* when you were waiting for 10 minutes to pass?
  - How many times did you begin to reposition yourself without thinking about it?
  - How did the pressure areas feel when you completed the 10 minutes? What color was the area?
  - How will this exercise affect your care of persons who cannot move?

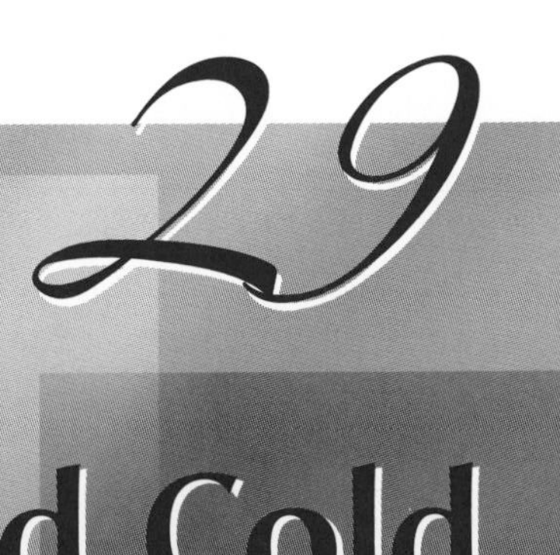

Heat and Cold Applications

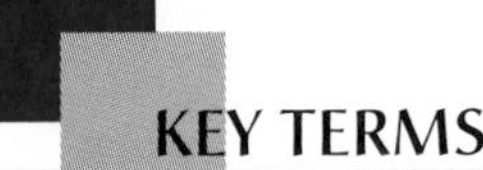

KEY TERMS

Compress
Constrict
Cyanosis
Dilate
Hyperthermia
Hypothermia Pack
Pack

Fill in the Blanks: Key Terms

1. A body temperature that is much higher than the person's normal range is ______________________.
2. ______________________ means to narrow.
3. A treatment that involves wrapping a body part with a wet or dry application is a ______________________.
4. A ______________________ is a soft pad applied over a body area.
5. ______________________ means to expand or open wider.
6. ______________________ occurs when the body temperature is very low.
7. Bluish skin color is ______________________.

Circle the BEST Answer

8. All of these are *true* about heat and cold applications *except*
   A. Heat and cold applications promote healing and comfort.
   B. Risk and complications can happen when heat and cold applications are used.
   C. Heat and cold applications have the same effects on the body.
   D. Heat and cold applications reduce tissue swelling.
9. Before you apply heat and cold applications, it is important to know whether
   A. A nurse is available to answer questions and to supervise you.
   B. Your state allows you to perform the procedure.
   C. The procedure is in your job description.
   D. All of the above statements are true.

10. When heat applications are applied at the correct temperature and for the correct time
    A. The blood vessels in the area dilate.
    B. The blood vessels in the area constrict.
    C. The skin looks pale.
    D. The person complains of pain.

11. Heat is not applied to a pregnant woman's abdomen because
    A. It may cause nausea and vomiting.
    B. The heat can affect fetal growth.
    C. She has difficulty sensing heat or pain.
    D. There are changes in the circulatory and nervous systems during pregnancy.

12. When heat is applied too long, a complication that occurs is
    A. Blood vessels dilate.
    B. Blood flow increases.
    C. Blood vessels constrict.
    D. More nutrients reach the area.

13. Why would an older person have a risk for burns with heat applications?
    A. Blood vessels dilate more easily.
    B. Heat penetrates the tissue more quickly.
    C. Skin is often thin and fragile.
    D. The nervous system reacts to the heat more quickly.

14. Moist heat applications have cooler temperatures than dry heat applications because
    A. Dry heat penetrates more deeply.
    B. Dry heat cannot cause burns.
    C. Heat penetrates deeper with a moist application.
    D. Moist heat stays at the desired temperature longer.

15. The care plan states that the person receives a heat application of 110° F. As a nursing assistant, you know that you should
    A. Measure the temperature carefully before applying to the person.
    B. Never apply an application that is above 106° F.
    C. Ask the person if the application is too warm.
    D. Apply the application, and remind the person not to remove the application.

16. When a hot or cold application is in place, you should check the area
    A. Every 15 to 20 minutes
    B. Every 5 minutes
    C. About every 30 minutes
    D. Once an hour

17. Heat and cold applications are applied for no longer than
    A. 1 hour
    B. 30 minutes
    C. 15 to 20 minutes
    D. 4 hours

18. When hot compresses are in place, you may apply an aquathermia pad over the compress to
    A. Keep the compress wet.
    B. Protect the area from injury.
    C. Measure the temperature of the compress.
    D. Maintain the correct temperature of the compress.

19. A hot soak is applied
    A. By putting the body part into water
    B. By applying a soft pad to a body part
    C. With a plastic wrap and bath towel as covers
    D. Only until the water temperature cools down

20. A sitz bath is given to a person with
    A. Muscle strains
    B. Rectal or female pelvic surgery
    C. A small area that needs a heat application
    D. An area that needs a cold application

21. When giving a sitz bath
    A. Pad the part of the tub in contact with the person.
    B. Observe for signs of weakness, faintness, or fatigue.
    C. Prevent the person from chills and burns.
    D. All of the above statements are true.

22. Hot packs may be heated by all of these methods *except*
    A. Boiling in water for a few minutes
    B. Squeezing, kneading or striking the pack
    C. Sterilizing in an autoclave
    D. Warming in a microwave oven

23. When you use an aquathermia pad
    A. The pad temperature will cool off after about 20 to 30 minutes.
    B. The temperature is maintained by the flow of water through the pad.
    C. You are applying a form of moist heat.
    D. You do not need to check the person as often as with other heat applications.

24. An aquathermia pad is placed
    A. Under the body part
    B. Directly against the skin
    C. In a flannel cover, towel, or pillowcase to insulate the pad
    D. On the body part and secured with pins

25. When a cold application is applied, the numbing effect helps to
    A. Reduce or relieve pain in the part
    B. Constrict blood vessels
    C. Decrease blood flow
    D. Cool the body part

26. Complications of cold applications include
    A. Burns and blisters
    B. Cyanosis
    C. Pain
    D. All of the above

27. Which of these cold applications is moist?
    A. Ice bag
    B. Cold compress
    C. Ice collar
    D. Ice glove

28. If the cover of a cold application becomes moist, you should
    A. Discard the cold pack, and get a new one.
    B. Leave it in place, and check the person more often.
    C. Remove the wet covering, and apply a dry cover.
    D. Remove it at once, and report this to the nurse.

29. When you need an ice bag in a home setting, you may use
    A. A disposable ice pack
    B. A bag of frozen peas or corn
    C. A plastic bag filled with ice
    D. All of the above

30. When cold applications are in place, which of these should be reported at once to the nurse?
    A. Slightly reddened skin
    B. Shivering
    C. Decrease in swelling of the part
    D. Decrease in pain at the site

31. When a person has hyperthermia, ice packs are applied to all of these areas *except* the
    A. Abdomen
    B. Head
    C. Underarms
    D. Groin

32. When hyperthermia or hypothermia has occurred, it is important to check often for changes in
    A. Vital signs
    B. Level of consciousness
    C. Skin temperature
    D. Complaints of pain

Fill in the Blanks

33. What are the effects of heat applications?

    A. ______________________________

    B. ______________________________

    C. ______________________________

    D. ______________________________

    E. ______________________________

34. When you are caring for a confused person and heat or cold is applied, how can you know whether they are in pain?

    ____

    ____

35. Fragile skin makes a person at risk for burns. Those with fragile skin include

    A. ______________________________

    B. ______________________________

    C. ______________________________

36. What are the advantages of dry heat applications?

    A. ______________________________

    B. ______________________________

37. When you are asked to apply heat or cold, what observations should be reported and recorded?

    A. ______________________________

    B. ______________________________

    C. ______________________________

    D. ______________________________

    E. ______________________________

    F. ______________________________

    G. ______________________________

38. What two methods can be used to keep a hot compress warm?

   A. ______________________________

   B. ______________________________

39. When the nurse asks you to prepare a warm soak, what is the temperature range that is correct?

   ____

40. When you are giving a sitz bath, what should you do if the person has a rapid pulse?

   ____

41. An aquathermia pad is used for

   ______________________________ heat.

42. When using an aquathermia pad, you should make sure the hoses do not have kinks or air bubbles to allow the water to

   ______________________________.

43. An aquathermia pad is usually set at what temperature?

   ______________________________ ° F

44. Name uses for cold applications.

   A. ______________________________

   B. ______________________________

   C. ______________________________

   D. ______________________________

   E. ______________________________

45. When you prepare an ice bag, collar, or glove, remove the excess air by

   ______________________________.

46. When a cold compress is in place, it usually needs to be changed every 5 minutes because it

   ______________________________.

47. When using a warming or cooling blanket with infants and children, what should be reported at once to the nurse?

   A. ______________________________

   B. ______________________________

Optional Learning Exercises

Your daughter, Sarah, age 3, falls and twists her ankle while out playing. You take her to the emergency room and are told to apply cold dry applications for the first day and then to apply heat as needed. Use the information you learned in this chapter to answer these questions about carrying out this treatment.

48. What are two purposes of the cold application for Sarah's injury?

   A. ______________________________

   B. ______________________________

49. The emergency room gives you a disposable ice pack to use. When it cools, what items in your home can be used to apply cold to the area?

   A. ______________________________

   B. ______________________________

50. How will you protect Sarah's skin?

   ____

51. How often do you check the application?

   ____

52. What signs and symptoms would indicate a complication of cold application?

   A. ______________________________

   B. ______________________________

   C. ______________________________

53. The cold application should stay in place for

   __________ minutes.

54. What happens if you leave a cold application in place too long?

____

____

55. After the first day, you apply heat to Sarah's ankle. This will

A. _______________________ is increased.

B. Tissues have more _______________________.

C. Excess fluid is _______________________.

56. At Sarah's age, you know she is at special risk for

_______________________________________.

Independent Learning Exercises

Role-play this situation with a classmate. One of you should act as the person, and one should act as the nursing assistant. Work together to answer the questions for each role.

Mr. Chavez is 45 years old and has a reddened area on his left calf. The doctor has ordered moist warm compresses to the area, and the nurse has delegated this task to you.

As the Nursing Assistant
- What questions would you ask the nurse before applying the compresses?
- What temperature range is used for this compress?
- How did you check the temperature of the compresses?
- How did you keep the compresses at the correct temperature?
- How often did you check the compress? What did you observe when you checked the area?

As Mr. Chavez
- How was the treatment explained to you?
- How were you positioned? How did the nursing assistant check to see whether you were comfortable?
- How did the compress feel? Was the temperature maintained? How?
- How often was the compress checked?

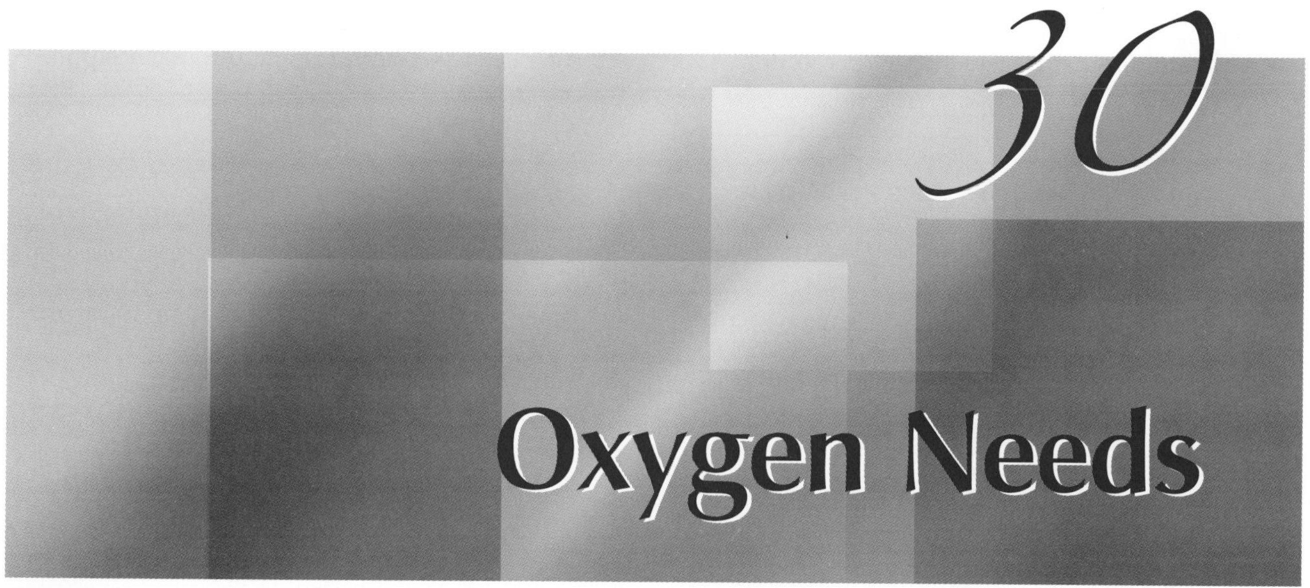

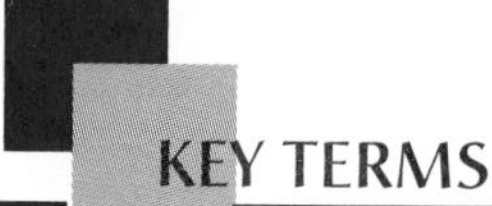

KEY TERMS

Allergy
Apnea
Biot's respirations
Bradypnea
Cheyne-Stokes
Dyspnea
Hemoptysis
Hemothorax
Hyperventilation
Hypoventilation
Hypoxemia
Hypoxia
Intubation
Kussmaul's respirations
Mechanical ventilation
Orthopnea
Orthopneic position
Oxygen concentration
Pleural effusion
Pneumothorax
Pollutant
Respiratory arrest
Respiratory depression
Tachypnea
Suction

Fill in the Blanks: Key Terms

1. ________________________ are rapid and deep respirations followed by 10 to 30 seconds of apnea.
2. Bloody sputum is called ________________________.
3. ________________________ is inserting an artificial airway.
4. Air in the pleural space is ________________________.
5. Rapid breathing where respirations are usually greater than 24 per minute is called ________________________.
6. An ________________________ is a sensitivity to a substance that causes the body to react with signs and symptoms.
7. Difficult, labored, or painful breathing is ________________________.
8. ________________________ is blood in the pleural space.
9. Being able to breathe deeply and comfortably only while sitting or standing is ________________________.

10. Respirations that are less than 12 per minute is slow breathing or ______________________________.

11. A reduced amount of oxygen in the blood is ______________________________.

12. ______________________________ describes slow, weak respirations that occur at a rate of fewer than 12 per minute.

13. The lack or absence of breathing is ______________________________.

14. ______________________________ is a pattern of respirations that are rapid and deeper than normal.

15. Using a machine to move air into and out of the lungs is ______________________________.

16. A harmful chemical or substance in the air or water is a ______________________________.

17. The process of withdrawing or sucking up fluid is ______________________________.

18. ______________________________ are respirations that gradually increase in rate and depth and then become shallow and slow. Breathing may stop for 10 to 20 seconds.

19. The ______________________________ is sitting up and leaning forward over a table.

20. The escape and collection of fluid in the pleural space is ______________________________.

21. ______________________________ occurs when breathing stops.

22. Very deep and rapid respirations that occur in diabetic coma is called ______________________________.

23. ______________________________ is the amount of hemoglobin that contains oxygen.

24. Cells that do not have enough oxygen have ______________________________.

25. ______________________________ occurs when respirations are slow, shallow, and sometimes irregular.

Circle the BEST Answer

26. Oxygen and carbon dioxide are exchanged in the
    A. Alveoli
    B. Larynx
    C. Trachea
    D. Bronchioles

27. Oxygen needs increase when the person
    A. Is older
    B. Is taking any drugs
    C. Has fever or pain
    D. Has good nutrition

28. Respiratory depression can occur when the person
    A. Exercises
    B. Has allergies
    C. Is taking narcotic drugs in large doses
    D. Smokes

29. Restlessness is an early sign of
    A. Hypoxia
    B. Apnea
    C. Hyperventilation
    D. Bradypnea

30. Signs of hypoxia should be reported at once because
    A. The person is in pain.
    B. Hypoxia is life threatening.
    C. It may cause pneumonia.
    D. The person may have chronic obstructive pulmonary disease (COPD).

31. An abnormal breathing pattern that is common when death is near is
    A. Kussmaul's respirations
    B. Biot's respirations
    C. Cheyne-Stokes respirations
    D. Tachypnea

32. When you prepare a person for a chest x-ray, you should
    A. Make sure the person does not eat for several hours before the test.
    B. Help the person to remove all clothing and jewelry from the neck to the waist.
    C. Tell the person not to drink any fluids before the x-ray.
    D. All of the above statements are true.

33. When a person has had a bronchoscopy, he or she is to receive nothing by mouth (NPO) until
    A. Complaints of nausea and vomiting are gone.
    B. The person wakes up.
    C. The gag and swallow reflex returns.
    D. The person tells you he or she is hungry.

34. You are caring for a person who just had a pulmonary function test performed. You would expect the person to
    A. Report chest pain
    B. Be very tired
    C. Have hemoptysis
    D. Complain of nausea and vomiting

35. If a pulse oximeter is being used, which of these sites would be best?
    A. A toe in the foot that is swollen
    B. A finger with a fake nail
    C. A toe with an open wound
    D. An earlobe

36. When you are delegated to place a pulse oximeter on a person, you should report to the nurse if
    A. The person is sleeping.
    B. The person's pulse does not equal the pulse on the display.
    C. You remove nail polish from the nail on the site used.
    D. You tape the oximeter in place.

37. When a person has breathing difficulties, breathing is usually easier when the person is
    A. In the supine position
    B. Lying on one side for long periods
    C. In the semi-Fowler's or Fowler's position
    D. In the prone position

38. Coughing and deep-breathing exercises
    A. Help prevent pneumonia and atelectasis
    B. Decrease pain after surgery or injury
    C. Are performed once a day
    D. Causes mucus to form in the lungs

39. If you are assisting a child with coughing and deep-breathing exercises, you might find it useful to use
    A. An incentive spirometer
    B. A mechanical ventilator
    C. Paper blowouts, horns, or pinwheels
    D. A pulse oximeter

40. When assisting with coughing and deep breathing, you should ask the person to
    A. Take deep breaths through the mouth.
    B. Hold the breath for 30 seconds.
    C. Exhale slowly through pursed lips.
    D. Repeat the exercise one or two times.

41. When a person uses an incentive spirometer, it allows the person to
    A. Take shallow breaths
    B. See air movement when inhaling
    C. See air movement when exhaling
    D. Exhale quickly

42. If a person is receiving oxygen, you may
    A. Set the flow rate.
    B. Start and maintain the therapy.
    C. Set up the system.
    D. All of the above statements are true.

43. If you are caring for a person with oxygen therapy, you may *not*
    A. Start and maintain oxygen therapy.
    B. Remove the mask for meals.
    C. Tell the nurse if the rate is too high or too low.
    D. Check for irritation from the device.

44. If a person receives oxygen through a nasal cannula, it is important to look for irritation
    A. On the nose, ears, and cheekbones
    B. Under the mask
    C. In the throat
    D. All of the above

45. If a person receives oxygen with a mask, the mask may be removed
    A. At bedtime
    B. For eating
    C. When the person is walking around
    D. When the person is talking

46. If you are asked to set up for oxygen administration, you will do all of these *except*
    A. Collect the device with connecting tubing.
    B. Attach the flow meter to the wall outlet or tank.
    C. Apply the oxygen administration device to the person.
    D. Fill the humidifier with distilled water.

47. When you care for a person receiving oxygen, you should know the oxygen flow rate. You should get this information from the
    A. Doctor
    B. Nurse and care plan
    C. Respiratory therapist
    D. Chart

48. If the oxygen administration setup has a humidifier, you should report if
    A. The container is half full of water.
    B. The humidifier is bubbling.
    C. The humidifier is not bubbling.
    D. Moisture collects under the mask.

49. Which of these would *not* be a sign of hypoxia?
    A. Disorientation and confusion
    B. Decrease in pulse rate and respirations
    C. Apprehension and anxiety
    D. Cyanosis of the skin, mucous membranes, and nail beds

50. When oxygen is in use, remove alcohol, nail polish remover, oils, and greases from the room because they
    A. Can ignite easily
    B. Make breathing more difficult
    C. Cause static electricity
    D. Make the oxygen less effective

51. If you are caring for a person with an artificial airway, your care should always include
    A. Removing the device to clean it
    B. Comforting and reassuring the person that the airway helps breathing
    C. Suctioning to maintain the airway
    D. Ensuring the person never takes a tub bath

52. When you are caring for a person who has an artificial airway, tell the nurse at once if the
    A. Person needs frequent oral hygiene.
    B. Person feels as if he or she is gagging
    C. Person cannot speak.
    D. Airway comes out or is dislodged.

53. When a person has a tracheostomy, the stoma is
    A. Uncovered when the person is outdoors
    B. Covered with plastic to prevent air from entering
    C. Covered when shaving
    D. Covered with a loose gauze dressing.

54. If you are caring for a child with a tracheostomy, you would tell the nurse if
    A. The child is crying.
    B. You can slide your finger under the ties that hold the tracheostomy in place.
    C. You cannot slide your finger under the ties that hold the tracheostomy in place.
    D. The child is sleeping in a supine position.

55. If you are caring for a person with a mechanical ventilator and the alarm sounds, you should first
    A. Get the nurse.
    B. Reset the alarms.
    C. Reassure the person.
    D. Check to see whether the person's tube is attached to the ventilator.

56. To avoid upsetting the person or family when a mechanical ventilator is being used
    A. Avoid eye contact.
    B. Work quietly, and do not talk to the person.
    C. Watch what you say and do when around the person and the family.
    D. Stay out of the room as much as possible.

57. If a person has chest tubes, Petrolatum gauze is kept at the bedside to
    A. Cover the insertion site if a chest tube comes out.
    B. Lubricate the site of the chest tube.
    C. Cleanse the skin around the chest tube.
    D. Apply to any open areas that occur.

Fill in the Blanks

58. As a person ages, the risk of pneumonia increases because
    A. Respiratory muscles ____________________
    B. Strength for ____________________

59. Smoking causes two diseases that affect oxygen needs. They are
    A. ____________________
    B. ____________________

60. Body positions that can be signs of altered respiratory function are
    A. ____________________
    B. ____________________

61. When a person used these body positions, the abnormal breathing pattern used is called ______________________.

62. Adults normally have ______________ respirations per minute. If the person has tachypnea, the respirations are ______________ per minute.

63. After a thoracentesis is done, the person is often checked for these respiratory signs and symptoms.

A. ______________

B. ______________

C. ______________

D. ______________

E. ______________

F. ______________

G. ______________

64. A pulse oximeter measures ______________________.

65. The normal range for this measurement is ______________________.

66. When recording the results of a pulse oximeter, you use SpO_2. This means

A. S = ______________

B. p = ______________

C. O_2= ______________

67. The pulse oximeter alarm sounds if

A. ______________

B. ______________

C. ______________

68. Coughing and deep-breathing exercises help prevent atelectasis, which is the ______________________.

69. If you are assisting a person with coughing and deep-breathing exercises, how can you help the person support the incision?

A. ______________

B. ______________

70. What is the goal of using an incentive spirometer?

____

This goal is met by

A. Air moves ______________

B. Secretions ______________

C. O_2 and CO_2 ______________

71. Oxygen needs to be humidified because it is a ______________ and dries the airway's ______________.

72. If you are asked to set up for oxygen administration, what information do you need from the nurse?

A. ______________

B. ______________

C. ______________

73. When you are caring for a person who is suctioned, immediately tell the nurse if these occur

A. ______________

B. ______________

C. ______________

D. ______________

74. When would you check the person's pulse, respirations, and pulse oximeter when assisting the nurse with suctioning?

____

75. If a person has mechanical ventilation, where do you find a plan for communication?

____

76. Why is it important for everyone to use the same signals for communication?

____

Crossword Puzzle

Fill in the crossword puzzle by answering the clues with words from this list.

ABG
bronchoscopy
COPD
hypoxemia
oxygen
pneumonia
RBC
spirometer
sputum
thoracentesis

Across

1. A test during which a scope is passed into the trachea and bronchi
3. Amount of oxygen in the blood that is less than normal
6. Mucus from the respiratory system
7. Procedure during which air or fluid is removed from the pleural sac
8. Machine that measures the amount of air inhaled
10. Chronic obstructive pulmonary disease

Down

2. Gas with no taste, odor, or color that is necessary for life
4. Inflammation of the lung
5. Arterial blood gases
9. Red blood cells

Optional Learning Exercises

You are caring for Mr. Reynolds, age 84 years old, who has COPD. Answer these questions about caring for Mr. Reynolds.

77. What position would make it easier for Mr. Reynolds to breathe when he is in bed?

____

78. When Mr. Reynolds is sitting up in a chair or on the side of the bed, what can you do to make him more comfortable?

____

Mrs. Fagan is receiving oxygen through a nasal cannula at 2 liters per minute. Her respirations are unlabored at 16 per minute, unless she is walking around or performing personal care activities, during which her respirations are 28 per minute and difficult. Answer these questions about her care.

79. Why is there no humidifier with the oxygen setup for Mrs. Fagan?

____

80. Where should you check for signs of irritation from the cannula?

A. _______________________________________

B. _______________________________________

C. _______________________________________

81. What are the abnormal respirations that Mrs. Fagan has with activity called?

____

Independent Learning Activities

Work with a classmate, and carry out these exercises. They will help you to understand how it feels to a person with breathing problems.

- Have your partner count your respirations while you are at rest. Then exercise by running or jogging in place for at least 2 minutes. Now have your partner check your respirations again. How have they changed? What is the rate, rhythm, or pattern? Are your respirations easy or labored?
- While you exercise, first try to breathe only through your nose. Then try breathing through your mouth. Which way makes you feel you are getting enough air?
- Place a drinking straw in your mouth and close your lips tightly around it. Now breathe only through the straw while at rest and during exercise. When you are at rest, how comfortable does this feel? Are you getting enough air? How is your air supply during exercise?
- Take a drinking straw, and place small pieces of paper in one end so that it is fairly tight. Now try breathing through the straw at rest and exercise. What is the difference between the open and blocked straw? Imagine if every breath you take feels like it does with the blocked straw. This is how many people with breathing problems feel all the time.

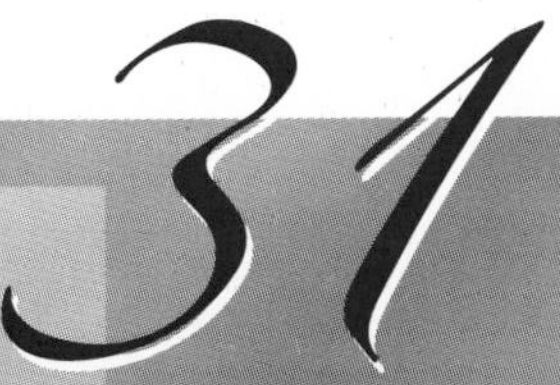

31 Rehabilitation and Restorative Care

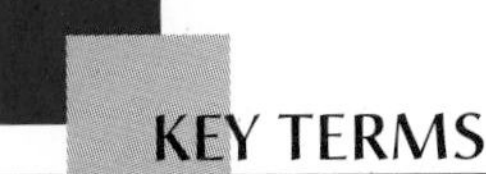

KEY TERMS

Activities of daily living
Disability
Prosthesis
Rehabilitation
Restorative aide
Restorative nursing care

Fill in the Blanks: Key Terms

1. A nursing assistant with special training in restorative nursing and rehabilitation skills is a ________________.

2. ________________ are those self-care activities performed daily to remain independent and to function in society.

3. An artificial replacement for a missing body part is a ________________.

4. Care that helps persons regain their health, strength, and independence is ________________.

5. A ________________ is any lost, absent, or impaired physical or mental function.

6. The process of restoring the disabled person to the highest possible level of physical, psychological, social, and economic functioning is ________________.

Circle the BEST Answer

7. The focus of rehabilitation is to
   A. Improve the person's abilities.
   B. Restore function to normal.
   C. Help the person regain health and strength.
   D. Prevent injury.

8. Restorative nursing helps the person regain
   A. Self-care, elimination, and positioning abilities
   B. Mobility, communication, and cognitive functions
   C. Health, strength, and independence
   D. All previous abilities

9. If you are a restorative aide, it means you have
   A. Taken special training in restorative nursing and rehabilitation skills
   B. Taken the required training for restorative aides
   C. Passed a special test to show you can perform these duties
   D. Earned the most seniority at the facility

10. When assisting with rehabilitation and restorative care, it is important to
   A. Give complete care to prevent exertion by the person.
   B. Make sure you do everything for the person.
   C. Encourage the person to perform ADL to the extent possible.
   D. Complete care quickly.

11. Which of these would be most helpful for a person receiving rehabilitative care?
   A. Give the person pity or sympathy when tasks are difficult.
   B. Remind the person not to try new skills or those that are difficult.
   C. Give praise when even a little progress is made.
   D. Encourage the person to perform ADL quickly.

12. When do rehabilitation services begin?
   A. When the person seeks health care
   B. After discharge from the hospital
   C. Only when ordered by the doctor
   D. When the person returns home

13. Complications can be prevented by
   A. Good alignment, turning and repositioning, and range-of-motion exercises
   B. Prolonged bed rest
   C. Incontinence
   D. Prolonged illnesses

14. Self-help devices help meet the goal of
   A. Recovery of all normal abilities
   B. Self-care
   C. Living alone
   D. Dependence on others

15. When dysphagia occurs after a stroke, a person may need
   A. Exercises to improve swallowing
   B. A gastrostomy tube
   C. A dysphagia diet
   D. All of the above

16. The care plan for a person in rehabilitation gives information to meet only
   A. Physical care needs
   B. ADL
   C. Physical, psychological, and social needs
   D. Psychological and social needs

17. The rehabilitation team meets to discuss the person's progress
   A. Every 9 days
   B. As often as needed to change the rehabilitation plan
   C. Every week
   D. Only when requested by the family or person

18. The rehabilitation team assesses the person's home to
   A. Make sure the person will be safe
   B. Determine whether the person will be able to move around in the home
   C. Recommend changes that are needed
   D. All of the above

19. OBRA requires that nursing centers
   A. Have a full-time physical therapist
   B. Provide services required by the person's comprehensive care plan
   C. Provide physical care only
   D. Employ full-time occupational and speech therapists

20. You can promote quality of life and encourage personal choice by
   A. Protecting the person from unkind remarks
   B. Letting the person decide when a bath is given
   C. Keeping the door closed when the person relearns new skills
   D. Asking the nurse to suggest ways to help control your feelings

Fill in the Blanks

21. Rehabilitation and restorative nursing programs do the following

   A. ______________________________

   B. ______________________________

22. Restorative nursing involves measures that promote

    A. ______________________

    B. ______________________

    C. ______________________

    D. ______________________

    E. ______________________

    F. ______________________

23. Rehabilitation takes longer in which age group?

    ____

    What are reasons for this?

    A. Chronic ______________________

    B. Risk ______________________

    C. Programs are ______________________

24. If a child has a disability from birth defects,

    normal ______________________ and

    ______________________ may be affected.

25. ADL include

    A. ______________________

    B. ______________________

    C. ______________________

    D. ______________________

    E. ______________________

    F. ______________________

26. If a person has difficulty feeding himself or herself, what eating devices can be used?

    A. ______________________

    B. ______________________

    C. ______________________

27. The goal for a prosthesis to is

    A. ______________________

    B. ______________________

28. When you are assisting with rehabilitation and restorative care, why should you practice the task that the person must perform?

    ____

    ____

29. When assisting with rehabilitation and restorative care, what complications can be prevented if you report early signs and symptoms?

    A. ______________________

    B. ______________________

    C. ______________________

Optional Learning Exercises

Mrs. Mercer is 82 years old. She is a resident in a rehabilitation unit because she had a stroke that has caused weakness on her right side. She is right-handed and needs to learn to use several self-help devices as she relearns ways to carry out ADL. She often becomes angry or depressed. Answer these questions about Mrs. Mercer and her care.

30. Mrs. Mercer is having difficulty with controlling urinary and bowel elimination. What would be the goal of her care for these problems?

    ____

    ____

    Her plan of care would include programs for

    ______________________ and

    ______________________.

31. Why does Mrs. Mercer need help at mealtime

    and to brush her teeth?

    ____

32. Mrs. Mercer needs help to get in and out of bed. When helping her to transfer, you remember to position the chair on her _________________________ side.

33. When Mrs. Mercer becomes discouraged because progress is slow, how can you help her? You can stress _________________________ and focus on _________________________.

Independent Learning Activities

Role-play the following situation with a classmate. Answer the questions about how you felt when you played Mrs. Leeds to understand how a person with a disability feels. Use your nondominant hand to attempt the activities she must do.

- Mary Leeds is 62 years old and had a stroke last month. She has weakness on her dominant side and has been admitted to a rehabilitation unit to relearn ADL. She is practicing eating by using a spoon to place fluids and food in her mouth. She is also learning to button clothing. How well could you hold the spoon with your nondominant hand?
  - What problems did you have controlling the spoon?
  - How rapidly could you eat? What type of food was easier to eat?
  - How well were you able to button your clothing? What techniques did you find that made you more successful?
  - How did this experience make you feel? How will it affect the way you interact with persons who have similar disabilities?

- With your instructor's permission, borrow a wheelchair from your school to use for 1 to 2 hours. Have a classmate push you around in the chair in a grocery store, mall, or school. You must stay in the chair for the entire time to experience the feelings of a person who must use a wheelchair. Use a handicap-equipped bathroom during this experience.
  - How comfortable was the wheelchair? Did you use any special padding or cushion in the seat?
  - What difficulties were encountered while moving around? While going through doorways?

- When encountering steps? While going down aisles? While moving through crowds? How did you deal with these difficulties?
  - How accessible was the handicap-equipped bathroom? How much room was available for you to transfer from the wheelchair to the toilet?
  - How did other people treat you? How many spoke to you? How many talked to your classmate and avoided you?
  - How did this experience make you feel? How will it affect the way you interact with a person in a wheelchair?

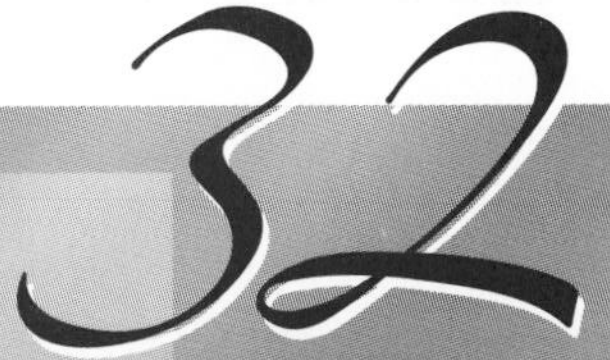

Hearing and Vision Problems

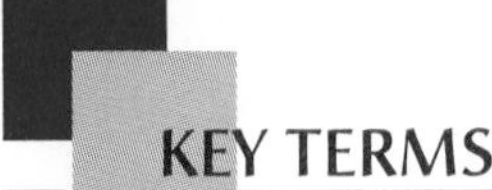

KEY TERMS

Braille
Cerumen
Deafness
Hearing loss
Tinnitus
Vertigo

Fill in the Blanks: Key Terms

1. Another name for earwax is

 ______________________________.

2. ____________________ is a writing system that uses raised dots for each letter of the alphabet.

3. When a person has difficulty hearing normal conversations, it is called a

 ______________________________.

4. Dizziness is called ____________________.

5. Hearing loss in which it is impossible for the person to understand speech through hearing alone is called ____________________.

6. ______________________________ is ringing in the ears.

Circle the BEST Answer

7. When an infant has otitis media, the baby may
 A. Have diarrhea
 B. Pull at the ears
 C. Roll the head from side to side
 D. All of the above

8. If a person has chronic otitis media, the person may develop
 A. Vertigo
 B. Permanent hearing loss
 C. Diarrhea
 D. Nausea and vomiting

9. If you are caring for a person who has Ménière disease, it is important to
 A. Prevent falls.
 B. Assist the person to move quickly.
 C. Keep the lights in the room very bright.
 D. Encourage the person to be active.

10. When you are caring for a person with a hearing loss, which of these would *not* help communication?
    A. Gain the person's attention by lightly touching the person's arm.
    B. Speak as loudly as possible.
    C. Do not cover your mouth or eat while talking.
    D. Use gestures and facial expressions to give useful clues.

11. A person with a hearing loss may
    A. Give wrong answers or responses.
    B. Think others are talking about them.
    C. Shun social events to avoid embarrassment.
    D. All of the above statements are true.

12. If an infant has hearing loss, the baby often
    A. Speaks in a very soft voice
    B. Avoids playing with other children
    C. Fails to start talking
    D. Becomes suspicious of others

13. When you are caring for a person with a hearing aid, check with the nurse before
    A. Turning the hearing aid off at night
    B. Inserting a new battery if needed
    C. Washing a hearing aid
    D. Removing the battery at night

14. When a person has glaucoma, he or she may have difficulty seeing objects
    A. That are far away
    B. To the right or left of the person
    C. Directly in front of the person
    D. That are bright colors

15. Cataracts are most commonly caused by
    A. Aging
    B. Injury
    C. Increased pressure in the eye
    D. Surgery

16. Report to the nurse if
    A. The person complains of eye pain or blurred vision.
    B. Glasses need to be cleaned.
    C. The person asks for equipment to clean contact lenses.
    D. The person asks for help to clean an artificial eye.

17. A person who is blind
    A. Is totally unable to see anything
    B. May sense some light but has no usable vision
    C. May have some usable vision but cannot read newsprint
    D. All of the above

18. When you enter the room of a blind person, you should first
    A. Touch the person to let him or her know you are there.
    B. Speak loudly to make sure the person knows you are there.
    C. Make sure the lights are bright.
    D. Identify yourself, and give your name, title, and reason for being there.

19. When a person is blind, you should avoid
    A. Rearranging furniture and equipment
    B. Using words such as "see," "look," or "read"
    C. Letting the person move about
    D. Letting the person perform self-care activities

20. When you assist a blind person to walk, it is best if you
    A. Walk slightly behind the person.
    B. Walk slightly ahead of the person.
    C. Grasp the person's arm firmly to guide him or her.
    D. Walk very slowly to allow the person to take small steps.

Fill in the Blanks

21. Otitis media is most common between the ages

    of ______________________________

    and ______________________________.

22. When a person has Ménière disease, attacks last

    ______________________________ or

    ______________________________.

23. With Ménière disease, the person should not

    walk alone in case

    ______________________________.

24. When age-related changes occur in the inner ear,

    it is harder for the person to hear

    ______________________________.

25. What are examples of noises that can cause hearing loss?

A. ______________________

B. ______________________

C. ______________________

D. ______________________

E. ______________________

26. When persons are 85 years of age or older, over ______________________ have a hearing loss.

27. Symptoms of hearing loss in children and adults include

A. ______________________

B. ______________________

C. ______________________

D. ______________________

E. ______________________

28. If a woman is speaking to a hearing-impaired person, why should she adjust the pitch of her voice?

____

29. Symptoms of glaucoma include

A. ______________________

B. ______________________

C. ______________________

30. The goal of treatment with glaucoma is to ______________________.

31. When you are caring for a person after cataract surgery, an eye shield is worn as directed and ______________________.

32. When cleaning plastic lenses in eyeglasses, it is important to use special cleaning solutions, tissues, and cloths because ______________________.

33. When caring for a person with an artificial eye, the eye socket is washed with ______________________.

34. The legally blind person sees at 20 feet what a person with normal vision sees at ______________________.

35. When you orient a person to the room, why do you let the person move around the room?

____

Labeling

36. Look at the sign language examples. What is the person telling you?

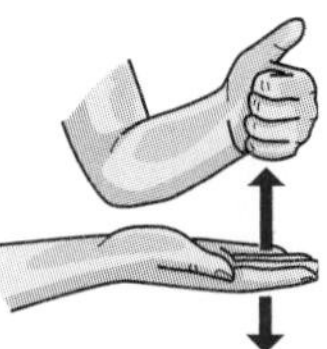

____

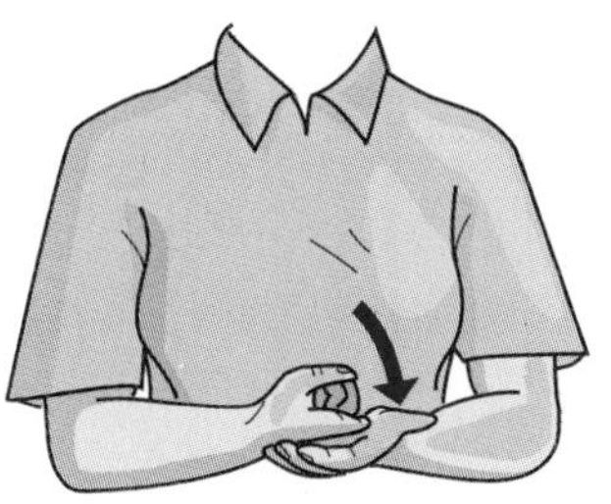

____

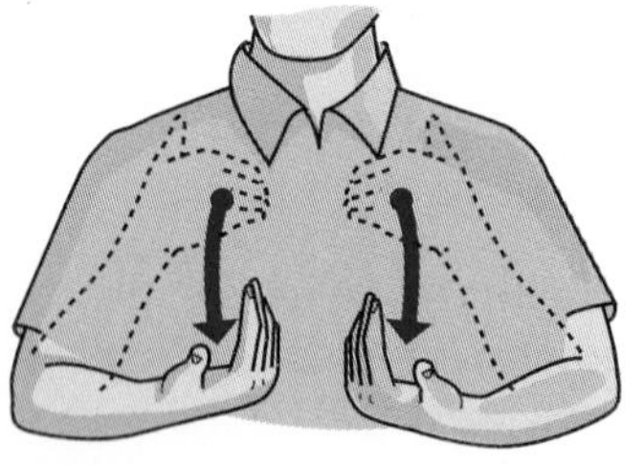

____

37. Look at the letters signed with the manual alphabet. What is the person telling you?

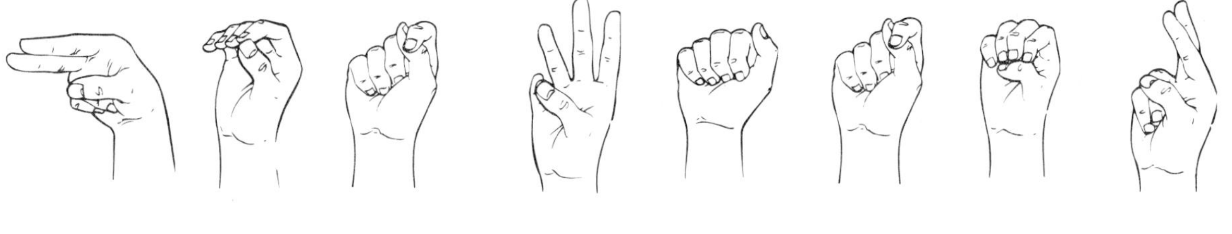

Crossword Puzzle

Fill in the crossword puzzle by answering the clues with words from this list.

cataract
choroid
cochlea
cornea
eardrum
glaucoma
incus
iris
lens
malleus
ossicles
pupil
retina
sclera
stapes

Across

1. Disorder in which fluid pressure increases in the eye and causes vision loss with eventual blindness.
3. Ossicle in the middle ear, which looks like a hammer.
7. Transparent part of the outer layer of the eye.
8. White of the eye.
9. Receptor for vision and the nerve fibers of the optic nerve are in this structure.
11. Second layer of the eye.
13. Ossicle in the middle ear, which is shaped like a stirrup.
14. Ossicle in the middle ear, which resembles an anvil.
15. Lies behind the pupil and reflects light to the retina.

Down

2. Part of the inner ear that looks like a snail shell.
4. Tympanic membrane in the ear.
5. Disorder in which the lens of the eye becomes cloudy. Vision blurs and dims.
6. Three small bones in the middle ear.
10. Opening in the middle of the iris that constricts and dilates.
12. Part of the choroid in the eye that gives the eye its color.

Optional Learning Exercises

Mr. Herman is an 85-year-old man with a hearing loss that has developed as he has gotten older. Answer these questions about his care.

38. Two nursing assistants are caring for Mr. Herman, a man and a woman. They notice that he answers questions asked by the male nursing assistant more quickly. What is the likely reason for this?

    ____

39. The nursing assistants have found that Mr. Herman is alert and oriented. They are surprised when Joan, another nursing assistant, tells them he is "senile." Why would Joan make this statement?

    ____

40. Mr. Herman says he is too tired to go to the gameroom for a party. He says no one likes him, and they talk about him. What are some reasons for his actions and statements?

    A. Tired because

    ____

    B. No one likes him

    ____

41. When giving care, the nursing assistant turns off the television and radio in Mr. Herman's room. Why is this done?

    ____

You are caring for Mrs. Sanchez, who is legally blind because of glaucoma. Answer the questions about her care.

42. When you enter the room, you notice that Mrs. Sanchez is looking at her mail with a magnifying glass. How is this possible since you thought she was blind?

    ____

43. When you enter the room, Mrs. Sanchez asks you to adjust the blinds. Why?

    ____

44. When you are helping Mrs. Sanchez to move around the room, you are careful not to leave her in the middle of the room. Why?

    ____

45. Mrs. Sanchez asks you to help her with her dinner tray. What can you do to help her?

    A. ______________________________

    B. ______________________________

Independent Learning Activities

- Cover your ears so that you cannot hear clearly. Use one of these methods or one that you have devised.
  - Commercial earplugs
  - Cotton plugs in ears
  - Cover ears with earmuffs or similar devices

- Keep your ears covered and hearing muffled for at least 1 hour as you go about your daily activities. A wise student will not wear earplugs during class time! Answer the following questions about the experience.
  - How did you find yourself compensating for the hearing loss? Did you turn up the television or radio? Ask others to write out information? Did you Stay away from others? Get angry or frustrated?
  - When you could not understand someone, what did you do? Did you ask him or her to repeat what was said? Ask him or her to speak louder? Did you answer even though you were unsure of what was said, or did you choose not to respond at all?
  - If you answered when unsure, what was your response? Did you tend to agree or disagree with the speaker? Why?
  - What methods listed in the chapter were helpful? What other methods did you use to understand what was being said? Watch the speaker? Cup your hand around ears?
  - How will this experience assist you when you care for a person with a hearing loss?

- Cover your eyes with a blindfold so you cannot see. Keep the blindfold on for at least 1 hour as you perform your normal activities. Have someone act as a guide during this time. In addition to your normal activities, include the activities listed. Answer the questions about the experience.
  - Go outside with your guide, and cross a street.
  - Visit a store or restaurant with your guide.
  - Eat a simple snack or meal.
  - Go to the toilet, wash your hands, and comb your hair.
  - Have your guide take you to a public area, place you in a chair or on a bench, and leave you alone for 5 to 10 minutes.

- You may wish to carry out this exercise using the blindfold and this alternate method. If you wear glasses, cover the lenses with a heavy coating of petroleum jelly. This will simulate the vision experienced by a person with cataracts. Answer the questions for both experiences.
  - How did you feel when you were unable to see what was going on around you? What noises or other sensory stimulants did you notice?
  - When you were crossing the street, how did you feel? Safe? Frightened?
  - When you were in a public area, what did you notice? How did you feel? How did others respond to you?
  - How comfortable were you about eating when you could not see the food? How were you able to locate the food? What problems did you have?
  - How did you manage in the bathroom? Were you able to find the equipment you needed? How competent did you feel about carrying out hand hygiene and grooming without seeing?
  - What were your feelings when left alone in a public area for 5 to 10 minutes? How much time seemed to pass before your guide returned? What concerns did you have? Safety? Fear of injury? Desertion?
  - How will both experiences help you when caring for a person with a vision loss?

- Have a group discussion with your classmates who have all carried out the exercises to simulate vision and hearing problems. Answer these questions.
  - Which disability did you find the most difficult to tolerate? Why?
  - If you had to live with one of these disabilities, which one would you choose? Why?
  - During these exercises, what happened that surprised you about being unable to see or hear? How does this discovery change your attitude about disabilities?

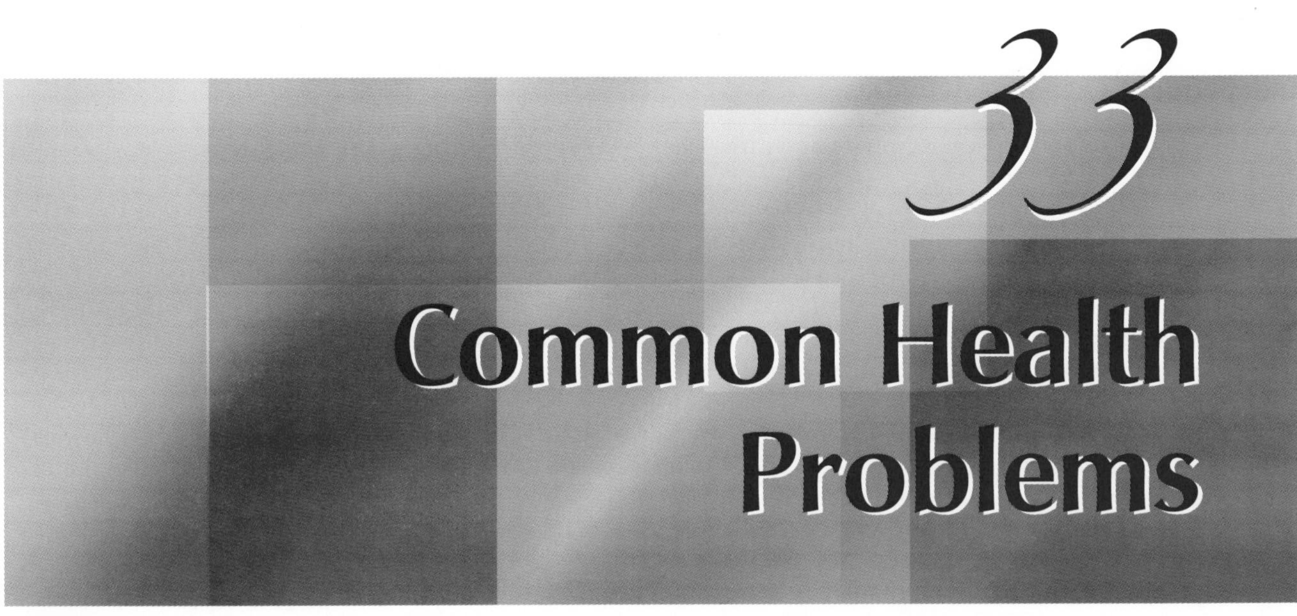

33 Common Health Problems

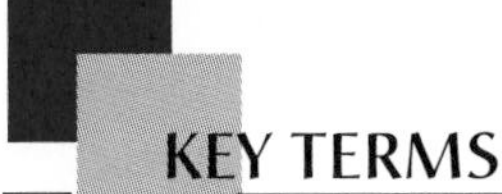

KEY TERMS

Amputation
Aphasia
Arthritis
Arthroplasty
Benign tumor
Cancer
Closed fracture
Compound fracture
Expressive aphasia
Expressive-receptive aphasia
Fracture
Gangrene
Hemiplegia
Hyperglycemia
Hypoglycemia
Malignant tumor
Metastasis
Open fracture
Paraplegia
Quadriplegia
Receptive aphasia
Simple fracture
Stomatitis
Tumor
Ureterostomy

Fill in the Blanks: Key Terms

1. The surgical creation of an artificial opening between the ureter and abdomen is a ______________________.
2. An ______________________ occurs when a broken bone has come through the skin. It is also called a compound fracture.
3. Difficulty expressing or sending thoughts and difficulty receiving information is called ______________________.
4. The spread of cancer to other parts of the body is ______________________.
5. A new growth of abnormal cells is a ______________________.
6. ______________________ is a condition in which there is death of tissue.
7. When the bone is broken but the skin is intact, it is called a simple fracture or a ______________________.
8. ______________________ is joint inflammation.
9. Low sugar in the blood is ______________________.

10. An inflammation of the mouth is

_______________________.

11. A _______________________ is a tumor that grows slowly and within a local area.

12. When a person has difficulty expressing or sending thoughts, it is called

_______________________.

13. Paralysis from the neck down is

_______________________.

14. An _______________________ is the surgical replacement of a joint.

15. Another name for an open fracture is a

_______________________.

16. _______________________ means high sugar in the blood.

17. A malignant tumor is

_______________________.

18. An _______________________ is the removal of all or part of an extremity.

19. A _______________________ is a broken bone.

20. A tumor that grows rapidly and invades other tissues is cancer or a

_______________________.

21. Difficulty receiving information is

_______________________.

22. _______________________ is paralysis on one side of the body.

23. The inability to speak is

_______________________.

24. Paralysis from the waist down is

_______________________.

25. Another name for a closed fracture is

_______________________.

Circle the BEST Answer

26. Benign tumors
    A. Grow slowly and within a local area
    B. Invade healthy tissue
    C. Spread to other parts of the body
    D. Divide in an orderly and controlled way

27. Risk factors that cause cancer include all of these *except*
    A. Exposure to sun and tanning booths
    B. Smoking, chewing tobacco and snuff, and secondhand smoke
    C. A diet high in fresh fruits and vegetables
    D. Close relatives who have had certain types of cancer

28. If you are caring for a person who is receiving radiation therapy to treat cancer, you might expect the person to
    A. Have pain related to the therapy
    B. Need extra rest because of fatigue
    C. Be at risk for bleeding and infections
    D. Complain of influenza-like symptoms—fever, muscle aches—for example

29. Chemotherapy involves
    A. Aiming x-ray beams at the tumor
    B. Giving drugs that prevent the production of certain hormones
    C. Introducing therapy to help the immune system
    D. Giving drugs that kill cells

30. You are giving care to Mrs. Ferris, who is receiving chemotherapy. She tells you she is upset because her hair is falling out. You know that
    A. Hair loss is often a side effect when a person receives chemotherapy.
    B. Hair loss is a result of her illness.
    C. You should immediately report this to the nurse because it means her chemotherapy is not working.
    D. Change the subject to keep Mrs. Ferris from getting upset.

31. When hormone therapy is used to treat cancer, a woman may experience
    A. Blood clots
    B. Changes in fertility
    C. Weight gain, hot flashes, nausea and vomiting
    D. All of the above

32. A person with cancer may complain of constipation because of
    A. The side effects of pain relief drugs
    B. Pain
    C. Rest and exercise
    D. Fluids and nutrition

33. When a person who is receiving treatment for cancer expresses anger, fear, and depression, you can help the most by
    A. Telling the person not to worry or get upset
    B. Giving the person privacy and time alone
    C. Being there when needed and listening to them
    D. Changing the subject to distract them

34. The most common cancer in children is
    A. Colon cancer
    B. Brain cancer
    C. Leukemia
    D. Kidney cancer

35. Osteoarthritis differs from rheumatoid arthritis because osteoarthritis
    A. Is an inflammatory disease
    B. Occurs with aging, joint injury, and obesity
    C. Causes the person not to feel well
    D. Occurs on both sides of the body

36. The treatment of a person with osteoarthritis should include all of these *except*
    A. Encouraging the person to apply heat and to take warm baths to relieve pain
    B. Avoiding cold weather and dampness
    C. Avoiding all exercises
    D. Encouraging weight loss if he or she is obese

37. You are caring for a person who has rheumatoid arthritis. The person has a flare-up of the disease. You should do all of these *except*
    A. Make sure the person exercises more frequently.
    B. Position the person in good body alignment.
    C. Make sure the person uses walking aids as needed.
    D. Apply splints to support affected joints.

38. When a child has juvenile rheumatoid arthritis, it can affect
    A. Mental functions
    B. Growth and development
    C. The digestive system
    D. The urinary system

39. Which of these will help strengthen bones in a person at risk for osteoporosis?
    A. Bed rest
    B. Decreased calcium intake
    C. Exercise and activity
    D. Smoking and alcohol.

40. Which of these is *not* a sign or symptom of a fracture?
    A. Full range of motion in the affected limb
    B. Bruising and color change in the skin in the area
    C. Pain and tenderness
    D. Swelling

41. When a person has a newly applied plaster cast, it will dry in
    A. 2 to 4 hours
    B. 3 to 4 days
    C. 24 to 48 hours
    D. 12 to 24 hours

42. You can prevent flat spots on the cast by
    A. Positioning the cast on a hard surface
    B. Supporting the entire cast with pillows
    C. Using your fingertips to lift the cast
    D. Covering the cast with a blanket

43. If a person complains of numbness in a part that is in a cast, you should
    A. Tell the person to move the limb a little to relieve the numbness.
    B. Reposition the person to help the numbness.
    C. Gently rub the exposed toes or fingers to relieve the numbness.
    D. Immediately report the complaint because numbness may mean pressure on a nerve or reduced blood flow to the part may exist.

44. If a person is in traction and you are giving care, it would be correct to
    A. Put bottom linens on the bed from the top down.
    B. Remove the weights while you are giving care.
    C. Turn the person from side to side to change the bed and give care.
    D. Assist the person to use the commode chair to avoid walking very far.

45. When caring for a person who has had surgery to repair a hip fracture, the operated leg should be
    A. Abducted at all times
    B. Adducted at all times
    C. Exercised with range-of-motion exercises every 4 hours
    D. Positioned to keep the hip in external rotation

46. If you assist a person to get up to a chair after hip surgery, you should
    A. Place the chair on the affected side.
    B. Have the person stand on the operative side.
    C. Place the person in a low, soft chair.
    D. Remind the person not to cross his or her legs.

47. For 6 to 8 weeks after hip surgery, the person should avoid
    A. Lying on the unaffected side
    B. Bending to put on shoes and socks or stockings
    C. Walking
    D. Sitting in a straight chair with arms

48. If a person complains of pain in the amputated part, you should
    A. Immediately report the complaint to the nurse.
    B. Tell the person that he or she is confused.
    C. Reassure the person that pain is a normal reaction.
    D. Tell the person that this feeling will go away shortly.

49. Which of these people are at higher risk for stroke?
    A. A 79-year-old white man with hypertension
    B. A 50-year-old woman who smokes and is slightly overweight
    C. A 60-year-old African-American man who has high blood pressure and diabetes
    D. A 75-year-old Asian man who is inactive and has normal blood pressure and diabetes

50. If a person who has had a stroke ignores the weaker side of the body, it is probably because the person has
    A. Lost movement on the weaker side
    B. Lost feeling on the weaker side
    C. Lost vision on the weaker side
    D. All of the above

51. When a person who has had a stroke has urinary incontinence, bladder training
    A. Will restore normal function
    B. Is always successful
    C. Will help the person regain the highest possible level of function
    D. Is not helpful and should not be done

52. You are caring for a person who has had a stroke. When giving care, the person easily follows your directions but cannot tell you what he or she wants when trying to talk. The person has
    A. Expressive aphasia
    B. Receptive aphasia
    C. Expressive-receptive aphasia
    D. Depressive aphasia

53. When a person has expressive aphasia, you can help with communication by
    A. Give all care without asking any questions.
    B. Ask the person to write out any questions.
    C. Limit questions to those that have "yes" or "no" answers.
    D. Avoid talking to avoid confusing the person.

54. A safety concern for a person with Parkinson's disease would be
    A. Changes in speech
    B. Swallowing and chewing problems
    C. Masklike expression
    D. Emotional changes

55. A person with relapsing-remitting multiple sclerosis is likely to
    A. Recover quickly from the disease
    B. Have mild symptoms that affect the nervous system
    C. Have a series of attacks that may cause more symptoms to occur
    D. Be given medication to cure the disease

56. A person who has a spinal cord injury in the lumbar region will likely have
    A. Quadriplegia
    B. Paraplegia
    C. Hemiplegia
    D. Some movement in all extremities

57. If a person with paralysis is unable to use the call bell
    A. Someone should stay in the room at all times.
    B. Tell the person to call you as loudly as possible.
    C. Check the person often.
    D. Check the person every 2 hours.

58. The most common cause of chronic bronchitis and emphysema is
    A. Family history
    B. Infections
    C. Smoking
    D. Exercise

59. When a person has COPD, the body cannot
   A. Exchange carbon dioxide and oxygen in the lungs
   B. Get nutrients from the bloodstream
   C. Absorb carbon monoxide
   D. Circulate blood in the lungs

60. When a person has pneumonia, fluid intake is increased to
   A. Decrease the amount of bacteria in the lungs
   B. Dilute medication given to treat the disease
   C. Thin mucous secretions
   D. Decrease inflammation of the breathing passages

61. Breathing is easier for a person with pneumonia when the person is positioned in
   A. Semi-Fowler's or Fowler's position
   B. Side-lying position
   C. Supine position
   D. A soft chair

62. When you are caring for a person with tuberculosis, you should
   A. Practice hand hygiene techniques if you have contact with sputum.
   B. Flush tissues down the toilet.
   C. Remind the person to cover the mouth and nose with tissues when coughing and sneezing.
   D. All of the above statements are true.

63. Hypertension (high blood pressure) is a condition in which
   A. The systolic pressure is 120 mm Hg or higher, and the diastolic is 70 mm Hg or higher.
   B. The systolic pressure is 100 mm Hg or higher, and the diastolic is 60 mm Hg or higher.
   C. The systolic pressure is 140 mm Hg or higher, and the diastolic is 90 mm Hg or higher.
   D. The systolic pressure is 140 mm Hg or higher, and the diastolic is 60 mm Hg or higher.

64. A risk factor for hypertension that cannot change is
   A. Stress
   B. Being overweight
   C. Age
   D. Lack of exercise

65. The leading cause of death in the United States is
   A. Coronary artery disease
   B. Hypertension
   C. Cancer
   D. COPD

66. When a person has angina pectoris, the chest pain occurs when
   A. Oxygen does not reach the lungs.
   B. The heart needs more oxygen.
   C. The blood pressure is too high.
   D. The heart muscle dies.

67. If a person has angina, it will usually be relieved by
   A. Resting for about 3 to15 minutes
   B. Taking narcotic drugs.
   C. Using oxygen therapy.
   D. Getting up and walking.

68. If a person takes a nitroglycerin tablet when an angina attack occurs, you should
   A. Give them a large glass of water to swallow the pill.
   B. Take the pills back to the nurse's station.
   C. Make sure the person tells the nurse a pill was taken.
   D. Encourage the person to walk around.

69. When a myocardial infarction occurs, it means that
   A. A part of the heart muscle dies.
   B. The heart muscle is not receiving enough oxygen.
   C. Blood flow to the heart increases.
   D. Blood backs up into the lungs.

70. If a person complains of pain that radiates to the neck, jaw, and teeth, you should get help because the person may be having
   A. An angina attack
   B. Indigestion
   C. A heart attack
   D. A stroke

71. When heart failure occurs, the person may have
   A. Fluid in the lungs
   B. Swelling in the feet and ankles
   C. Confusion, dizziness, and fainting
   D. All of the above

72. An older person with heart failure is at risk for
   A. Contractures
   B. Skin breakdown
   C. Fractures
   D. Urinary tract infections

73. Women have a higher risk of urinary tract infections because of
   A. Hormone levels in the body
   B. Short female urethra
   C. Bacteria
   D. Prostrate gland secretions

74. If a person has cystitis, you should
   A. Restrict fluid intake.
   B. Assist the person to ambulate frequently.
   C. Keep the person on bed rest.
   D. Encourage the person to drink 2000 ml per day.

75. When a person wears a ureterostomy pouch, you may assist the person to
   A. Replace the pouch every 3 to 5 days.
   B. Remove the pouch before showering or bathing.
   C. Replace the pouch anytime it leaks.
   D. Use sterile technique when changing the pouch.

76. If you are caring for a person with renal calculi, you will be expected to
   A. Restrict fluids.
   B. Keep the person on bed rest.
   C. Strain all urine.
   D. Give complete care to avoid any movement.

77. When you care for a person with acute renal failure, the care plan will likely include a plan to
   A. Increase fluid intake to 2000 to 3000 cc per day.
   B. Measure and record urine output every hour.
   C. Make sure the person does not drink any fluids.
   D. Measure person's weight once every week.

78. Chronic renal failure
   A. Occurs suddenly
   B. Generally improves with kidney function returning to normal within 1 year
   C. Occurs when nephrons of the kidney are destroyed over many years
   D. Has very little effect on the person's overall health

79. An obese 50-year-old woman with hypertension is newly diagnosed with diabetes. She most likely has
   A. Type 1
   B. Type 2
   C. Gestational
   D. None of the above

80. A person with diabetes complains of thirst and frequently urinates. You notice the person has a flushed face and slow, deep, and labored respirations. It is likely the person has
   A. Hyperglycemia
   B. Hypoglycemia
   C. Diabetic coma
   D. An infection

81. A child has diabetes and must carefully follow a diet. Why is the child allowed to carry snacks to school?
   A. Because he or she will have snacks like his friends
   B. Because the child does not like the school lunch provided
   C. Because his blood sugar level may drop while at school
   D. Because he is rapidly growing and needs extra food

82. Risk factors for diverticular disease include
   A. High-fiber diet
   B. Frequent diarrhea
   C. Low-fiber diet
   D. Inactivity

83. Vomiting can be life threatening when it
   A. Is caused by an infection
   B. Is aspirated and obstructs the airway
   C. Contains undigested food
   D. Has a bitter taste

84. All of these communicable childhood diseases may be transmitted by airborne contact *except*
   A. Poliomyelitis
   B. Rubella (German measles)
   C. Mumps
   D. Chickenpox

85. When hepatitis is contracted by eating or drinking food or water contaminated by feces, it is
   A. Hepatitis A
   B. Hepatitis B
   C. Hepatitis C
   D. Hepatitis D and E

86. A person with hepatitis will need good skin care because
   A. Muscle aches exist.
   B. The person often has itching and skin rash.
   C. Nausea and vomiting is present.
   D. Diarrhea or constipation occurs.

87. Why is hepatitis A more common in preschool and school-age children?
   A. Children do not often wash their hands after defecating.
   B. The immune system of children is immature.
   C. Children have not yet developed an immunity to the disease.
   D. Children often have open cuts and can transmit the disease to one another.

88. HIV is not spread by
    A. Blood
    B. Semen
    C. Sneezing or coughing
    D. Breast milk

89. To protect yourself from HIV and AIDS, you should
    A. Avoid all body fluids when giving care.
    B. Refuse to care for persons diagnosed with these diseases.
    C. Follow Standard Precautions and the Bloodborne Pathogen Standard when giving care.
    D. Always use sterile techniques when giving care.

90. A woman who complains of a frothy, thick, foul-smelling yellow vaginal discharge most likely has
    A. Gonorrhea
    B. Genital warts
    C. Syphilis
    D. Trichomoniasis

Matching

Match the form of COPD with the related symptom.

91. ________ Person develops a barrel chest.

92. ________ Mucus and inflamed breathing passages obstruct airflow.

93. ________ Alveoli become less elastic.

94. ________ Air passages narrow.

95. ________ First symptom is often a smoker's cough in morning.

96. ________ Normal O_2 and CO_2 exchange cannot occur in affected alveoli.

97. ________ Allergies and emotional stress are common causes.

A. Chronic bronchitis
B. Emphysema
C. Asthma

Match the symptom listed with either hypoglycemia or hyperglycemia.

98. ________ Trembling; shakiness

99. ________ Sweet breath odor

100. ________ Blurred vision

101. ________ Cold, clammy skin

102. ________ Slow, deep, and labored respirations

103. ________ Dizziness

104. ________ Flushed face

105. ________ Frequent urination

A. Hypoglycemia
B. Hyperglycemia

Match the type of hepatitis with the correct statement.

106. ________ Occurs in person infected with hepatitis B
107. ________ Caused by poor sanitation, crowded living conditions
108. ________ Caused by hepatitis B
109. ________ Person may have virus but no symptoms

A. Hepatitis A
B. Hepatitis B
C. Hepatitis C
D. Hepatitis D

Match the sexually transmitted disease with the correct statement.

110. ________ Surgically removed if ointment is not effective.
111. ________ Sores may have a watery discharge.
112. ________ Vaginal bleeding may exist.
113. ________ Urinary urgency and frequency occurs.
114. ________ Disease is treated with antiviral drugs.
115. ________ Person may not show symptoms.

A. Herpes
B. Genital warts
C. Gonorrhea
D. Chlamydia

Fill in the Blanks

116. Signs and symptoms of cancer include

A. ________________________________

B. ________________________________

C. ________________________________

D. ________________________________

E. ________________________________

F. ________________________________

G. ________________________________

H. ________________________________

117. When a person has radiation therapy, side effects at the treatment site can be

A. ________________________________

B. ________________________________

C. ________________________________

118. Chemotherapy has the following uses when treating cancer

A. ________________________________

B. ________________________________

C. ________________________________

119. When a person has cancer, preventing bowel problems is one of the person's needs. Explain why bowel problems occur.

A. Constipation occurs from

________________________________.

B. Diarrhea occurs from

________________________________.

120. If you are caring for a person with osteoarthritis, exercise is important because it

A. ________________________________

B. ________________________________

C. ________________________________

121. Rest and joint care are also used to treat osteo-arthritis. Explain how these treatments help.

A. Regular rest

____

B. Cane and walkers

____

C. Splints

____

122. Name the type of arthritis described in the following

A. More common in women in middle age

____

B. Joint injury and obesity are causes

____

C. Is an inflammatory disease

____

D. Occurs on both sides of the body

____

E. Often occurs in joints that bear the body's weight

____

123. List the risks factors to developing osteoporosis.

A. ______________________________

B. ______________________________

C. ______________________________

D. ______________________________

E. ______________________________

F. ______________________________

G. ______________________________

H. ______________________________

124. What diseases may cause a bone to fracture?

A. ______________________________

B. ______________________________

C. ______________________________

125. When fractured bone ends are brought together into a normal position, it is called ______________________________.

A. If the skin is not opened, this is called ______________________________.

B. When surgery is done to bring the bone into alignment, it is called ______________________________.

126. The skin is protected before casting with ______________________________.

127. If you are caring for a person with a cast, what signs and symptoms must be reported at once?

A. ______________________________

B. ______________________________

C. ______________________________

D. ______________________________

E. ______________________________

F. ______________________________

G. ______________________________

H. ______________________________

I. ______________________________

J. ______________________________

128. When you are caring for a person in traction, you should

A. Perform range-of-motion for

_______________.

B. Provide a _______________

for elimination.

C. Check pin, nails, wire, or tong sites for

_______________.

129. For 6 to 8 weeks after a hip prosthesis is implanted, the person avoids

A. _______________

B. _______________

C. _______________

D. _______________

E. _______________

130. What diseases increase the risk for stroke?

A. _______________

B. _______________

C. _______________

D. _______________

131. Which risk factors for stroke cannot be changed?

A. _______________

B. _______________

C. _______________

D. _______________

132. Which risk factors for stroke can be reduced by changes in personal habits?

A. _______________

B. _______________

C. _______________

D. _______________

E. _______________

133. What are the signs and symptoms of Parkinson's disease?

A. _______________

B. _______________

C. _______________

D. _______________

E. _______________

134. Which type of multiple sclerosis has a series of attacks and then has a lessening or disappearance of the symptoms. More flare-ups and more symptoms can occur.

____

135. Head trauma in newborns is the result of

_______________.

136. Where did the spinal cord injury occur in these examples?

A. Leg function is lost

____

B. Muscle function below the chest is lost

____

C. Muscle is lost in the arms, chest, and below the chest

____

137. When a person has a spinal cord injury, the goal is to have the person learn to function at

_______________.

138. A type of COPD that is triggered by allergies and emotional stress is

_______________.

139. How do these risk factors increase blood pressure?

A. Stress ______________________

B. Tobacco ______________________

C. High-salt diet ______________________

D. Excessive alcohol ______________________

E. Lack of exercise ______________________

140. Angina pain is relieved by

______________________.

141. Pain from a myocardial infarction is usually on the ______________________ and may radiate to the ______________________.

142. When left-sided heart failure occurs, blood ______________________. What effect does this have on the rest of the body?

A. Brain ______________________

B. Kidneys ______________________

C. Skin ______________________

D. Blood pressure ______________________

143. When right-sided heart failure occurs, what signs and symptoms happen to these areas?

A. Feet and ankles ______________________

B. Liver ______________________

C. Abdomen ______________________

144. Older persons with heart failure are at risk for pressure ulcers because of

A. ______________________

B. ______________________

C. ______________________

145. An older man may be at risk for a urinary tract infection because of an

______________________.

146. What are the risk factors of developing renal calculi?

A. Age, race, sex ______________________

B. ______________________

C. ______________________

D. ______________________

147. A person with renal calculi is encouraged to drink 2000 to 3000 ml of fluid a day to help

______________________.

148. When acute renal failure occurs, two phases occur. Name and explain these phases.

A. First phase ______________________

(i) Urine output is ______________________.

(ii) Phase lasts ______________________.

B. Second phase ______________________

(i) Urine output is ______________________.

(ii) Phase lasts ______________________.

149. Signs and symptoms of chronic renal failure appear when ______________________.

150. You may need to assist a person in chronic renal failure with nutritional needs. List what is needed in these areas.

A. Diet ______________________

B. Fluid intake ______________________

151. Name the type of diabetes described

A. ______________________ diabetes will be treated with healthy eating, exercise, and sometimes, oral drugs.

B. ______________________ diabetes will be treated with daily insulin therapy, healthy eating, and exercise.

152. Slow wound healing occurs in diabetes because of ______________________.

153. What can you do to make a person more comfortable after the person has vomited?

A. ______________________

B. ______________________

C. ______________________

D. ______________________

154. How are communicable diseases transmitted from one person to another?

A. ______________________

B. ______________________

C. ______________________

D. ______________________

E. ______________________

155. To protect yourself when caring for a person with hepatitis, you should follow ______________________.

156. AIDS is caused by a ______________________ that attacks the ______________________.

157. A threat to the health team when caring for a person with AIDS is from ______________________.

158. Why are older persons at risk for AIDS?

A. ______________________

B. ______________________

159. Sexually transmitted diseases (STDs) are spread by

A. ______________________

B. ______________________

C. ______________________

160. The use of ______________________ helps prevent the spread of STDs.

Optional Learning Exercises

Mrs. Myers is a 62 year old who is having chemotherapy to treat cancer. She has not been eating well and complains of feeling very tired. When you are assisting her with personal care, you notice a large amount of hair on her pillow. Answer the questions about Mrs. Myers and her care.

161. Mrs. Myers probably is not eating well because the chemotherapy ______________________ the gastrointestinal tract and causes ______________________ and ______________________.

162. She may also have ______________________, which is called stomatitis. You can help her to relieve the discomfort and to eat better when you provide good ______________________.

163. What is causing Mrs. Myers to lose her hair?

____

What is this condition called?

____

Mr. Miller is 78 years old. He has worked in construction for many years during which he performed heavy physical work. He complains about pain in his hips and right knee. His fingers are deformed by the arthritis and interfere with good range of motion.

Ms. Haxton is 40 years old. She has swelling, warmth, and tenderness in her wrists, in several finger joints on both hands, and in both knees. She tells you that she has had arthritis for 10 years and it "comes and goes." At present, Ms. Haxton is complaining about pain in the affected joints, has a temperature of 100.2° F, and states she is very tired. Answer the questions about these two persons with arthritis.

164. Mr. Miller has

_______________________________.

What time of day is he likely to have more joint stiffness?

____

165. It is cold and raining. Which of these persons is likely to be more affected?

____

166. Ms. Haxton has _______________________________.

She is likely to complain of not feeling well

because the arthritis affects

_______________________________ and joints.

You are caring for several persons with diabetes. They are
- 75-year-old African-American man
- 45-year-old white, obese woman
- 32-year-old pregnant woman
- 60-year-old Hispanic woman with hypertension
- 14-year-old girl who has lost 15 pounds

Answer the questions about these persons.

167. Which persons are most likely to have type 2 diabetes?

A. _______________________________

B. _______________________________

C. _______________________________

168. The 32-year-old woman probably has

_______________________________.

She is at risk to develop

_______________________________ later in life.

169. The 14-year-old girl probably has

_______________________________.

170. Which type of diabetes develops rapidly?

____

Independent Learning Exercises

- Many people have had a fracture at some time. If you have had a broken bone, answer these questions about the experience.
  - Did you know the bone was broken right away or several hours later? Days later? How did you find out?
  - What symptoms did you have? Describe the pain.
  - What treatment was done? A cast? Surgery? Pins, plates, screws, traction?
  - How did the fracture affect your day-to-day life? Work? School? Leisure activities?
  - What changes were needed for you to carry out ADL? How much help did you need from others? How did the need for help make you feel?
  - How was your mobility affected? How was your walking affected? How did the broken bone affect getting out of bed or out of a chair? Driving?
  - What discomfort did you have during the healing process? With the cast or surgical site?
  - What permanent or long-range problems occurred? Was periodic pain present? Did you experience limited mobility?

- If you have never had a fracture, try this experiment to get a small sample of how a fracture may interfere with your life. Make an immobilizer for your leg. Use one of the methods suggested, or devise one of your own.
  - Find four pieces of sturdy cardboard that are long enough to reach from the ankle to mid-thigh. Place them on the front, back, and sides of your leg, and secure with elastic bandages or cloth strips. You should not be able to bend your knee.
  - Use several layers of newspaper or magazines and wrap around your leg from ankle to knee. Secure with elastic bandages or cloth strips. You should not be able to bend the knee.

- After the "cast" is in place, leave it on for 1 to 2 hours and go about your normal routine. Answer the questions about what you experienced.
  - How much did the "cast" interfere with your routine?
  - How did the cast interfere with your ADL? Driving? Walking? Working?
  - What other problems did you have with the cast?
  - How did you feel when you were in the cast? Awkward? Embarrassed?
  - How do you think this short experience will help you care for someone with a cast?

- Try these experiments to understand how these diseases affect the body or the person.
  - **Osteoporosis** Fold a piece of standard 8½″ × 11″ paper in half the long way three times. (It will now be about 1″ x 11″) Try to tear it in half along the fold and along the 1″ edge. What happens? Unfold the paper once (it will be approximately 2″ × 11″), and cut pieces out along all of the edges. This step will make the paper porous much like the bone becomes with osteoporosis. Refold the paper to the 1″ × 11″ size and try to tear it again. What happens now?
  - **Coronary artery disease** Use a straw to drink water. Now, put small pieces of paper towel into the end of the straw and try to drink again. What happens? Add more paper and try to drink again. How does this experiment relate to coronary artery disease?

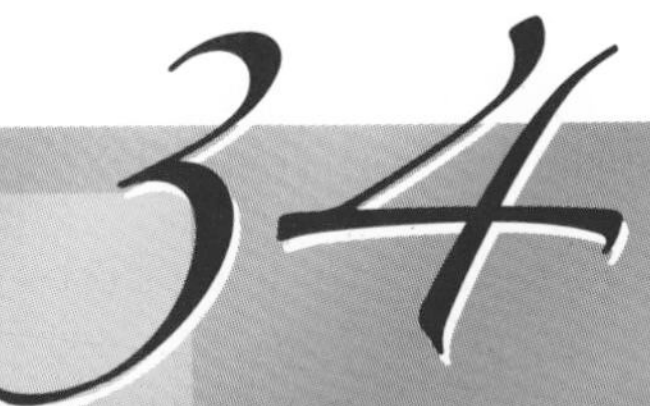

34 Mental Health Problems

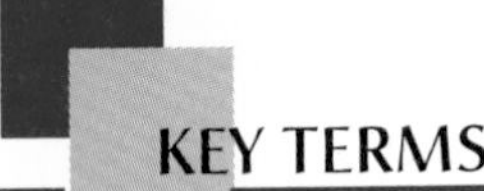

KEY TERMS

Affect
Anxiety
Compulsion
Conscious
Defense mechanism
Delusion
Delusion of grandeur
Delusion of persecution
Ego
Emotional illness
Hallucination
Id
Mental
Mental disorder
Mental health
Mental illness
Obsession
Panic
Paranoia
Personality
Phobia
Psychiatric disorder
Psychosis
Stress
Stressor
Subconscious
Superego
Unconscious

Fill in the Blanks: Key Terms

1. When a person has an exaggerated belief about one's own importance, wealth, power, or talents, it is called ______________________.
2. Mental illness, emotional disorder, or psychiatric disorder is also a ______________________.
3. A ______________________ is any factor that causes stress.
4. ______________________ is feelings and emotions.
5. ______________________ is the part of the personality dealing with reality. It deals with thoughts, feelings, good sense, and problem solving.
6. ______________________ is relating to the mind. It is something that exists in the mind or is performed by the mind.
7. A recurrent, unwanted thought or idea is an ______________________.

8. The part of the personality concerned with right and wrong is the ______________________.
9. The response or change in the body caused by any emotional, physical, social, or economic factor is ______________________.
10. ______________________ is a vague, uneasy feeling that occurs in response to stress.
11. ______________________ is another name for mental illness, mental disorder, or psychiatric disorder.
12. A ______________________ is fear, panic, or dread.
13. Awareness of the environment and experiences is ______________________. The person knows what is happening and can control thoughts and behaviors.
14. A false belief is a ______________________.
15. ______________________ is a disturbance in the ability to cope or adjust to stress; behavior and functioning are impaired. This condition is also called a mental disorder, emotional illness, or a psychiatric disorder.
16. Experiences and feelings that cannot be recalled is ______________________.
17. A state of severe mental impairment is ______________________.
18. A ______________________ is seeing, hearing, or feeling something that is not real.
19. ______________________ is a disorder of the mind. The person has false beliefs and suspicions about a person or situation.
20. The repeating of an act over and over is ______________________.
21. ______________________ is when the person copes with and adjusts to everyday stresses in ways accepted by society.
22. The set of attitudes, values, behaviors, and traits of a person is ______________________.
23. The ______________________ is memory, experiences, and thoughts of which the person is not aware. They are easily recalled.
24. ______________________ is a false belief that one is being mistreated, abused, or harassed.
25. An intense and sudden feeling of fear, anxiety, terror, or dread is ______________________.
26. ______________________ is another name for mental illness, mental disorder, or emotional disorder.
27. A ______________________ is an unconscious reaction that blocks unpleasant or threatening feelings.
28. The ______________________ is the part of the personality at the unconscious level. It is concerned with pleasure.

Circle the BEST Answer

29. The causes of mental health disorders include
    A. Physical illness
    B. Growth and development tasks
    C. Not being able to cope or adjust to stress
    D. Personality development

30. The part of the personality that deals with reality is the
    A. Ego
    B. Subconscious
    C. Id
    D. Superego

31. Which of these statements about anxiety is *not* true?
    A. Anxiety often occurs when needs are not met.
    B. Anxiety is always abnormal.
    C. Increases in pulse, respirations, and blood pressure may be the result of anxiety.
    D. The anxiety level depends on the stressor.

32. An unhealthy coping mechanism would be
    A. Talking about the problem
    B. Playing music
    C. Smoking
    D. Exercising

33. A student fails a test and blames a friend for not helping with studying. This is an example of a defense mechanism called
    A. Conversion
    B. Projection
    C. Repression
    D. Displacement

34. Panic is
    A. The highest level of anxiety
    B. A disorder that occurs gradually
    C. A psychosis
    D. A condition that continues for many months or years

35. When a person washes his hands over and over, it may be a sign of
    A. Schizophrenia
    B. Hallucinations
    C. Phobia
    D. Obsessive-compulsive disorder

36. A person you are caring for tells you that he is the president of the United States. He has a delusion of grandeur, which is a part of
    A. Obsessive-compulsive disorder
    B. A phobia
    C. Bipolar disorder
    D. Schizophrenia

37. A person with bipolar disorder may
    A. Be more depressed than manic
    B. Be more manic than depressed
    C. Alternate between depression and mania
    D. Have any of the above

38. A major safety risk of depression is that the person
    A. May be very sad
    B. Has thoughts of suicide and death
    C. Has depressed body functions
    D. Cannot concentrate

39. Depression may be overlooked in older persons because
    A. It does not occur often in older persons.
    B. Depression is very mild in older persons.
    C. The person may be diagnosed with a cognitive disorder.
    D. Physical problems are more important.

40. A person with an antisocial personality may
    A. Be suspicious and distrust others
    B. Have violent behavior
    C. See, hear, or feel something that is not real
    D. Blame others for actions and behaviors

41. All abused drugs
    A. Depress the nervous system
    B. Stimulate the nervous system
    C. Affect the mind and thinking
    D. Are illegal substances

42. When a young woman eats large amounts of food and then purges the body, she has
    A. Anorexia nervosa
    B. Depression
    C. Anxiety
    D. Bulimia nervosa

43. Safety measures are included in the care plan of a person with mental health problems if
    A. Communication is a problem
    B. The person is anxious
    C. Suicide is a risk
    D. The person does not learn from experiences or punishment

Fill in the Blanks

44. What are causes of mental health disorders?

 A. ______________________________

 B. ______________________________

 C. ______________________________

 D. ______________________________

 E. ______________________________

45. Name the defense mechanism being used in these situations.

 A. A girl fails a test. She blames another girl for not helping her study.

 ____

 B. A man does not like his boss. He buys the boss an expensive Christmas present.

 ____

 C. A girl complains of a stomachache, so she will not have to read aloud.

 ____

 D. A child is angry with his teacher. He hits his brother.

 ____

 E. A woman frequently misses work and is often late. She gets a bad evaluation. She says that the boss does not like her.

 ____

46. Below are examples of problems that occur with schizophrenia. Name each one.

 A. A man believes his neighbor is poisoning his water.

 ____

 B. A woman says that voices told her to set fire to her apartment.

 ____

 C. A man believes that he is a doctor.

 ____

 D. A woman tells you she owns three BMW cars and is the president of McDonald's.

 ____

Optional Learning Exercises

47. An infant wants to be fed immediately. At this stage of development, the part of the personality that is making the infant want to be satisfied almost right away is the

 ______________________________.

48. A teenager is with friends who are drinking alcohol, and he does not join them. What part of the personality is affecting his behavior?

 ____

49. Mr. Johnson is very worried about his surgery tomorrow. You notice that he is talking very fast and is sweating. You give him directions to collect a urine specimen. Five minutes later, he turns on his call light to ask you to repeat the directions. He tells you he is using the toilet "all the time" because he has diarrhea and frequent urination. The nurse tells you all of these things are signs and symptoms of what?

 ____

 ____

50. You are assigned to care for Mrs. Grand, a new resident. She is getting ready to go to the dining room. You help her get dressed, and she tells you she wants to wash her hands before going to the dining room. She goes to the bathroom and washes her hands for several minutes. As she leaves the room, she stops to turn off the light. She then tells you she must wash her hands again. She repeats washing her hands and turning the lights on and off four or five times. You report this to the nurse who tells you Mrs. Grand has what?

 ____

 ____

Independent Learning Activities

- Try this experiment with a group of classmates. Make up labels with various roles for "staff members" and "mentally ill" persons. A list is provided, but you may add or subtract according to the size of your group. Make sure that the group includes a mixture of people with mental health problems and staff or visitors.

Doctor	Person with bipolar disorder
Nurse	Person with delusions of grandeur
Visitor	Person with obsessive-compulsive disorder
Nursing assistant	Person with schizophrenia with paranoia
Recreational therapist	Person with hallucinations
Dietitian	Person with anorexia nervosa

- Attach a label to each person so that he or she cannot read it. (It may be placed on the back or on the forehead.) Have everyone move about the group and talk to each other based on how the person thinks he or she should approach the person with a particular label. Continue the experiment for about 15 minutes, and then use the questions to guide a group discussion.
  - How did you feel talking to a person with a mental health disorder?
  - How were the people with a mental health disorder approached? How quickly were the mentally ill persons able to sense that this was their label? What cues did they receive from others?
  - How quickly did staff members recognize the label they had? What cues did they receive from others?
  - In what ways did the approach of others cause people to respond in a way expected? Did the people with mental health problems show signs of the illness based on the reaction of others?
  - What did the group learn about approaching a person with a mental health problem?

- Consider the following situation, and answer the questions concerning how you would feel about caring for a person with a mental health problem.

  SITUATION: Marion Cross, 65 years old, is a patient in an acute care hospital with a diagnosis of pneumonia. The nurse tells you Mrs. Cross has a history of schizophrenia. You are assigned to provide AM care for Mrs. Cross.
  - How would you approach Mrs. Cross when you enter her room? How would your knowledge about her mental health problem affect your initial contact with her?
  - What would you do if Mrs. Cross told you she sees an elephant in the room? What would you say to her?
  - How would you react if Mrs. Cross told you that she owns Disney World and goes there free anytime she wants? How would you respond?
  - How would you provide good oral hygiene if Mrs. Cross refuses to cooperate because she is sure the staff is trying to poison her? What could you try that might be helpful?
  - What would you do if Mrs. Cross curls up in a tight ball and refuses to talk or cooperate during AM care? What could you do to maintain her hygiene?
  - How would you feel about caring for a person with abnormal behavior? Why?

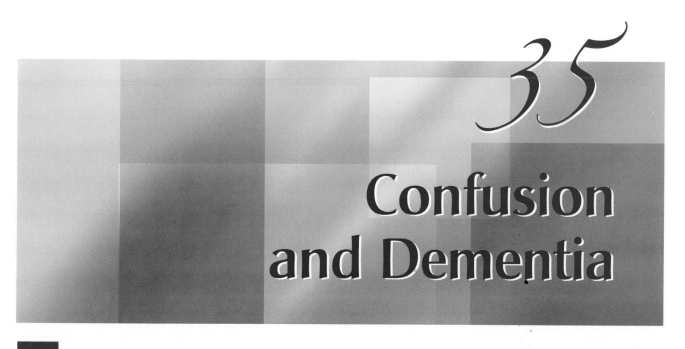

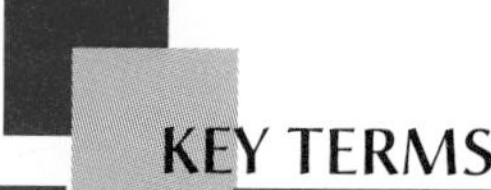

KEY TERMS

Delirium
Delusion
Dementia
Hallucination
Pseudodementia
Sundowning

Fill in the Blanks: Key Terms

1. A false belief is a ______________________.
2. Seeing, hearing, or feeling something that is not real is ______________________.
3. Increased signs, symptoms, and behavior of Alzheimer's disease (AD) during hours of darkness is ______________________.
4. ______________________ is a state of temporary but acute mental confusion that comes on suddenly.
5. The loss of cognitive function and social function caused by changes in the brain is ______________________.
6. ______________________ is false dementia.

Circle the BEST Answer

7. Confusion caused by aging
   A. Occurs suddenly
   B. Has reduced blood flow to the brain
   C. Can be cured
   D. Is usually temporary
8. Acute confusion
   A. Is usually temporary
   B. Is the result of aging
   C. Cannot be cured
   D. Is the result of physical changes
9. When a person is confused, it is helpful if you
   A. Repeat the date and time as often as necessary.
   B. Change the routine each day to stimulate the person.
   C. Keep the drapes pulled during the day.
   D. Give complex answers to questions.
10. Hearing and vision decrease with confusion, so you should
    A. Speak in a loud voice.
    B. Write out directions to the person.
    C. Face the person, and speak clearly and slowly.
    D. Keep the lighting dim in the room.

11. Dementia can be treated if it is caused by
    A. AIDS
    B. Depression
    C. Brain tumors
    D. AD

12. Dementia
    A. Is the same as changes in the brain that occur with aging
    B. Causes the person to have difficulty with common tasks
    C. Is always temporary and can be cured
    D. Affects most older people

13. The most common type of permanent dementia in older persons is
    A. AD
    B. Dementia
    C. Depression
    D. Delirium

14. If hypoglycemia occurs, it may cause
    A. AD
    B. Pseudodementia
    C. Delirium
    D. Depression

15. Depression is often overlooked in older persons because
    A. Signs and symptoms are similar to aging.
    B. Depression is rare in older persons.
    C. Depression is a temporary condition that passes without treatment.
    D. Depression is always the result of a physical problem.

16. The classic sign of AD is
    A. Mood and personality changes
    B. Gradual loss of short-term memory
    C. Acute confusion and delirium
    D. Wandering and sundowning

17. In stage 1 of AD, the person may
    A. Walk slowly with a shuffling gait
    B. Be totally incontinent
    C. Blame others for mistakes
    D. Become agitated and may be violent

18. As AD progresses to stage 2, the person
    A. Has difficulty performing every day tasks
    B. Needs assistance with ADL
    C. Is disoriented to time and place
    D. Has seizures

19. In stage 3 of AD, the person may
    A. Forget recent events
    B. Lose impulse control and use foul language or have poor table manners
    C. Be less interested in things or be less outgoing
    D. Be disoriented to person, time, and place

20. When a person with AD wanders, the major concern is
    A. The person's comfort
    B. Protecting the person from injury or life-threatening accidents
    C. Inconvenience of the family or facility
    D. Making sure the person gets enough rest and sleep

21. When a person with AD has symptoms of sundowning, it may be caused by
    A. Being tired or hungry
    B. Having poor judgment
    C. Having impaired vision or hearing
    D. Looking for something or someone

22. Too much stimuli from too many questions asked all at once can overwhelm a person and cause
    A. Delusions
    B. Catastrophic reactions
    C. Hallucinations
    D. Sundowning

23. A caregiver may cause agitation and restlessness by
    A. Calling the person by name
    B. Selecting tasks and activities specific to the person's cognitive abilities and interests
    C. Encouraging activity early in the day
    D. Insisting the person hurry to complete care quickly

24. When a person with AD screams, it may be because the person
    A. Has hearing and vision problems
    B. Is trying to communicate
    C. Has too much stimulation in the environment
    D. All of the above

25. When the person with AD has abnormal sexual behaviors, it may be the result of
    A. Disorientation to person, time, and place
    B. Poor hygiene
    C. Infection, pain, or discomfort in the urinary or reproductive systems
    D. All of the above

26. If a person with AD displays sexual behaviors, the nurse may tell you to
    A. Tell the person this behavior is not acceptable.
    B. Make sure the person has good hygiene to prevent itching.
    C. Avoid caring for the person.
    D. Ignore the behavior because the disease causes it.

27. What should you do when a person repeats the same motions or repeats the same words over and over?
    A. Remind the person to stop the repeating.
    B. Immediately report this to the nurse.
    C. Take the person for a walk, or distract the person with music or picture books.
    D. Isolate the person in his or her room until the repeating behavior stops.

28. A person with AD is encouraged to take part in therapies and activities that
    A. Increase the level of confusion
    B. Help the person feel useful, worthwhile, and active
    C. Prevent aggressive behaviors
    D. Improve physical problems such as incontinence and contractures

29. How do AD special care units differ from other areas of a care facility?
    A. Complete care is provided.
    B. Entrances and exits may be locked.
    C. Meals are served in the person's room.
    D. No activities are provided.

30. A person with AD no longer stays in a secured unit when
    A. The condition improves
    B. The family requests a move to another unit
    C. The person cannot sit or walk and is in bed
    D. Aggressive behaviors disrupt the unit

31. A family who cares for a person with dementia at home
    A. May feel anger and resentment toward the person
    B. May feel guilty
    C. Needs assistance from others to cope with the person
    D. All of the above

Fill in the Blanks

32. Cognitive functioning involves

    A. ______________________________

    B. ______________________________

    C. ______________________________

    D. ______________________________

    E. ______________________________

    F. ______________________________

33. What senses decrease with changes in the nervous system from aging?

    A. ______________________________

    B. ______________________________

    C. ______________________________

    D. ______________________________

    E. ______________________________

34. Some early warning signs of dementia affect these areas. Explain or give an example for each one.

    A. Recent memory

    ____

    B. Common tasks memory

    ____

    C. Language memory

    ____

    D. Judgment memory

    ____

35. What substances can cause dementia?

    A. ______________________________

    B. ______________________________

36. Pseudodementia can occur with

_______________ and

_______________.

37. Depression has signs and symptoms that are similar to signs and symptoms of

_______________ and

_______________. They are

A. _______________

B. _______________

C. _______________

D. _______________

E. _______________

F. _______________

G. _______________

H. _______________

I. _______________

J. _______________

38. AD damages brain cells that control these functions.

A. _______________

B. _______________

C. _______________

D. _______________

E. _______________

F. _______________

G. _______________

H. _______________

39. Certain behaviors are common with AD. Name the behavior for each of these examples.

A. The person becomes more anxious, confused, or restless during the night.

____

B. The person sits in a chair and folds the same napkin over and over.

____

C. The person begins to scream and cry when a visitor asks many questions.

____

D. The person walks away from home and cannot find the way back home.

____

E. The person begins to pace when he or she needs to eliminate or when he is hungry.

____

F. The person tells you he sees his dog sitting in the room, but you do not see anything.

____

G. The person hits and pinches the staff when a shower is given.

____

H. The person tries to hug and kiss other residents of the _______________.

Optional Learning Exercises

You are caring for Mr. Harris, a 78 year old who is confused. You know there are ways to help a person to be more oriented. Answer these questions about ways to help a confused person.

40. How can you help to orient Mr. Harris to who he is every time you are in contact with him?

____

41. What are two ways you can help to orient Mr. Harris to time?

    A. ______________________________

    B. ______________________________

42. What are ways you can maintain the day-night cycle?

    A. ______________________________

    B. ______________________________

    C. ______________________________

    D. ______________________________

You are caring for Mrs. Matthews, an 82-year-old resident. The nurse tells you she lived with her daughter for the last 2 years, but the family is now concerned for her safety. She left the home when the temperature was 35° F and was found 2 miles away wearing a light sweater. On another occasion, she turned on the gas stove and could not remember how to turn it off. Sometimes, she did not recognize her daughter and resisted getting a bath or changing clothes. Since admission to the care facility, she repeatedly tells everyone she must leave to go to her birthday party. She brushes her arms and legs and tells you "bugs" are crawling on her. Answer these questions about Mrs. Matthews and her care.

43. Mrs. Matthews is living in a special care unit in the nursing facility. What is the most important reason for this?

    ____

44. Mrs. Matthews is diagnosed with AD and is probably in stage ____________ of the disease. What activities would indicate she is in this stage?

    A. ______________________________

    B. ______________________________

    C. ______________________________

    D. ______________________________

    E. ______________________________

45. The nurse may encourage Mrs. Matthew's daughter to join a

    ______________________________ group.

    How can this be helpful to the daughter?

    A. ______________________________

    B. ______________________________

    C. ______________________________

Independent Learning Activities

Consider the following situation, and answer the questions about how you would feel.

- **SITUATION:** Imagine you are in a strange country in which people talk to you, but you do not understand what they are saying. They use strange tools to eat, and you cannot figure out how to use them. They try to feed you food that you do not recognize. Sometimes these people seem friendly and caring; at other times, they become angry because you are not doing what they ask you to do. You become frightened when they try to remove your clothes and take you in a room to shower you. You become frightened and upset because you do not know what will happen next. At times other strangers come to your room and bring gifts. They talk kindly to you, but you do not know them. They seem upset when you do not respond to their gifts and gestures. The doors and windows in this country are all locked, and you cannot find a way out so that you can go home.
    - How does this situation relate to the information in this chapter?
    - How would you react if you were the person in this situation? Why?
    - What methods might you use to try to communicate with the person in this situation?
    - Why would the person want to go home? What does "home" mean to him or her?
    - How will this exercise help you when you care for a person who is confused?

Consider the situation, and answer the questions about how you would care for a person who has dementia.

- **SITUATION:** You are assigned to care for Ronald Myers, 85 years old, who has AD. He often wanders from room to room and tries to open the outside doors. He frequently becomes agitated and restless, especially in the evening. Most of the time, Mr. Myers is unable to feed himself and is often incontinent. He keeps repeating, "Help me, help me" all day.
  - How do you feel about caring for a person like this? Frightened? Angry? Impatient? How do you deal with your feelings to enable you to give care to the person?
  - At what stage of AD is Mr. Myers? What signs and symptoms support your answer?
  - Why would it be ineffective to remind Mr. Myers of the date and time during your shift? Why is this a good technique with some confused persons and not with others?
  - Why does Mr. Myers become more agitated toward evening? What is this called?
  - What methods could you use to make sure Mr. Myers receives the care needed to maintain good personal hygiene? How could you get him to cooperate or participate in his care?
  - What parts of Mr. Myers behavior would be most difficult for you to tolerate? What would you do if you found yourself becoming irritated and angry with Mr. Myers?
  - What information in this chapter has helped you understand persons like Mr. Myers better? How will this information help you give better care to these persons and to maintain their quality of life?

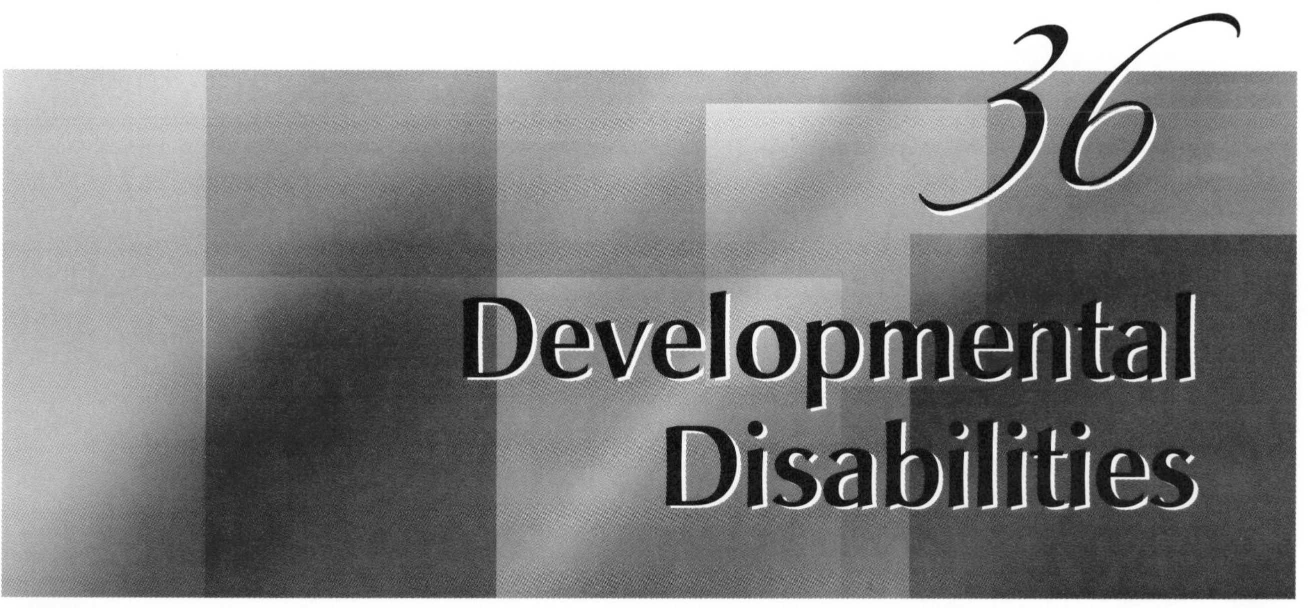

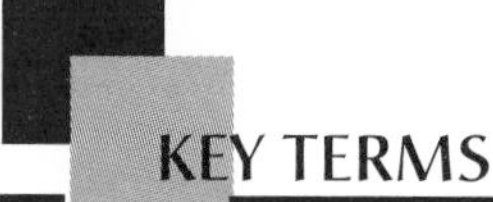

KEY TERMS

Convulsion
Developmental disability
Diplegia
Seizure
Spastic

Fill in the Blanks: Key Terms

1. When similar body parts are affected on both sides of the body, it is called ________________________.
2. The uncontrolled contractions of skeletal muscles is ________________________.
3. Another name for a seizure is a ________________________.
4. A severe, permanent physical or mental disability that occurs before 22 years of age is ________________________.
5. A ________________________ or a convulsion is the violent and sudden contractions or tremors of muscles.

Circle the BEST Answer

6. A developmental disability
   A. Always occurs at birth
   B. Is usually temporary
   C. Limits function in three or more life skills
   D. Is present before the age of 12
7. Developmentally disabled adults
   A. Need life-long assistance, support, and special services
   B. Can usually live independently after they become adults
   C. Always need to be in long-term care in special centers
   D. Generally outgrow the problems as they mature
8. A person is considered to have mental retardation if he or she
   A. Has an intelligence quotient (IQ) score below 70 to 75
   B. Has difficulty understanding the behavior of others
   C. Is limited in the skills needed to live, work, and play
   D. All of the above

9. The Arc of the United States is a national organization
   A. Related to Alzheimer's disease
   B. Dealing with mental retardation
   C. That provides care for people with physical disability
   D. For persons with cerebral palsy

10. Down syndrome (DS) is caused by
   A. An extra 21st chromosome
   B. Head injury during birth
   C. Diseases of the mother during pregnancy
   D. Lack of oxygen to the brain

11. A person with DS is at risk for
   A. Cerebral palsy
   B. Diplegia
   C. Alzheimer's disease after age 35
   D. Poor nutrition

12. Cerebral palsy is a group of disorders involving
   A. Mental retardation
   B. Muscle weakness or poor muscle control
   C. Abnormal genes from one or both parents
   D. Increased risk of developing leukemia

13. When a person has spastic cerebral palsy, the symptoms include
   A. Constant slow weaving or writhing motions
   B. Uncontrolled contractions of skeletal muscles
   C. Little or no eye contact
   D. Strong attachment to a single item, idea, activity, or person

14. A person with autism may have
   A. Frequent tantrums for no apparent reason
   B. Bladder and bowel control problems
   C. Generalized seizures
   D. Hemiplegia

15. An adult with autism may
   A. Need help to develop social and work skills
   B. Work and live independently
   C. Live in group homes or residential care centers
   D. All of the above

16. Seizures are caused by
   A. Diplegia
   B. Bursts of electrical energy in the brain
   C. Mental illness
   D. Spinal abnormalities

17. When epilepsy can be controlled, it usually
   A. Does not affect learning and ADL
   B. Is easily controlled with drugs
   C. Can be cured with medications
   D. Requires the person to have assistance to develop social and work skills

18. Spina bifida occurs
   A. At birth as a result of injury during delivery
   B. Because of traumatic injury in childhood
   C. During the first month of pregnancy
   D. As a result of child abuse

19. Which of these types of spina bifida cause the person to have leg paralysis and a lack of bowel and bladder control?
   A. Spina bifida cystica
   B. Myelomeningocele
   C. Spina bifida occulta
   D. Meningocele

20. A shunt placed in the brain of a child with hydrocephalus will
   A. Relieve pressure on the brain
   B. Drain fluid from the brain to the abdomen
   C. Reduce the mental retardation or neurological damage that may occur with hydrocephalus
   D. All of the above

Fill in the Blanks

21. A developmental disability is present when function is limited in three or more of these life skills

   A. ______________________________

   B. ______________________________

   C. ______________________________

   D. ______________________________

   E. ______________________________

   F. ______________________________

   G. ______________________________

22. What genetic conditions can cause mental retardation?

   A. ______________________________

   B. ______________________________

   C. ______________________________

23. Mental retardation may be caused after birth by

A. ______________________

B. ______________________

C. ______________________

D. ______________________

E. ______________________

F. ______________________

G. ______________________

24. According to the Arc of the United States, mental retardation involves a condition being present before ______________________.

25. The Arc believes that persons with mental retardation

A. ______________________

B. ______________________

C. ______________________

D. ______________________

26. If a child has DS, how are these areas affected?

A. Head ______________________

B. Eyes ______________________

C. Tongue ______________________

D. Nose ______________________

E. Hands and fingers ______________________

27. Persons with DS need therapy in these areas

A. ______________________

B. ______________________

C. ______________________

D. ______________________

28. The usual cause of cerebral palsy is a lack of

______________________.

29. The goal for a person with cerebral palsy is to be

______________________.

30. What skills are impaired with autism?

A. ______________________

B. ______________________

C. ______________________

D. ______________________

E. ______________________

F. ______________________

31. Explain the difference in seizures.

A. A partial seizure occurs in

______________________.

B. A generalized seizure involves the

______________________.

32. Spina bifida is a defect of the

______________________.

33. Children with spina bifida may have learning problems with

A. ______________________

B. ______________________

C. ______________________

D. ______________________

34. Spina bifida may place the person at risk for problems such as

A. ______________________

B. ______________________

C. ______________________

D. ______________________

E. ____________________

F. ____________________

G. ____________________

35. If hydrocephalus is not treated, the person may have

A. ____________________

B. ____________________

Optional Learning Exercises

Mr. Murphy is one of the residents you care for. He has DS. Answer the questions that relate to him.

36. Mr. Murphy is 40 years old. What disease is a risk for persons older than 35 years of age with DS?

____

37. Mr. Murphy is encouraged to eat a well-balanced, high-fiber diet and to attend regular exercise classes. Why are these important for a person with DS?

____

38. What types of therapies may help Mr. Murphy to communicate more clearly?

A. ____________________

B. ____________________

You care for Mary Reynolds who has cerebral palsy. Answer these questions about Ms. Reynolds.

39. It is difficult to feed Ms. Reynolds because she drools, grimaces, and moves her head constantly. You know that she does this because she has a type of cerebral palsy called ____________________.

40. Because Ms. Reynolds remains in bed or a special chair all the time, she is at special risk for ____________________ because of immobility. She needs to be repositioned at least every ____________________.

Mr. Calhoun was in an automobile accident and now has epilepsy. Answer these questions about his care.

41. Mr. Calhoun has frequent seizures. He asks you how long he will continue to have these. You report this to the nurse, and she tells Mr. Calhoun that seizures cannot be ____________________ at this time. What may be done to control his seizures?

____

42. At this time, Mr. Calhoun's seizures are not controlled and can occur at any time. What limits may be placed on Mr. Calhoun when he returns home?

A. ____________________

B. ____________________

43. Because Mr. Calhoun is at risk for accidents and injuries, he will need to have safety measures in what areas?

A. ____________________

B. ____________________

C. ____________________

D. ____________________

Independent Learning Activities

- Many communities have services available to families with children and adults who are developmentally disabled. Some communities have sheltered workshops, day care, sheltered living centers, or physical and occupational therapy programs. If your community offers these services, ask permission to visit them and observe the persons being served there. Answer these questions when you observe in the agency.
  - What age groups are served in this program?
  - What activities are available to the group?
  - What training is required for the people who work there?
  - How do the persons in the program act? Are they happy? Bored? Withdrawn? List any other reactions?
  - What other services are available to these individuals in the agency? In the community?
  - Where do the persons in this program live? With family? As residents of in-group homes? Other?

- Do you know a family who has a developmentally disabled family member? Ask the family if they will answer these questions about living with this person.
  - How old is the developmentally disabled person? Where does the person live?
  - What abilities does the person have? What disabilities interfere with the ADL for the person?
  - What therapies are being done to help the person reach his or her highest level of function?
  - What community programs have been helpful for the person?
  - How does this person's disability affect the family? Physically? Emotionally? Financially? How does the disability affect the family's day-to-day activities?

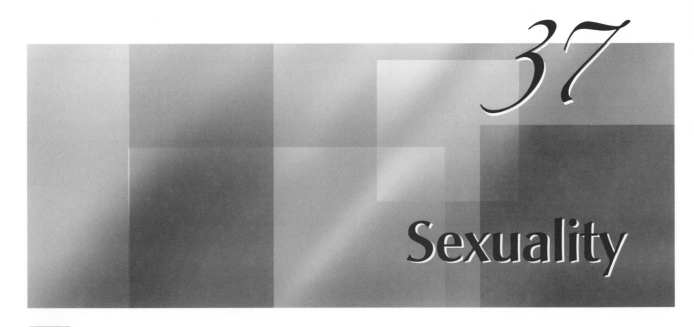

KEY TERMS

Bisexual
Erectile dysfunction
Heterosexual
Homosexual
Impotence
Menopause
Sex
Sexuality
Transsexual
Transvestite

Fill in the Blanks: Key Terms

1. ______________________ is the time when menstruation stops.
2. Another name for impotence is ______________________.
3. ______________________ is the physical, psychological, social, cultural, and spiritual factors that affect a person's feelings and attitudes about his or her sex.
4. A ______________________ is a person who becomes sexually excited by dressing in the clothes of the other sex.
5. A person attracted to both sexes is ______________________.
6. A ______________________ is a person who believes that he or she is really a member of the other sex.
7. A ______________________ is a person who is attracted to members of the same sex.
8. The physical activities involving the organs of reproduction is ______________________.
9. A person who is attracted to members of the other sex is ______________________.
10. The inability of the man to have an erection is erectile dysfunction or ______________________.

Circle the BEST Answer

11. Sexuality
    A. Involves the personality and the body
    B. Is the physical activities involving reproductive organs
    C. Is unimportant in old age
    D. All of the above

12. A woman who is attracted to men is
    A. Homosexual
    B. Heterosexual
    C. Lesbian
    D. Bisexual

13. Transvestites are often
    A. Homosexual
    B. Transsexual
    C. Married and heterosexual
    D. Bisexual

14. Diabetes, spinal cord injuries, and multiple sclerosis may cause
    A. Impotence
    B. Menopause
    C. Sexual aggression
    D. Heterosexuality

15. All of these are *true* about sexuality and older persons *except*
    A. An orgasm is less forceful in older persons than in younger persons.
    B. Arousal takes longer.
    C. Hormone production increases in men and women.
    D. Love, affection, and intimacy are needed throughout life.

16. When older adult couples are living in a nursing center, they
    A. Can share the same room
    B. Are placed in separate rooms
    C. Are not encouraged to be intimate
    D. Cannot share a bed

17. When a person in a nursing center is sexually aggressive, it may be
    A. Caused by changes in mental function
    B. A way to gain your attention
    C. Caused by genital soreness or itching
    D. All of the above

18. If a person touches you in the wrong way, you should
    A. Ignore it and realize the person is not responsible.
    B. Tell the person you do not like him or her.
    C. Tell the person that those behaviors make you uncomfortable.
    D. Refuse to give care to the person.

19. If you do not share a person's sexual attitudes, values, practices, or standards, you should
    A. Not judge or gossip about the person.
    B. Avoid the person.
    C. Tell him or her your feelings.
    D. Discuss the person's relationships with other staff members.

Fill in the Blanks

20. Sexuality develops when the baby is

    ______________________________.

21. Children know their own sex at age

    ______________________________.

22. Name the sexual relationship in the follow example

    A man dresses in female clothing

    ____

23. Sexual ability may be affected by

    A. ______________________________

    B. ______________________________

    C. ______________________________

    D. ______________________________

24. As aging occurs, hormones decrease. These hormones are

    A. Men ______________________________

    B. Women ______________________________

25. Some older people do not have intercourse. They may express their sexual needs or desires by

    ______________________________.

26. When you are assisting persons, what grooming practices will promote sexuality for residents?

 A. Men ______________________________

 B. Women ______________________________

27. What can you do to allow privacy for a person and a partner?

 A. Close

 ____

 B. Remind the person about

 ____

 C. Tell other

 ____

 D. Knock

 ____

Optional Learning Exercises

Mr. and Mrs. Davis are 78 year-old residents in a nursing center and share a room. They need assistance with ADL but are mentally alert. They are an affectionate couple and care deeply for each other. Answer these questions about meeting their sexuality needs.

28. Mr. Davis has diabetes and high blood pressure. What effect can these disorders have on sexuality?

 ____

29. Mrs. Davis tells you that she and her husband are still sexually active, but that "it is not the same" as when they were younger. What changes occur with aging that can affect sexual performance?

 A. Men ______________________________

 B. Women ______________________________

30. Because of the changes, what do you think would be an important thing you could do when they ask for privacy?

 ____

Independent Learning Activities

- Consider this situation about a sexually aggressive person, and answer the questions about how you would respond.
 SITUATION: John James is 72 years old and has paraplegia because of an accident several years ago. His caregivers report that he has recently begun to make sexually suggestive remarks. While you are giving his morning care, he touches you several times in private areas and makes frequent sexually suggestive remarks. The other nursing assistants tell you they just ignore him or joke around with him about the actions.
 - What would you say to Mr. James when he touched you in private areas?
 - How would you respond to his suggestive remarks?
 - What would you say to your colleagues who suggest that you ignore or joke with Mr. James?
 - Has this type of situation ever occurred to you? How did you handle it? What would you do differently after studying this chapter?

- Consider this situation about caring for a person who is gay. Answer the questions about how you would respond.
 SITUATION: Bobbie Freeman is 45 years old and has had gallbladder surgery. While assisting her to ambulate, she begins to talk about her friend, Judy. She tells you that they have been lovers for 15 years.
 - What would you say to a person who tells you she is gay?
 - What effect would this information have on the care you provide for the person?
 - Has this type of situation ever occurred when you were caring for a person? How did you respond? How would you respond after studying this chapter?

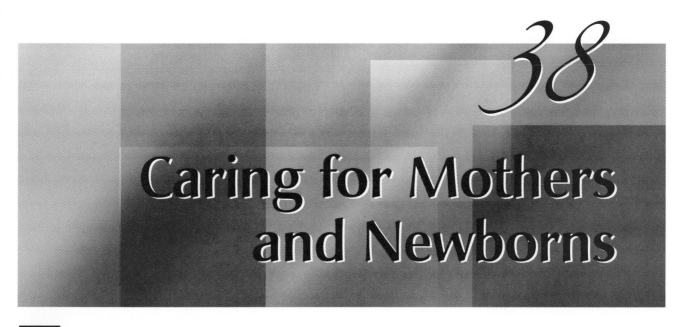

38 Caring for Mothers and Newborns

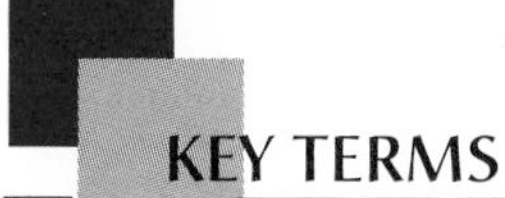

KEY TERMS

Circumcision
Episiotomy
Lochia
Postpartum
Umbilical cord

Fill in the Blanks: Key Terms

1. An ________________________ is an incision into the perineum.
2. After childbirth is called ________________________.
3. ________________________ is the surgical removal of foreskin from the penis.
4. The vaginal discharge that occurs after childbirth is ________________________.
5. The structure that carries blood, oxygen, and nutrients from the mother to the fetus is the ________________________.

Circle the BEST Answer

6. You lift a newborn by
   A. The arms
   B. Using only one hand
   C. Supporting the head and upper back
   D. Using two hands to support the back and buttocks
7. Babies cry when they
   A. Are hungry
   B. Are uncomfortable, wet, frightened, or tired
   C. Want attention
   D. All of the above
8. Babies should not be placed on an adult or child's bed because
   A. The beds will not provide enough support.
   B. The baby can get trapped between the bed and the wall or between the bed and another object.
   C. Babies must sleep on their backs.
   D. The beds are too firm for comfort.

9. When a crib is checked for safety, which of these is *not* correct?
   A. There should be less than a two-finger width between the edge of the mattress and crib side.
   B. Drop-side latches cannot be easily released by the baby.
   C. Slats are spaced no more than 3 inches apart.
   D. There are no cutouts in the headboard or footboard to allow head entrapment.

10. Toys or pacifiers can safely have
    A. Ball-shaped ends or squeakers
    B. Ribbons, strings, or cords attached
    C. Small parts that can be detached for the baby to chew on
    D. Large handles or a shield that are too large to lodge in the baby's throat

11. Which of these should be reported to the nurse at once?
    A. The baby has rectal temperature of 99.6° F.
    B. The baby has a soft, unformed stool after being breast-fed.
    C. The baby turns his or her head to one side or puts a hand to one ear.
    D. The baby cries when the diaper is wet or when he or she is hungry.

12. A breast-fed baby generally nurses
    A. Every 2 to 3 hours
    B. Every 8 to 12 hours
    C. About once an hour for very short periods
    D. On a very strict schedule

13. When a mother is breast-feeding, she should avoid
    A. Drinking whole milk
    B. Eating spicy and gas-forming foods
    C. Foods that are high in calories or calcium
    D. Moderate amounts of foods with caffeine

14. When the mother is breast-feeding, she should
    A. Position the baby by using a pillow to prop the baby
    B. Stroke the baby's cheek with her nipple
    C. Nurse only from one breast at each feeding
    D. Lay the baby on his or her stomach after feeding

15. When preparing bottles for feeding babies, you should
    A. Prepare bottles that can be used within 24 hours.
    B. Sterilize the bottles by boiling them.
    C. Rinse bottles and nipples that have been used only in cool water.
    D. Never use any soap when cleaning the equipment because soap can cause serious stomach and intestinal irritation.

16. When preparing to give a bottle to a baby
    A. Take the bottle from the refrigerator without heating.
    B. Warm the bottle in lukewarm water.
    C. Set the bottle out of the refrigerator, and allow it to warm.
    D. Heat the bottle in a microwave oven.

17. When diapering a baby, report to the nurse if the
    A. Stool is soft and unformed.
    B. Stool is hard and formed or watery.
    C. Diaper is wet six to eight times a day.
    D. Baby has three stools in one day.

18. The umbilical cord stump falls off
    A. At birth
    B. Within 2 to 3 days after birth
    C. Within 2 to 3 weeks after birth
    D. None of the above

19. Circumcision care includes
    A. Washing the area with mild soap and water
    B. Cleaning the area with a sterile solution
    C. Applying a snug dressing to the area
    D. Cleaning the area once a day

20. Sponge baths are given
    A. To protect the dry skin of an infant
    B. Until the cord site and circumcision are healed
    C. Because it is unsafe to give a baby a tub bath
    D. Until the baby is able to support the head without assistance

21. When giving a bath to a baby, the water should be
    A. Room temperature
    B. 75° to 80° F
    C. 100° to 105° F
    D. 110° to 115° F

22. An important safety measure when giving a bath to a baby is to
    A. Apply lotion when the bath is finished.
    B. Clean the ears and nostrils with cotton swabs.
    C. Use a mild soap when bathing the baby.
    D. Always keep one hand on the baby if you must look away.

23. When a baby is breast-fed, the baby is weighed
    A. Once a day
    B. Before and after each breast-feeding
    C. After every diaper change
    D. Once a week

24. When a mother breast-feeds, she
    A. Can expect a menstrual period within 3 to 8 weeks
    B. Cannot get pregnant as long as she continues to breast-feed
    C. Needs to use birth control measures to prevent pregnancy
    D. Will have difficulty losing weight gained during the pregnancy

25. You are caring for a mother who had a baby 4 weeks ago. She tells you she is concerned because she has whitish vaginal drainage. You know that this is
    A. Abnormal and should be reported to the nurse at once
    B. Unusual, because her discharge should be pinkish brown in color
    C. Normal at this time after having a baby
    D. A sign that she has an infection

26. A mother may have emotional swings after having a baby, which are caused by
    A. Hormonal changes
    B. Lifestyle changes
    C. Lack of sleep
    D. All of the above

Fill in the Blanks

27. When lifting or holding a baby, you must support the ______________________ and ______________________.

28. You should not place pillows, quilts, or soft toys in the crib because they may cause ______________________.

29. Babies are *not* placed on their stomachs for sleep, because this position can ______________________.

30. A toy chest should have no latch so the child cannot be ______________________.

31. What signs or symptoms related to each of these may indicate the baby is ill?
    A. Skin color ______________________
    B. Respirations ______________________
    C. Eyes ______________________
    D. Stools ______________________

32. When a mother is breast-feeding, if the baby finished the last feeding at the right breast, the baby starts the next feeding at the ______________________ breast.

33. The baby is burped at least twice when breast-feeding. Burping is done
    A. ______________________
    B. ______________________

34. When planning meals or grocery shopping for a mother who is breast-feeding, what should you know about her diet?
    A. Calories
    ____
    B. Milk, yogurt, and cheese group
    ____
    C. Calcium
    ____
    D. What foods should be avoided?
    ____
    Why? ______________________
    E. What foods are used in moderation?
    ____
    ____
    Why? ______________________

35. Why is it important to rinse baby bottles, caps, and nipples thoroughly to remove all soap?

____

36. You can prevent having air in the neck of the bottle or in the nipple by

_______________.

37. When you are burping a baby, you should support the _______________ for the first _______________.

38. If you are using cloth diapers, rinse the soiled diaper in _______________.

39. When changing a baby's diaper, what observations should be reported and recorded?

A. _______________

B. _______________

C. _______________

D. _______________

40. When diapering a newborn, what should you do if the baby has an unhealed circumcision or a cord stump still attached?

A. Circumcision

____

B. Cord Stump

____

41. The base of the cord stump is wiped with

_______________.

This promotes _______________.

42. When caring for the umbilical cord, you should report to the nurse if you see

A. _______________

B. _______________

43. Petrolatum gauze dressing or jelly is applied to an unhealed circumcision to

A. _______________

B. _______________

44. To protect an infant during a bath, what safety measures are followed?

A. Room temperature

____

B. Bath water temperature

____

C. _______________

D. _______________

E. _______________

45. What steps are used to wash a baby's head?

A. _______________

B. _______________

C. _______________

D. _______________

E. _______________

46. To protect a baby from falling when you weigh him or her, always keep

_______________.

47. Describe the vaginal discharge that occurs after childbirth.

A. Lochia rubra _______________

It is seen during the _______________.

B. Lochia serosa _______________

It lasts about _______________

C. Lochia alba _______________

It continues for _______________

48. What signs and symptoms of postpartum complications should be reported to the nurse at once?

A. ______________________________

B. ______________________________

C. ______________________________

D. ______________________________

E. ______________________________

F. ______________________________

G. ______________________________

H. ______________________________

I. ______________________________

J. ______________________________

K. ______________________________

Optional Learning Exercises

You are caring for Marilyn Hansen and her newborn son, Samuel, at home. Answer the questions about their care.

49. Ms. Hansen asks you if the playpen she was given is safe. What safety guidelines are important for a playpen?

A. ______________________________

B. ______________________________

C. ______________________________

D. ______________________________

E. ______________________________

F. ______________________________

G. ______________________________

50. Ms. Hansen is breast-feeding. When she strokes the baby's cheek with her nipple, what does the baby do?

____

This is called the

____

51. Ms. Hansen is having difficulty in removing Samuel from her breast. You tell her to break the suction she can

____

____

52. You notice that the nipples are dry and cracking. What are two things Ms. Hansen can do to prevent this from occurring?

A. ______________________________

B. ______________________________

53. When you are changing Samuel's diaper, clean the genital area from

______________________________.

54. The cord stump is still in place. Ms. Hansen asks you when it will fall off. You tell her it dries up and falls off in ______________________________.

55. Samuel has been circumcised and Ms. Hansen is concerned because the penis looks red, swollen, and sore. You know that this is

______________________________. However, you should observe the circumcision for signs of

A. ______________________________

and ______________________________.

B. There should be no

______________________________.

56. Ms. Hansen asks whether she should bathe Samuel in the morning or in the evening. You tell her an evening bath might help Samuel sleep longer because a bath is

______________________________.

Independent Learning Activities

- Many communities offer baby care classes, parenting classes, and breast-feeding classes. Find out what is available in your community and ask permission to attend one or more of these classes. Answer these questions about what you learned.
  - Where were the classes offered? How many classes were offered for each topic?
  - What new information did you get from attending the classes? How did studying this chapter help you when you went to the classes?

- Talk with a friend or family member who has recently had a baby. Ask the following questions.
  - How did the mother learn about caring for herself and a newborn? Did she attend classes? Talk with family members? With friends?
  - How did she feel when she brought the new baby home? What help did she have from her family or friends? How did she cope when she felt tired or overwhelmed?
  - How did she care for the umbilical cord? How long was the cord stump attached? What problems did she have with cord care? What signs and symptoms did she know were signs of a problem?
  - If the baby was a boy, was he circumcised? What care did she give to the circumcision? What problems did she have with the circumcision?
  - How did she feed the baby—breast or bottle? What were the reasons she chose the method she used? If breast-feeding was her choice, how long did she continue to breast-feed? What were the advantages of the method chosen? What were the disadvantages?

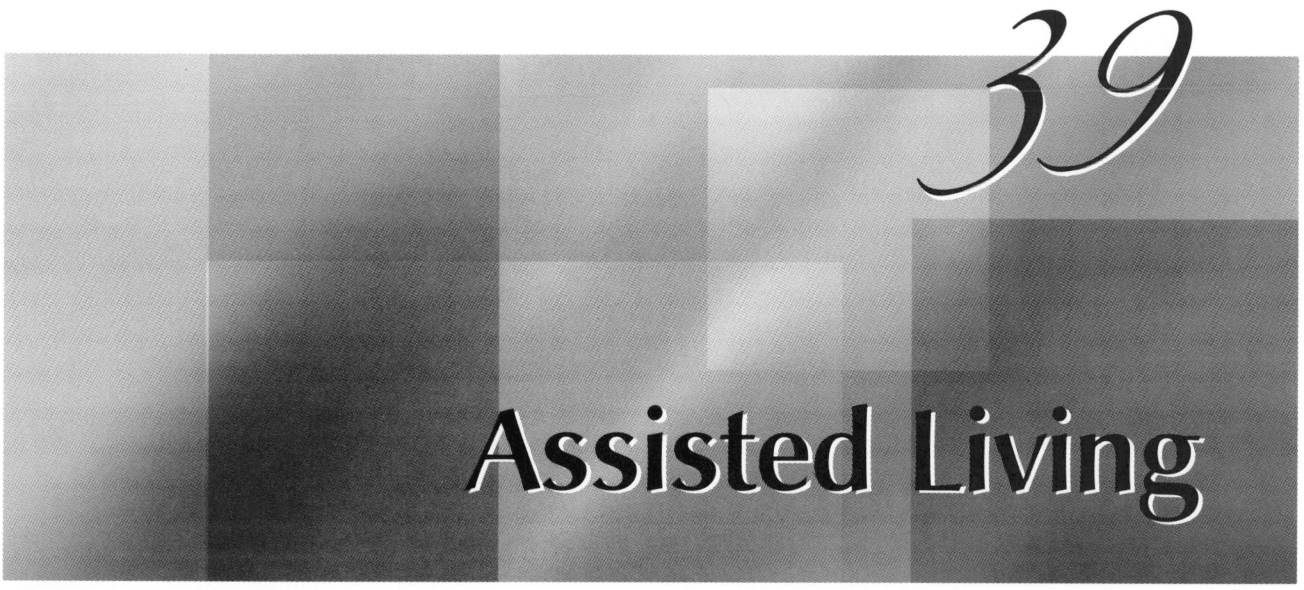

39 Assisted Living

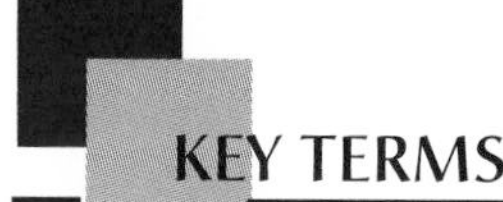

KEY TERMS

Assisted living residence
Medication reminder
Service plan

Fill in the Blanks: Key Terms

1. A ________________________ is reminding the person to take drugs, observing that they were taken as prescribed, and charting that they were taken.
2. A written plan that lists the services needed by the person and who provides them is a ________________________.
3. An ________________________ provides housing, support services, and health care to persons needing help with ADL.

Circle the BEST Answer

4. Which of these persons would *not* be living in assisted living?
   A. Someone who needs help taking drugs.
   B. A person who has problems thinking, reasoning, and with judgment.
   C. A person who must stay in bed all the time because of failing health.
   D. Someone who is lonely and wants to live with people.

5. When a person lives in an assisted living unit, one requirement is that the unit must have
   A. At least two rooms and a bath
   B. Both a bathtub and a shower
   C. A door that locks, and the person keeps the key
   D. A double- or queen-sized bed

6. Environmental requirements in assisted living units include
   A. Common bathrooms have toilet paper, soap, and cloth towels or a dryer.
   B. Pets or animals must be kept in kennels.
   C. Hot water temperatures are between 110° F and 130° F.
   D. Garbage is stored in covered containers lined with plastic bags that are removed at least once a day.

7. An Alzheimer's special care unit provides
   A. Programs that rehabilitate the person to normal function
   B. Activities that provide stimulation and promote the highest level of function
   C. Each person with a private room that locks
   D. A private apartment with cooking facilities

8. A nursing assistant in an assisted living facility may have training in all of these areas *except*
   A. Assisting with medications
   B. Early signs of illness and the need for health care
   C. Food preparation, service, and storage
   D. Measuring and giving medications

9. Which of these do not describe a resident in assisted living?
   A. The person must be able to leave the building in an emergency.
   B. The person must have stable health.
   C. The person may need some limited health care or treatment.
   D. The person needs help with complex medical problems and requires skilled nursing care.

10. A service plan for a person in assisted living
    A. Is reviewed every 90 days
    B. Lists the services needed by the person and who provides them
    C. States the medications that the person takes each day
    D. Is reviewed and revised only when needs changed

11. Meals in an assisted living facility
    A. Are served in the person's room
    B. Include the noon meal only
    C. Are posted in a weekly menu
    D. Cannot meet special dietary needs

12. When you assist with housekeeping, you will be expected to
    A. Clean the tub or shower after each use
    B. Put out clean towels and washcloths every week
    C. Use a disinfectant or water and detergent to clean bathroom surfaces once a week
    D. Dust furniture every day

13. A measure you should follow when handling, preparing, or storing foods is
    A. Use leftover food within 4 or 5 days.
    B. Wash all pots and pans in a dishwasher.
    C. Date and refrigerate containers of leftovers, and refrigerate as soon as possible.
    D. Clean kitchen appliances, counters, tables, and other surfaces once a day.

14. When assisting with laundry, a guideline to follow is
    A. Sort items according to the amount of soil on the items.
    B. Wear gloves when handling soiled laundry.
    C. Use hot water to wash all items.
    D. Use the highest setting on the dryer to sanitize the items.

15. When you assist a person with medications, it may involve
    A. Opening containers for the person who cannot do so.
    B. Measuring the medications for the person.
    C. Explaining to a person the action of the medication.
    D. Preparing a pill organizer for the person each week.

16. If a drug error occurs, you should
    A. Tell the person not to do it again.
    B. Make sure the person takes the correct medication at the next scheduled time.
    C. Report the error to the RN.
    D. Immediately take away all medications from the person.

17. An attendant is needed in an assisted living unit 24 hours a day to
    A. Give care to those who need it.
    B. Make sure medications are dispensed when ordered.
    C. Assist those who need help if an emergency occurs.
    D. Provide activities for the residents.

18. A resident can be transferred, discharged, or evicted from the facility if
    A. The facility closes
    B. The person is a threat to the health and safety of self or others
    C. The person fails to pay for services as agreed
    D. All of the above

19. Which of these is not a right of a resident in assisted living?
    A. Right to privacy and dignity, especially during personal care or services
    B. Right to have overnight guests whenever the resident wishes
    C. Right to perform work for the facility if it consents and if the agreed upon work arrangement is part of the service plan
    D. Right to request to relocate or refuse to relocate within the facility

Fill in the Blanks

20. When working in an assisted living setting, you should follow ______________________ when contact with blood, body fluids, secretions, excretions, or potentially contaminated items is likely.

21. According to the American Association of Retired Persons (AARP), most persons in assisted living settings need help with

    A. ______________________

    B. ______________________

    C. ______________________

    D. ______________________

    E. ______________________

    F. Almost half are ______________________

22. A bathroom in assisted living must provide privacy and

    A. ______________________

    B. ______________________

    C. ______________________

    D. ______________________

    E. ______________________

23. If you are assigned to work on an Alzheimer's care unit, you know the staff must have training about ______________________. Many states require ______________________.

24. The assisted living facility cannot employ a person with a ______________________.

25. The service plan relates to these services needed by the person

    A. ______________________

    B. ______________________

    C. ______________________

    D. ______________________

    E. ______________________

    F. ______________________

    G. ______________________

26. A 24-hour emergency communication system is provided so the person can use it for an ______________________.

27. The time between the evening meal and breakfast is usually no more than ______________________. It can be longer if ______________________.

28. When eating and cooking items are washed by hand, what is the order in which they are washed?

    A. ______________________ and ______________________

    B. ______________________

    C. ______________________

    D. ______________________

    E. ______________________ and ______________________

29. Eating and cooking items are placed in a drainer to dry after washing because ______________________.

30. If you are assisting the person with taking medications, you should know the five rights of drug administration. They are

A. ______________________

B. ______________________

C. ______________________

D. ______________________

E. ______________________

31. If a person is taking his or her drugs and states that a pill looks different, what should you do?

____

32. If a person needs a medication reminder, it means reminding the person

A. ______________________

B. ______________________

C. ______________________

33. If you are assisting in drug administration, you should report any drug error to the RN. Errors would include

A. ______________________

B. ______________________

C. ______________________

D. ______________________

E. ______________________

F. ______________________

Optional Learning Exercises

You are working in an assisting living facility. What would you do in these situations?

34. You are providing housekeeping assistance to Mrs. Miller who lives alone in an assisted living facility. The stove is on and a pan has burning food in it. Mrs. Miller tells you she did not put the pan on the stove. What should you do?

____

____

What is a likely reason for her behavior?

____

35. A resident in the facility has lived there for 2 years and has needed little assistance. He recently had a stroke and now needs care for all of his ADL. Why is he being moved to a nursing facility?

____

36. Mrs. Jenkins tells you she is expecting an important phone call and wants to eat her lunch in her room. What should you do?

____

37. Mr. Shante asks you to get his medicines ready for him to take. What assistance are you allowed to give when the nurse has trained you?

A. ______________________

B. ______________________

C. ______________________

D. ______________________

E. ______________________

F. ______________________

G. ______________________

H. ______________________

38. When you are assisting Mrs. Clyde with her medicines, you notice two of the labels have an expired date. What should you do?

____

____

39. Mrs. Johnson asks you when the next meeting of the quilting group will be. She also asks what days the community craft fair is planned. Where would you direct her to find this information?

____

____

Independent Learning Activities

- Find out if your community has any assisted living facilities. They may be part of another facility or may be an independent facility. Visit the facility to answer these questions.
  - What services are offered in the facility? Who provides the services? Nursing assistants? Other assistants? What training is required?
  - What kinds of living quarters are provided? What belongings can the person bring from home?
  - What activities are scheduled? How are residents given information about these activities?
  - How do the residents act? Happy? Withdrawn? Sad? How do the staff members act?

- Find out what laws in your state apply to assisted living facilities. Answer these questions about the laws.
  - What type of license is required for an assisted living facility? Do the laws apply to independent facilities, as well as those attached to other facilities?
  - What laws apply to staff training for these facilities? Does the state require workers to be nursing assistants with special training?
  - What does the state law say about assisting with medications? What non-licensed persons can assist with medications? What training is required?

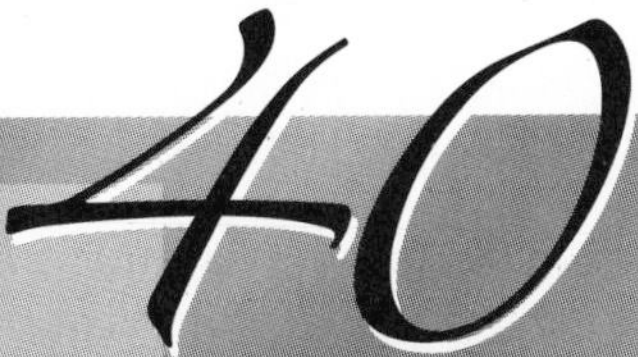

Basic Emergency Care

KEY TERMS

Anaphylaxis
Cardiac arrest
Convulsion
Fainting
First aid
Hemorrhage
Respiratory arrest
Seizure
Shock

Fill in the Blanks: Key Terms

1. In ______________________, breathing stops but the heart still pumps for several minutes.
2. The sudden loss of consciousness from an inadequate blood supply to the brain is ______________________.
3. When the heart and breathing stops without warning, it is ______________________.
4. ______________________ is a condition that results when not enough blood is supplied to organs and tissues.
5. Emergency care that is given to an ill or injured person before medical help arrives is ______________________.
6. A convulsion may also be called a ______________________.
7. ______________________ is the excessive loss of blood in a short period.
8. Violent and sudden contractions or tremors of muscles is a seizure or a ______________________.
9. A life-threatening sensitivity to an antigen is ______________________.

Circle the BEST Answer

10. When an emergency occurs in long-term care, the nurse will
    A. Call the doctor for orders.
    B. Decide when to activate the emergency medical service (EMS).
    C. Call the supervisor.
    D. Assist the person to bed.

11. If you find a person lying on the floor, you should
    A. Keep the person lying down.
    B. Help the person back to bed.
    C. Elevate the head.
    D. Help the person to a chair.

12. If the nurse instructs you to activate the EMS, you should do all of these *except*
    A. Tell the operator your location.
    B. Explain to the operator what has happened.
    C. Describe aid that is being given.
    D. Hang up as soon as you have finished giving the information.

13. When cardiac arrest occurs, it is important to restore breathing and circulation quickly because
    A. The lungs will be damaged.
    B. The person will lose consciousness.
    C. Permanent brain damage will occur.
    D. Hemorrhage will occur.

14. In respiratory arrest, breathing must be restored to prevent
    A. Lung damage
    B. Cardiac arrest
    C. A decrease in the pulse and blood pressure
    D. An increase in pulse and respiration

15. Which of these steps is *not* part of the pediatric "Chain of Survival?"
    A. Early access to the emergency response system
    B. Early cardiopulmonary resuscitation (CPR)
    C. Early defibrillation
    D. Early advanced care

16. Which of these is *not* a major sign of cardiac arrest?
    A. Complaints of chest pain
    B. No pulse
    C. No breathing
    D. No response

17. The purpose of the head-tilt/chin-lift maneuver is to
    A. Make the person more comfortable.
    B. Open the airway.
    C. Practice Standard Precautions.
    D. Stimulate the heart to beat.

18. To determine breathlessness, you should
    A. Ask the person if he or she can take a deep breath.
    B. Pinch the person's nostrils shut with your thumb and index finger.
    C. Look to see whether the person's chest rises and falls.
    D. Remove the person's dentures.

19. When you use mouth-to-mouth breathing, you should
    A. Allow the person's chin to relax against the neck.
    B. Place your mouth loosely over the person's mouth.
    C. Blow into the person's mouth slowly. You should see the chest rise.
    D. Apply pressure on the chin to close the mouth.

20. Mouth-to-nose breathing is used when you
    A. Cannot ventilate through the person's mouth
    B. Want to avoid contact with body fluids
    C. Are giving rescue breaths to a child
    D. Do not need to give chest compressions

21. A mouth-to-barrier device is used to
    A. Make a better seal when giving rescue breathing
    B. Give CPR to a person who has a mouth injury
    C. Giving CPR to a young child or infant only
    D. Prevent contact with the person's mouth and blood, body fluids, secretions, or excretions

22. If mouth-to-mouth breathing is not possible, you
    A. Cannot give any rescue breathing
    B. May use mouth-to-nose or mouth-to-stoma breathing
    C. May only give chest compressions
    D. Can use an Ambu bag

23. When CPR is started, you first give
    A. 5 chest compressions
    B. 2 breaths
    C. 5 breaths
    D. 15 chest compressions

24. The purpose of chest compressions is to
    A. Deflate the lungs
    B. Increase oxygen in the blood
    C. Force blood through the circulatory system
    D. Help the heart work more effectively

25. For chest compressions to be effective, the person must be
    A. In the prone position
    B. On a soft surface
    C. In the supine position on a hard, flat surface
    D. In a semi-Fowler's position

26. When preparing to give chest compressions, locate the hands
    A. Midway on the sternum
    B. On the lower half of the sternum
    C. Side by side over the sternum
    D. Slightly below the end of the sternum

27. When giving chest compressions to an adult, depress the sternum
    A. About 1 to $1^1/_2$ inches
    B. About $^1/_2$ to 1 inch
    C. About 2 to $2^1/_2$ inches
    D. About $1^1/_2$ to 2 inches

28. CPR is performed when the person
    A. Does not respond when you shout, "Are you OK?"
    B. Is not breathing
    C. Is unconscious
    D. Does not respond, is not breathing, and has no pulse

29. If the person is not breathing or not breathing adequately, give two breaths that last
    A. About 2 seconds each
    B. About 5 seconds each
    C. 5 to 10 seconds each
    D. 15 seconds each

30. When performing one-rescuer CPR, chest compressions are given at a rate of
    A. 15 compressions per minute
    B. 100 compressions per minute
    C. 60 compressions per minute
    D. 12 compressions per minute

31. When performing one-rescuer CPR, he or she checks for a carotid pulse, breathing, coughing, and moving after
    A. 5 minutes
    B. 100 compressions
    C. One cycle of 15 compressions and 2 breaths
    D. Four cycles of 15 compressions and 2 breaths

32. Two-rescuer CPR is performed at the rate of
    A. 5 compressions and 1 breath
    B. 10 compressions and 1 breath
    C. 10 compressions and 2 breaths
    D. 15 compressions and 2 breaths

33. When checking for a pulse on an infant, you should use the
    A. Apical pulse
    B. Carotid pulse
    C. Brachial pulse
    D. Radial pulse

34. To perform rescue breathing on an infant
    A. Use mouth-to-nose breathing
    B. Use mouth-to-mouth breathing
    C. Cover the infant's nose and mouth with your mouth
    D. Always use mouth-to-barrier breathing

35. One-rescuer infant CPR is performed at the rate of
    A. 5 chest compressions followed by 1 breath
    B. 10 chest compressions followed by 1 breath
    C. 15 chest compressions followed by 1 breath
    D. 15 chest compressions followed by 2 breaths

36. When giving chest compressions on an infant, the sternum is compressed
    A. About 1 to $1^1/_2$ inches
    B. $^1/_2$ to 1 inch
    C. $1^1/_2$ to 2 inches
    D. $^1/_2$ to $^3/_4$ inch

37. A person with a foreign body obstructed airway (FBOA)
    A. Can move some air in and out of the lungs
    B. Can remove the object with forceful coughing
    C. Cannot breathe, speak, or cough
    D. Does not lose consciousness

38. The Heimlich maneuver is used when the person is
    A. Standing, sitting, or lying
    B. Conscious
    C. Unconscious
    D. All of the above

39. If a person is very obese or pregnant, an FBOA is relieved with
    A. The Heimlich maneuver
    B. Chest thrusts
    C. CPR
    D. A finger sweep

40. When performing the Heimlich maneuver, a fist is placed
    A. In the middle of the abdomen above the navel and below the end of the sternum
    B. On the lower part of the sternum
    C. In the middle of the sternum
    D. On the lower part of the abdomen below the navel

41. If a person with an FBOA loses consciousness, lower the person to the floor, activate the EMS, and then
   A. Perform the Heimlich maneuver.
   B. Do a finger sweep to check for a foreign object.
   C. Give two slow rescue breaths.
   D. Open the airway using the head-tilt/chin-lift method.

42. If you find an unconscious adult, you should
   A. Assume the person is choking, and perform the Heimlich maneuver.
   B. Begin CPR immediately.
   C. Open the airway, and check for breathing.
   D. Do the finger sweep maneuver to check for foreign objects.

43. Which of these is *not* a sign of FBOA in infants and children?
   A. High-pitched, noisy, or wheezing sounds with inspiration
   B. Cyanosis
   C. Cannot speak or cry
   D. Harsh, coughing with vomiting

44. If an infant or child has respiratory infection that causes an airway obstruction
   A. The child needs immediate emergency care in a hospital.
   B. You should follow the procedure to relieve an FBOA.
   C. It will be relieved as part of the treatment for the illness.
   D. The child will go into cardiac arrest.

45. To relieve an FBOA in an infant, you will
   A. Use abdominal thrusts.
   B. Use only back blows.
   C. Give five back blows, followed by five chest thrusts.
   D. Do a finger sweep even if you do not see an object.

46. If a child is responsive and has an FBOA, you should use
   A. Five back blows, followed by five chest thrusts
   B. Chest compressions similar to those used in CPR
   C. Only back blows until the object is dislodged
   D. The Heimlich maneuver as used with an adult

47. If you find an unresponsive infant or child, you should first
   A. Check for breathing.
   B. Do a finger sweep to see if you can find an object.
   C. Check for a pulse.
   D. Give abdominal thrusts.

48. Side-lying position is the recovery position when the person is breathing and has a pulse but is not responding because the position
   A. Helps keep the airway open
   B. Allows fluids to drain from the mouth
   C. Prevents the tongue from falling toward the back of the throat
   D. All of the above

49. When an automated external defibrillator (AED) is used, it
   A. Stops the heart
   B. Slows the heartbeat down
   C. Stops ventricular fibrillation and restores a regular heart beat
   D. Starts the heartbeat

50. Which of these is a sign of internal hemorrhage?
   A. Steady flow of blood from a wound
   B. Pain, shock, vomiting blood or coughing up blood
   C. Bleeding that occurs in spurts
   D. Dried blood at the site of an injury

51. To control external bleeding, you should do all of these *except*
   A. Remove any objects that have pierced or stabbed the person.
   B. Place a sterile dressing directly over the wound.
   C. Apply pressure with your hand directly over the bleeding site.
   D. Bind the wound when bleeding stops.

52. If a person is in shock, it is helpful if you
   A. Have the person sit in a chair.
   B. Keep the person cool by removing some of the clothing.
   C. Stay calm. This helps the person feel more secure.
   D. Give the person something to drink or eat.

53. If a person has anaphylactic shock, you should
   A. Give the person a cool drink.
   B. Keep the person warm.
   C. Apply cool compresses to reddened areas.
   D. Activate the EMS immediately.

54. When a person has a seizure, you should
   A. Place an object between the teeth.
   B. Distract the person to stop the seizure.
   C. Position the person in bed.
   D. Move furniture, equipment, and sharp objects away from the person.

55. If you are assisting a person with burns, it is correct to
   A. Remove burned clothing.
   B. Cover the burn wounds with a clean, cool, moist covering.
   C. Give the person plenty of fluids.
   D. Apply oils or ointments to the burns.

56. If a person tells you he or she feels faint, it is best if you
   A. Have the person lie down in a supine position.
   B. Let the person walk around to increase circulation.
   C. Have the person sit or lie down before fainting occurs.
   D. Ask the person to raise his or her head with pillows if the person is lying down.

57. When a stroke occurs, position the person in the recovery position
   A. On the affected side
   B. On the unaffected side
   C. In the supine position
   D. In a semi-Fowler's position

Fill in the Blanks

58. When you activate the EMS, what information should you give to the operator?

   A. ____________________

   B. ____________________

   C. ____________________

   D. ____________________

   E. ____________________

   F. ____________________

59. "Chain of Survival" actions are

   A. ____________________

   B. ____________________

   C. ____________________

   D. ____________________

60. CPR means ____________________.

61. CPR has three basic parts. They are

   A. ____________________

   B. ____________________

   C. ____________________

62. When performing the head-tilt/chin-lift maneuver, explain how you tilt the head and lift the chin.

   A. Tilt ____________________

   B. Place ____________________

   C. Lift ____________________

63. When you are trying to determine breathlessness, explain what you do when you

   A. Look ____________________

   B. Listen ____________________

   C. Feel ____________________

64. When you perform mouth-to-mouth breathing, it is likely you will have contact with ____________________.

65. If a person has a mouth that is severely injured and you need to perform rescue breathing, you will use ____________________.

66. To find the carotid pulse, place ____________________. Slide your fingers down ____________________.

67. The major causes of cardiac arrest in children are ____________________ and ____________________.

68. If you suspect a child in cardiac arrest has an injury, turn the child on his or her back by

_______________.

69. When performing chest compressions on an infant, you press the sternum down with

_______________.

70. When performing chest compressions on a child, you press the sternum down with the

_______________.

71. Common causes of choking that place older persons at risk are

A. _______________
B. _______________
C. _______________
D. _______________

72. When a pregnant or very obese person chokes, you may be able to dislodge the object by doing

_______________. This is done by

A. _______________
B. _______________
C. _______________
D. _______________
E. _______________

73. Children can choke on small objects such as

A. _______________
B. _______________
C. _______________
D. _______________
E. _______________
F. _______________
G. _______________
H. _______________
I. _______________
J. _______________

74. Abdominal thrusts are not given to infants because they can cause

_______________.

75. If you choke, you can perform the Heimlich maneuver on yourself by

A. _______________
B. _______________
C. _______________
D. _______________
E. _______________
F. _______________

76. List the signs and symptoms of shock.

A. _______________
B. _______________
C. _______________
D. _______________
E. _______________
F. _______________
G. _______________

77. Describe the two phases of a generalized tonic-clonic seizure.

A. Tonic phase _______________
B. Clonic phase _______________

78. _______________ seizures are more common in children.

79. Describe the two types of burns.

A. Partial-thickness burns involve

______________________________.

B. Full-thickness burns involve

______________________________.

80. A partial thickness burn is very painful because

______________________________.

81. Common causes of fainting are

A. ______________________________

B. ______________________________

C. ______________________________

D. ______________________________

82. When a person has a stroke, the affected side

______________________________.

83. When an emergency occurs, what rights are protected when you do the following?

A. Do not expose the person unnecessarily.

____

B. Do not discuss information about the person's care, treatment, and condition.

____

C. The person is allowed to choose a hospital to receive care.

____

Optional Learning Exercises

You are eating in a fast-food restaurant when a man at the next table begins choking and gasping for air. Answer the questions about this situation.

84. What should you do first?

____

85. You determine the man is not able to breath in air. What would you do?

____

86. You are unsuccessful in dislodging the food and the man becomes unresponsive. After you lower the man to the floor, you should first

______________________________.

87. Before beginning rescue breathing, you need to

______________________________.

88. Open the airway with the

______________________________.

89. Give ______________________________ rescue breaths and ______________________________ abdominal thrusts.

You are visiting a neighbor and she is washing dishes. As she washes a glass, it shatters and she sustains a deep cut on her wrist. Answer the questions about how you would respond.

90. How would you know whether the bleeding was from an artery or vein?

____

91. Your neighbor is crying and walking around the room. What is the best thing you can do to help her?

____

92. Clean rubber gloves are lying on the counter. How can they be useful to you?

____

93. What materials in the home could be used to place over the wound?

____

94. Your neighbor is restless, and has a rapid and weak pulse. You notice her skin is cold, moist and pale. These signs indicate she may be in

______________________________.

95. Her wound is still bleeding, and she loses consciousness. What should you do before you continue to give first aid?

____

Independent Learning Activities

- You have learned some basic emergency care in this chapter. Find out where a more advanced first aid course is available in your community. Answer these questions about the course.
  - What agency or agencies offer a course in first aid?
  - How long does the course last? How much does it cost?
  - Who may take the course? The public? Medical personnel? Others such as police and firefighters?
  - What subjects are covered in the course?
  - Would taking this course help you on your job? In your family? In your community?

- Most health care facilities require employees to take a course in basic CPR. You may be required to take CPR as part of this course. Answer these questions about CPR training in your community.
  - What agency or agencies offer CPR courses?
  - How long does the course take? How much does it cost?
  - Who can take the courses? The public? Medical personnel? Are different classes offered to the medical personnel? If so, what is the difference?
  - How often does the person need to be re-certified? How does the re-certification course differ from the beginning class?

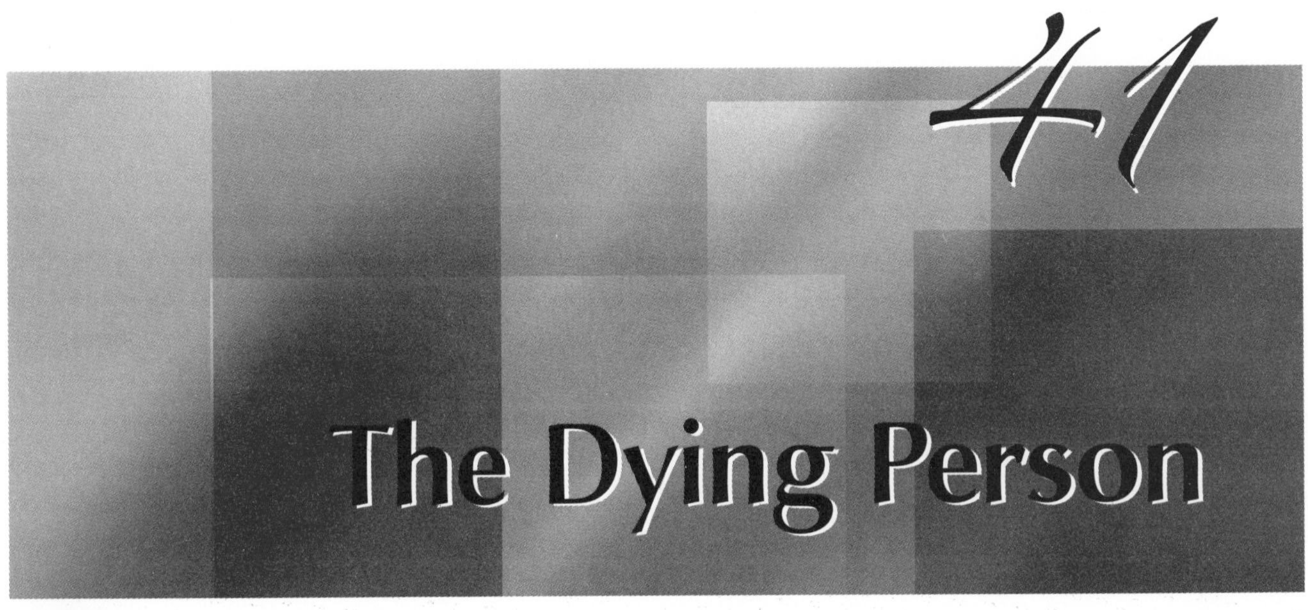

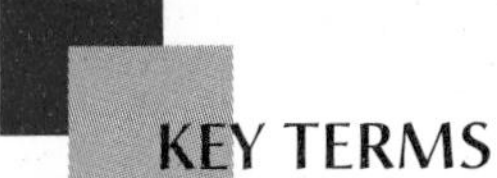

KEY TERMS

Advance directive
Postmortem
Reincarnation
Rigor mortis
Terminal illness

Fill in the Blanks: Key Terms

1. The stiffness or rigidity of skeletal muscles that occurs after death is ________________________.
2. An ________________________ is a document stating a person's wishes about health care when that person cannot make his or her own decisions.
3. After death is ________________________.
4. An illness or injury for which there is no reasonable expectation of recovery is a ________________________.
5. ________________________ is the belief that the spirit or soul is reborn in another human body or in another form of life.

Circle the BEST Answer

6. When a person has a terminal illness
   A. The doctor is able to predict accurately when the person will die.
   B. Modern medicine can cure the disease.
   C. He or she often lives longer than expected because of a strong will to live.
   D. He or she will die when expected.

7. Practices and attitudes among people from India include
   A. Placing small pillows under the body's neck, feet, and wrists
   B. Wearing white clothing for mourning
   C. Providing a time and place for prayer for the family and the person
   D. Having an aversion to death

8. A group that believes in reincarnation would be
   A. Hindus
   B. Chinese
   C. Christians
   D. Jewish people

9. Children between ages 3 and 5 years see death as
   A. Final
   B. Punishment for being bad
   C. Suffering and pain
   D. A reunion with those who have died

10. Older persons see death as
   A. A temporary state
   B. Freedom from pain, suffering, and disability
   C. Something that happens to other people
   D. Something that affects plans, hopes, dreams, and ambitions

11. In which stage of dying does the person make promises and make "just one more" request?
   A. Acceptance
   B. Anger
   C. Depression
   D. Bargaining

12. If a dying person begins to talk about worries and concerns, you should
   A. Call a spiritual leader
   B. Tell the nurse
   C. Be there and listen quietly
   D. Change the subject to more pleasant topics

13. When a person is dying, care should be given
   A. Only if the person requests it
   B. To meet basic needs
   C. Often to keep the person active
   D. Only while the person is conscious

14. Because vision fails as death approaches, you should
   A. Explain what you are doing to the person when you are in the room.
   B. Have the room very brightly lit.
   C. Turn out all the lights.
   D. Keep the eyes covered at all times.

15. Hearing is one of the last functions lost, so it is important to
   A. Speak in a normal voice.
   B. Offer words of comfort.
   C. Provide reassurance and explanations about care.
   D. All of the above statements are true.

16. As death nears, oral hygiene is
   A. Routinely given
   B. More frequently given when taking oral fluids is difficult
   C. Very infrequently to avoid disturbing the person
   D. Never given because the person cannot swallow

17. Which of these does not occur as death nears?
   A. The body temperature rises.
   B. The skin becomes cool, pale, and mottled.
   C. Perspiration decreases.
   D. Circulation fails.

18. Because of breathing difficulties, the dying person is generally more comfortable in
   A. The supine position
   B. A side-lying position
   C. A prone position
   D. The semi-Fowler's position

19. When a person is dying, you can help the family by
   A. Allowing the family to stay as long as they wish
   B. Staying away from the room and delaying the giving of care
   C. Telling the family that they need to leave so you can give care
   D. Telling the family that the person who is dying is not in pain

20. The goal of hospice is to
   A. Curing the person
   B. Improving the dying person's quality of life
   C. Providing life-saving measures
   D. Helping the family seek hospitals or clinics that specialize in the disease of the dying person

21. If a person has a living will, it instructs doctors
   A. Not to start measures that will save the person's life
   B. To start CPR whenever necessary
   C. Not to start measures that prolong dying
   D. Never to activate the EMS

22. If the doctor writes a "Do not resuscitate" (DNR) order, it means that
   A. The person will not be resuscitated.
   B. The person will be resuscitated if it is an emergency.
   C. The doctor will decide whether to resuscitate.
   D. The RN may decide that in a particular situation, resuscitation is needed.

23. A sign that death is near would be
    A. Deep, rapid respirations begin.
    B. Blood pressure begins to fall.
    C. Muscles tense and contract in spasms.
    D. Peristalsis increases.

24. When the family wishes to see the body after death, it should be
    A. Positioned in normal alignment
    B. Positioned to appear comfortable and natural
    C. Soiled areas are bathed and cleaned
    D. All of the above

25. When you are assisting with postmortem care, you should
    A. Place the body in good alignment in the supine position without pillows.
    B. Tape all jewelry in place.
    C. Gently pull eyelids over the eyes.
    D. Dress the person in regular clothing.

26. An identification tag is attached to the big toe or
    A. Wrist
    B. Ankle
    C. Upper arm
    D. Upper leg

27. The dying person's Bill of Rights includes all of these *except*
    A. The right to have my questions answered honestly
    B. The right to be free from pain
    C. The right to participate in resident and family groups
    D. The right to participate in decisions concerning my care

Fill in the Blanks

28. It is important to examine your own feelings about death because they will affect ____________________.

29. When you understand the dying process, you can approach the dying person with ____________________.

30. Religious beliefs strengthen when dying, and they often provide ____________________.

31. Adults fear death because they fear
    A. ____________________
    B. ____________________
    C. ____________________
    D. ____________________
    E. ____________________
    F. ____________________

32. Name the five stages of dying.
    A. ____________________
    B. ____________________
    C. ____________________
    D. ____________________
    E. ____________________

33. When caring for a dying person, do not ask questions that need long answers because ____________________.

34. Because crusting and irritation of the nostrils can occur, you should ____________________.

35. What kinds of elimination problems can occur in the dying person?
    A. ____________ and ____________
    B. ____________________
    C. ____________________

36. You can promote comfort by providing
    A. ____________________
    B. ____________________
    C. ____________________
    D. ____________________
    E. ____________________

37. Hospice care focuses on these needs of the dying person and families.

A. ______________________________

B. ______________________________

C. ______________________________

D. ______________________________

38. The Patient Self-Determination Act and OBRA give two rights that affect the rights of a dying person. They are

A. ______________________________

B. ______________________________

39. A living will instructs doctors to

A. ______________________________

B. ______________________________

40. When a person cannot make health care decisions, the authority to do so is given to the person with ______________________________.

41. What are the signs that death is near?

A. ______________________________

B. ______________________________

C. ______________________________

D. ______________________________

E. ______________________________

F. ______________________________

42. The signs of death include no ______________________________. The pupils are ______________________________ and ______________________________.

43. When assisting with postmortem care, you need this information from the nurse.

A. ______________________________

B. ______________________________

C. ______________________________

D. ______________________________

44. Under OBRA, the right to confidentiality before and after death provides that

____

____

Optional Learning Exercises

You are assigned to care for Mrs. Adams, who is dying. Answer the questions regarding this situation.

45. You find Mrs. Adams crying in her room. When you ask her what is wrong, she tells you that no one gave her fresh water this morning and that she has not yet had her bath. She tells you just to go away. What stage of dying is she displaying?

____

46. Later in the day, Mrs. Adams tells you she cannot wait until she is better to go home and plant her garden. She states that she knows the tests done last week were wrong and that she will quickly recover from her illness. What stage is she displaying?

____

Why is she displaying two different stages so rapidly?

____

47. A minister comes to visit Mrs. Adams while you are giving care. What should you do?

____

48. You are working one night and find Mrs. Adams awake during the night. She asks you to sit with her. She begins to talk about her fears, worries, and anxieties. What are two things you can do to convey caring to her?

____

49. As Mrs. Adams becomes weaker, a family member is always at her bedside. When he or she asks to assist with her care, you know that this is acceptable because ______________________.

50. Mrs. Adams has very irregular breathing that becomes deeper and then stops for a period. This pattern of breathing, called ______________________, occurs because the ______________________ fails as death nears.

51. Mrs. Adams dies while you are working, and the nurse asks you to assist with postmortem care. As you clean soiled areas, you assist the nurse to turn the body and air is expelled. This occurs because ______________________.

52. You wear gloves during postmortem care to protect you from ______________________.

Independent Learning Activities

- It is important to explore your own beliefs about death and dying before you care for persons who are dying. Answer these questions to understand your own feelings.
  - Have you attended a funeral or visited a funeral home? How did you feel?
  - Has anyone close to you died? How did you assist with any of the funeral arrangements? What kinds of preparation did the family do?
  - What cultural or religious practices in your family affect death and funeral arrangements? How do you think these practices will affect you when you care for those who are dying?
  - Have you ever been present when someone died? In your personal life? As a student? At your job? How did you respond? What were you asked to do in this situation?
  - What is your personal belief about a living will? How will you respond if a person or family refuses a feeding tube or a ventilator? How will you respond if they ask to have these measures discontinued and the person dies?
  - What is your personal belief about a DNR order? How would you feel if a person you are caring for has this order? How will you respond when the person dies and no effort is made to help the person?

Procedure Checklists

Using a Fire Extinguisher

QUALITY OF LIFE

Name: ______________________

Date: ______________________

Remembered to:
- ◆ Knock before entering the person's room
- ◆ Address the person by name
- ◆ Introduce yourself by name and title

Procedure	S	U	Comments
1. Pulled the fire alarm.	_____	_____	__________
2. Got the nearest fire extinguisher.	_____	_____	__________
3. Carried the extinguisher upright.	_____	_____	__________
4. Took the extinguisher to the fire.	_____	_____	__________
5. Removed the safety pin.	_____	_____	__________
6. Directed the hose at the base of the fire.	_____	_____	__________
7. Pushed the top handle down.	_____	_____	__________
8. Swept the hose slowly back and forth at the base of the fire.	_____	_____	__________

Applying Restraints

QUALITY OF LIFE

Name: ______________________

Date: ______________________

Remembered to:
- ◆ Knock before entering the person's room
- ◆ Address the person by name
- ◆ Introduce yourself by name and title

Pre-Procedure	S	U	Comments
1. Followed Delegation Guidelines for applying restraints.	_____	_____	__________
2. Collected the following as instructed by the nurse:			
• Correct type and size of restraint	_____	_____	__________
• Padding for bony areas	_____	_____	__________
• Bed rail pads or gap protectors, if necessary	_____	_____	__________
3. Practiced hand hygiene.	_____	_____	__________
4. Identified the person. Checked the identification bracelet against the assignment sheet. Called the person by name.	_____	_____	__________
5. Explained the procedure to the person.	_____	_____	__________
6. Provided for privacy.	_____	_____	__________

Procedure

	S	U	Comments
7. Made sure the person was comfortable and in good body alignment.	_____	_____	__________
8. Applied the bed rail pads or gap protectors on the bed, if needed. Followed the manufacturer's instructions.	_____	_____	__________
9. Padded bony areas according to nurse's instructions.	_____	_____	__________
10. Read the manufacturer's instructions. Noted the front and back of the restraint.	_____	_____	__________
11. For wrist restraints:			
a. Applied first restraint following the manufacturer's instructions. Placed the soft part toward the skin.	_____	_____	__________
b. Secured the restraint to ensure that it was snug but not tight. Slid one or two fingers under the restraint. Followed the manufacturer's instructions.	_____	_____	__________
c. Tied the straps to the movable part of the bed frame out of the person's reach. Used an agency-approved tie. Left 1 to 2 inches of slack in the straps.	_____	_____	__________
d. Applied second restraint following the manufacturer's instructions. Placed the soft part toward the skin.	_____	_____	__________
e. Secured the second restraint to ensure that it was snug but not tight. Slid one or two fingers under the restraint. Followed the manufacturer's instructions.	_____	_____	__________
f. Tied the second restraint straps to the movable part of the bed frame out of the person's reach. Used an agency-approved tie. Left 1 or 2 inches of slack in the straps.	_____	_____	__________

Procedure—cont'd	S	U	Comments
12. For mitt restraints:			
a. Made sure the person's hands were clean and dry.	_____	_____	_______________
b. Applied the first mitt restraint. Followed the manufacturer's instructions.	_____	_____	_______________
c. Tied the straps to the movable part of the bed frame. Used an agency-approved tie. Left 1 to 2 inches of slack in the straps.	_____	_____	_______________
d. Made sure the restraint was snug. Slid a finger between the restraint and the wrist. Adjusted the straps as needed. Rechecked for snugness.	_____	_____	_______________
e. Applied the second mitt restraint. Followed the manufacturer's instructions.	_____	_____	_______________
f. Tied the straps to the movable part of the bed frame. Used an agency-approved tie. Left 1 to 2 inches of slack in the straps.	_____	_____	_______________
g. Made sure the restraint was snug. Slid a finger between the restraint and the wrist. Adjusted the straps as needed. Rechecked for snugness.	_____	_____	_______________
13. For a belt restraint:			
a. Assisted the person to a sitting position.	_____	_____	_______________
b. Applied the restraint with free hand. Followed the manufacturer's instructions.	_____	_____	_______________
c. Removed wrinkles or creases from the front and back of the restraint.	_____	_____	_______________
d. Brought the tie through the slots in the belt.	_____	_____	_______________
e. Helped the person lie down, if in bed.	_____	_____	_______________
f. Made sure the person was comfortable and in good body alignment.	_____	_____	_______________
g. Secured the straps to the movable part of the bed frame out of the person's reach or to the chair or wheelchair. Used an agency-approved tie. Left 1 to 2 inches of slack in the straps.	_____	_____	_______________
14. For a vest restraint:			
a. Assisted the person to a sitting position.	_____	_____	_______________
b. Applied the restraint with your free hand. Followed the manufacturer's instructions. Crossed the V part of the vest in the front.	_____	_____	_______________
c. Made sure the vest was free of wrinkles in the front and back.	_____	_____	_______________
d. Helped the person lie down, if in bed.	_____	_____	_______________
e. Brought the straps through the slots.	_____	_____	_______________
f. Made sure the person was comfortable and in good body alignment.	_____	_____	_______________
g. Secured the straps to the chair or to the movable part of the bed frame at waist level out of the person's reach. Used an agency-approved tie. Left 1 to 2 inches of slack in the straps.	_____	_____	_______________

Procedure—cont'd

	S	U	Comments
h. Made sure the vest was snug. Slid an open hand between the restraint and the person. Adjusted the restraint as needed. Rechecked for snugness.	_____	_____	__________
15. For a jacket restraint:			
a. Assisted the person to a sitting position.	_____	_____	__________
b. Applied the restraint with your free hand. Followed the manufacturer's instructions. Remembered that the jacket opening goes in the back.	_____	_____	__________
c. Closed the back with the zipper, ties, or hook and loop closures.	_____	_____	__________
d. Made sure the side seams were under the arms. Removed any wrinkles in the front and back.	_____	_____	__________
e. Helped the person lie down, if in bed.	_____	_____	__________
f. Made sure the person was comfortable and in good body alignment.	_____	_____	__________
g. Secured the straps to the chair or to the movable part of the bed frame at waist level out of the person's reach. Used an agency-approved knot. Left 1 to 2 inches of slack in the straps.	_____	_____	__________
h. Made sure the jacket was snug. Slid an open hand between the restraint and the person. Adjusted the restraint as needed. Rechecked for snugness.	_____	_____	__________
16. For elbow restraints:			
a. Wrapped the restraint around the child's first elbow. Followed the manufacturer's instructions.	_____	_____	__________
b. Secured the restraint. Followed the manufacturer's instructions. Left 1 to 2 inches of slack in the straps.	_____	_____	__________
c. Wrapped the restraint around the child's second elbow. Followed the manufacturer's instructions.	_____	_____	__________
d. Secured the restraint. Followed the manufacturer's instructions. Left 1 to 2 inches of slack in the straps.	_____	_____	__________

Post-Procedure

	S	U	Comments
17. Positioned the person as the nurse directed.	_____	_____	__________
18. Placed the call bell within the person's reach.	_____	_____	__________
19. Raised or lowered bed rails. Followed the care plan and the manufacturer's instructions for the restraint.	_____	_____	__________
20. Unscreened the person.	_____	_____	__________
21. Decontaminated your hands.	_____	_____	__________
22. Checked the person and the restraint at least every 15 minutes. Reported and recorded your observations.	_____	_____	__________
a. For wrist and mitt restraints: Checked the pulse, color, and temperature of the restrained part.	_____	_____	__________
b. For vest, jacket, and belt restraints: Checked the person's breathing. Called for the nurse at once if the person was not breathing or was having difficulty breathing. Made sure the restraint was properly positioned in the front and back.	_____	_____	__________

Post-Procedure—cont'd	S	U	Comments
23. Performed the following at least every 2 hours:			
• Removed the restraint.	____	____	____________
• Repositioned the person.	____	____	____________
• Met food, fluid, hygiene, and elimination needs.	____	____	____________
• Gave skin care.	____	____	____________
• Performed range-of-motion exercises or ambulated the person. Followed the care plan.	____	____	____________
• Reapplied the restraints.	____	____	____________
24. Reported and recorded your observations and the care given.	____	____	____________

Handwashing

Quality of Life

Name: ____________________

Date: ____________________

Remembered to:
- ◆ Knock before entering the person's room
- ◆ Address the person by name
- ◆ Introduce yourself by name and title

Procedure	S	U	Comments
1. Viewed Safety Alert: Hand Hygiene.			
2. Made sure you had soap, paper towels, orange stick or nail file, and wastebasket. Collected missing items.			
3. Pushed your watch up 4 to 5 inches. Also pushed up uniform sleeves.			
4. Stood away from the sink. Made sure that clothes did not touch the sink. Stood so the soap and faucet were easy to reach.			
5. Turned on and adjusted the water until it felt warm.			
6. Wet your wrists and hands. Kept your hands lower than your elbows.			
7. Applied about 1 teaspoon of soap to your hands.			
8. Rubbed your palms together and interlaced your fingers. Worked up a good lather. Performed this step for at least 15 seconds.			
9. Washed each hand and wrist thoroughly. Cleaned well between the fingers.			
10. Cleaned under the fingernails. Rubbed your fingertips against your palms.			
11. Cleaned under fingernails with a nail file or an orange stick if first handwashing of the day or if hands were highly soiled.			
12. Rinsed wrists and hands well. Water flowed from the arms to the hands.			
13. Repeated application of 1 teaspoon of soap to your hands.			
14. Rubbed your palms together and interlaced your fingers, worked up a good lather. Performed this step for 15 seconds.			
15. Washed each hand and wrist thoroughly. Cleaned well between the fingers.			
16. Dried your wrists and hands with paper towels. Patted dry, starting at finger tips.			
17. Discarded the paper towels.			
18. Turned off each faucet with a clean, dry paper towel.			
19. Discarded paper towels.			

Removing Gloves

Quality of Life

Name: ______________________

Date: ______________________

Remembered to:
- ◆ **Knock before entering the person's room**
- ◆ **Address the person by name**
- ◆ **Introduce yourself by name and title**

Procedure	S	U	Comments
1. Made sure that glove only touched glove.	____	____	____________
2. Grasped a glove on the outside just below the cuff.	____	____	____________
3. Pulled the glove down over your hand so that it was inside out.	____	____	____________
4. Held the removed glove with your other gloved hand.	____	____	____________
5. Reached inside the other glove. Used the first two fingers of the ungloved hand.	____	____	____________
6. Pulled the glove down (inside out) over your hand and the other glove.	____	____	____________
7. Discarded the gloves. Followed agency policy.	____	____	____________
8. Decontaminated your hands.	____	____	____________

Wearing a Mask

QUALITY OF LIFE

Name: ______________________

Date: ______________________

Remembered to:
- Knock before entering the person's room
- Address the person by name
- Introduce yourself by name and title

Procedure	S	U	Comments
1. Completed hand hygiene.	_____	_____	__________
2. Picked up the mask by its upper ties. Did not touch the part that covers your face.	_____	_____	__________
3. Placed the mask over your nose and mouth.	_____	_____	__________
4. Placed the upper strings above your ears. Tied them at the back of your head.	_____	_____	__________
5. Tied the lower strings at the back of your neck. The lower part of the mask was under your chin.	_____	_____	__________
6. Pinched the metal band around your nose. Top of the mask was snug over your nose. If glasses were worn, the mask was snug under the bottom of the glasses.	_____	_____	__________
7. Decontaminate your hands.	_____	_____	__________
8. Provided care. Avoided coughing, sneezing, and unnecessary talking.	_____	_____	__________
9. Changed the mask when it became moist or contaminated.	_____	_____	__________
10. Removed the mask as follows:			
a. Removed the gloves.	_____	_____	__________
b. Decontaminated your hands.	_____	_____	__________
c. Untied the lower strings.	_____	_____	__________
d. Untied the top strings.	_____	_____	__________
e. Held the top strings. Removed the mask.	_____	_____	__________
f. Brought the strings together. Folded the inside of the mask together, and did not touch the inside of the mask.	_____	_____	__________
11. Discarded mask. Followed agency policy.	_____	_____	__________
12. Decontaminated your hands.	_____	_____	__________

Donning and Removing a Gown

QUALITY OF LIFE

Name: ____________________

Date: ____________________

Remembered to:
- Knock before entering the person's room
- Address the person by name
- Introduce yourself by name and title

Procedure	S	U	Comments
1. Removed watch and all jewelry.	___	___	___
2. Rolled up uniform sleeves.	___	___	___
3. Completed hand hygiene.	___	___	___
4. Positioned facemask if required.	___	___	___
5. Held a clean gown out in front of you. Allowed it to unfold. Did not shake the gown.	___	___	___
6. Placed your hands and arms through the sleeves.	___	___	___
7. Made sure that the gown covered the front of your uniform and that it fit snug at the neck.	___	___	___
8. Tied the strings at the back of the neck.	___	___	___
9. Overlapped the back of the gown. Made sure it snuggly covered your uniform.	___	___	___
10. Tied the waist strings at the back.	___	___	___
11. Put on the gloves.	___	___	___
12. Provided care.	___	___	___
13. Removed and discarded the gloves. Decontaminated your hands.	___	___	___
14. Removed the gown as follows:			
a. Untied the waist strings.	___	___	___
b. Decontaminated your hands.	___	___	___
c. Untied the neck strings. Did not touch the outside of the gown.	___	___	___
d. Pulled the gown down from the shoulders.	___	___	___
e. Turned the gown inside out as it was removed. Held it at the shoulder seams, and brought your hands together.	___	___	___
15. Rolled up the gown away from you. Kept it inside out.	___	___	___
16. Discarded the gown. Followed agency policy.	___	___	___
17. Decontaminated your hands.	___	___	___
18. Removed the facemask. Discarded it. Followed agency policy.	___	___	___
19. Decontaminated your hands.	___	___	___
20. Opened the door using a paper towel. Discarded it as you left.	___	___	___

Double Bagging

QUALITY OF LIFE

Name: ______________________

Date: ______________________

Remembered to:
- **Knock before entering the person's room**
- **Address the person by name**
- **Introduce yourself by name and title**

Procedure	S	U	Comments
1. Asked a co-worker to assist. Co-worker stood outside of the room.	____	____	____________
2. Placed soiled linen, reusable items, disposable supplies, and trash in the correct containers. Containers were lined with leak-proof BIOHAZARD bags.	____	____	____________
3. Securely sealed the bags with ties.	____	____	____________
4. Asked your co-worker to make a wide cuff on the clean bag to protect your hands from contamination. Held it wide open.	____	____	____________
5. Placed the contaminated bag into the clean bag. Did not touch the outside of the clean bag.	____	____	____________
6. Asked co-worker to seal bag. Made sure it was labeled according to agency policy.	____	____	____________
7. Had the co-worker use separate bags as needed for other contaminated bags.	____	____	____________
8. Asked co-worker to take or send the bags to the appropriate department for disposal, disinfection, or sterilization.	____	____	____________

Sterile Gloving

QUALITY OF LIFE

Name: ______________________

Date: ______________________

Remembered to:
- ◆ **Knock before entering the person's room**
- ◆ **Address the person by name**
- ◆ **Introduce yourself by name and title**

Procedure	S	U	Comments
1. Followed Delegation Guidelines: Assisting With Sterile Procedures. Viewed Safety Alerts: Surgical Asepsis and Sterile Gloving.	____	____	________
2. Completed hand hygiene.	____	____	________
3. Arranged a sterile field.	____	____	________
4. Inspected the package for sterility:			
a. Checked the expiration date.	____	____	________
b. Confirmed that the package was dry.	____	____	________
c. Checked for tears, holes, punctures, and watermarks.	____	____	________
5. Arranged a work surface:			
a. Made sure there was enough room.	____	____	________
b. Arranged the work surface at waist level and within vision.	____	____	________
c. Cleaned and dried the work surface.	____	____	________
d. Did not reach over the work surface. Did not turn back on the work surface.	____	____	________
6. Opened the package. Grasped the flaps. Gently peeled back the flaps.	____	____	________
7. Removed the inner package. Placed it on work surface.	____	____	________
8. Read the manufacturer's instructions on the inner package if labeled with left, right, up, and down.	____	____	________
9. Arranged the inner package for left, right, up, and down. Left glove was on your left. Right glove was on your right. The cuffs were near you with the fingers pointing away.	____	____	________
10. Grasped the folded edges of the inner package. Used your thumb and index finger of each hand.	____	____	________
11. Folded back the inner package to expose the gloves. Made sure not to touch or otherwise contaminate the inside of the package or gloves. (Inside of the inner package is a sterile field.)	____	____	________
12. Noted that each glove had a cuff 2 to 3 inches wide. (Cuffs and inside of gloves are not considered sterile.)	____	____	________
13. Put on the right glove if you are right handed *or* put on the left glove if you are left handed.			
a. Picked up the glove with your other hand. Used your thumb, index, and middle fingers.	____	____	________
b. Touched only the cuff and inside of the glove.	____	____	________
c. Turned the hand to gloved palm side up.	____	____	________
d. Lifted the cuff up. Slid your fingers and hand in the glove.	____	____	________
e. Pulled the glove over your hand. If some fingers got stuck, left them that way until the other glove was on.	____	____	________
f. Left the cuff turned down.	____	____	________

Procedure—cont'd	S	U	Comments
14. Used your gloved hand to put on the other glove.			
a. Reached under the cuff of the second glove. Used the four fingers of your gloved hand. Kept your gloved thumb close to your gloved palm.	_____	_____	____________
b. Pulled on the second glove. Your gloved hand did not touch the cuff or any surface. Held the thumb of your first gloved hand away from your gloved palm.	_____	_____	____________
15. Adjusted each glove with the other hand until smooth and comfortable.	_____	_____	____________
16. Slid your fingers under the cuffs to pull them up.	_____	_____	____________
17. Touched only sterile items.	_____	_____	____________
18. Removed the gloves.	_____	_____	____________
19. Decontaminated your hands.	_____	_____	____________

Raising the Person's Head and Shoulders

QUALITY OF LIFE

Name: ____________________

Date: ____________________

Remembered to:
- Knock before entering the person's room
- Address the person by name
- Introduce yourself by name and title

Pre-Procedure

	S	U	Comments
1. Followed Delegation Guidelines: Lifting and Moving Persons in Bed. Viewed Safety Alert: Lifting and Moving Persons in Bed.			
2. Asked co-worker to assist, if needed.			
3. Completed hand hygiene.			
4. Identified the person. Checked the identification bracelet against the assignment sheet. Called the person by name.			
5. Explained the procedure to the person.			
6. Provided for privacy.			
7. Locked the bed wheels.			
8. Raised the bed for body mechanics. Bed rails were up, if used.			

Procedure

	S	U	Comments
9. Asked co-worker to stand on the other side of bed. Lowered bed rails if up.			
10. Asked the person to put the near arm under your near arm and behind your shoulder. Person's hand rested on top of your shoulder. Worker on the person's right side had the person's right hand rested on your right shoulder. The person did the same with the co-worker on the left side, person's left hand rested on co-worker's left arm.			
11. Placed your arm nearest the person under the person's arm. Your hand was placed on the person's shoulder. Your co-worker placed his or her arm nearest the person under the person's arm. Co-worker hand was on the person's shoulder.			
12. Placed your free arm under the person's neck and shoulders. Co-worker placed his or her free arm under the person's neck and shoulders.			
13. Helped the person pull up to a sitting or semi-sitting position on the count of "3."			
14. Used the arm and hand that supported the person's neck and shoulders to give care. Co-worker supported the person.			
15. Helped the person lay down. Provided support with your locked arms. Supported person's neck and shoulders with your other arm.			

Post-Procedure	S	U	Comments
16. Provided for comfort. Positioned the person in good body alignment.	_____	_____	____________________
17. Placed the call bell within reach.	_____	_____	____________________
18. Raised or lowered bed rails. Followed plan of care.	_____	_____	____________________
19. Lowered the bed to its lowest position.	_____	_____	____________________
20. Unscreened the person.	_____	_____	____________________
21. Decontaminated your hands.	_____	_____	____________________
22. Reported and recorded your observations.	_____	_____	____________________

Moving the Person Up in Bed

QUALITY OF LIFE

Name: ______________________

Date: ______________________

Remembered to:
- **Knock before entering the person's room**
- **Address the person by name**
- **Introduce yourself by name and title**

Pre-Procedure	S	U	Comments
1. Followed Delegation Guidelines: Lifting and Moving Persons in Bed. Viewed Safety Alert: Lifting and Moving Persons in Bed.	____	____	____
2. Ask co-worker to assist, if needed.	____	____	____
3. Completed hand hygiene.	____	____	____
4. Identified the person. Checked the identification bracelet against the assignment sheet. Called the person by name.	____	____	____
5. Explained the procedure to the person.	____	____	____
6. Provided for privacy.	____	____	____
7. Locked the bed wheels.	____	____	____
8. Raised the bed for body mechanics. Raised bed rails if used.	____	____	____

Procedure

	S	U	Comments
9. Lowered the head of the bed to a level appropriate for the person. It was as flat as possible.	____	____	____
10. Stood on one side of the bed. Co-worker stood on the other side.	____	____	____
11. Lowered the bed rail near you. Co-worker lowered the bed rail near him or her.	____	____	____
12. Placed the pillow against the headboard if person could be without to prevent the person's head from hitting the headboard when moved up in bed.	____	____	____
13. Stood with a wide base of support. Pointed the foot nearest the head of the bed toward the head of the bed. Faced the head of the bed.	____	____	____
14. Bent your hips and knees. Kept your back straight.	____	____	____
15. Placed one arm under the person's shoulder and one arm under the thighs. Co-worker did the same. Grasped each other's forearms.	____	____	____
16. Asked the person to grasp the trapeze, if present.	____	____	____
17. Had the person flex both knees.	____	____	____
18. Explained that you will move on the count of "3." If able, the person pushed against the bed with his or her feet.	____	____	____
19. Moved the person to the head of the bed on the count of "3." Shifted your weight from your rear leg to your front leg.	____	____	____
20. Repeated until the person was appropriately positioned.			
a. Stood with a wide base of support. Pointed the foot nearest the head of the bed toward the head of the bed. Faced the head of the bed.	____	____	____
b. Bent your hips and knees. Kept your back straight.	____	____	____

Procedure—cont'd	S	U	Comments
c. Placed one arm under the person's shoulder and one arm under the thighs. Co-worker did the same. Grasped each other's forearms.	____	____	________
d. Asked the person to grasp the trapeze, if present.	____	____	________
e. Had the person flex both knees.	____	____	________
f. Explained that you will move on the count of "3." The person pushed against the bed with their feet if able.	____	____	________
g. Moved the person to the head of the bed on the count of "3". Shifted your weight from your rear leg to your front leg.	____	____	________

Post-Procedure

	S	U	Comments
21. Placed the pillow under the person's head and shoulders. Straightened the linens.	____	____	________
22. Provided for comfort. Positioned the person in good body alignment.	____	____	________
23. Placed the call bell within reach.	____	____	________
24. Raised or lowered bed rails. Followed the care plan.	____	____	________
25. Raised the head of the bed to a level that was appropriate for the person.	____	____	________
26. Lowered the bed to its lowest position.	____	____	________
27. Unscreened the person.	____	____	________
28. Decontaminated your hands.	____	____	________
29. Reported and recorded your observations.	____	____	________

Moving the Person Up in Bed

QUALITY OF LIFE

Name: ______________________

Date: ______________________

Remembered to:
- **Knock before entering the person's room**
- **Address the person by name**
- **Introduce yourself by name and title**

Pre-Procedure	**S**	**U**	**Comments**
1. Followed Delegation Guidelines: Lifting and Moving Persons in Bed. Viewed Safety Alert: Lifting and Moving Persons in Bed.	____	____	____________
2. Asked co-worker to assist, if needed.	____	____	____________
3. Completed hand hygiene.	____	____	____________
4. Identified the person. Checked the identification bracelet against the assignment sheet. Called the person by name.	____	____	____________
5. Explained the procedure to the person.	____	____	____________
6. Provided for privacy.	____	____	____________
7. Locked the bed wheels.	____	____	____________
8. Raised the bed for body mechanics. Bed rails were up, if used.	____	____	____________
Procedure			
9. Lowered the head of the bed to a level appropriate for the person. It was as flat as possible.	____	____	____________
10. Stood on one side of the bed. Co-worker stood on the other side.	____	____	____________
11. Lowered the bed rails if up.	____	____	____________
12. Placed the pillow against the headboard if the person could be without it.	____	____	____________
13. Stood with a broad base of support. Pointed the foot nearest the head of the bed toward the head of the bed. Faced the head of the bed.	____	____	____________
14. Rolled the sides of the lift sheet up close to the person.	____	____	____________
15. Firmly grasped the rolled up lift sheet near the person's shoulders and buttocks. Supported the head.	____	____	____________
16. Bent your hips and knees.	____	____	____________
17. Moved the person up in bed on the count of "3." Shifted your weight from your rear leg to your front leg.	____	____	____________
18. Repeated until person was appropriately positioned.			
a. Stood with a broad base of support. Pointed the foot nearest the head of the bed toward the head of the bed. Faced the head of the bed.	____	____	____________
b. Rolled the sides of the lift sheet up close to the person.	____	____	____________
c. Firmly grasped the rolled up lift sheet near the person's shoulders and buttocks. Supported the person's head.	____	____	____________
d. Bent your hips and knees.	____	____	____________
e. Moved the person up in bed on the count of "3." Shifted your weight from your rear leg to your front leg.	____	____	____________

Post-Procedure	S	U	Comments
19. Unrolled the lift sheet.			
20. Placed the pillow under the person's head and shoulders. Straightened linens.			
21. Provided for comfort. Positioned the person in good body alignment.			
22. Placed the call bell within reach.			
23. Raised or lowered the bed rails. Followed the care plan.			
24. Raised the head of the bed to a level appropriate for the person.			
25. Lowered the bed to its lowest position.			
26. Unscreened the person.			
27. Decontaminated your hands.			
28. Reported and recorded your observations.			

Moving the Person to the Side of the Bed

QUALITY OF LIFE

Name: ______________________

Date: ______________________

Remembered to:
- **Knock before entering the person's room**
- **Address the person by name**
- **Introduce yourself by name and title**

Pre-Procedure	**S**	**U**	**Comments**
1. Followed Delegation Guidelines: Lifting and Moving Persons in Bed. Viewed Safety Alert: Lifting and Moving Persons in Bed and Moving the Person to the Side of the Bed.	_____	_____	__________
2. Asked co-worker to assist, if needed.	_____	_____	__________
3. Completed hand hygiene.	_____	_____	__________
4. Identified the person. Checked the identification bracelet against the assignment sheet. Called the person by name.	_____	_____	__________
5. Explained the procedure to the person.	_____	_____	__________
6. Provided for privacy.	_____	_____	__________
7. Locked the bed wheels.	_____	_____	__________
8. Raised the bed for body mechanics. Raised bed rails if used.	_____	_____	__________

Procedure

9. Lowered the head of the bed to a level appropriate for the person. It was as flat as possible.	_____	_____	__________
10. Stood on the side of the bed to which you will move the person.	_____	_____	__________
11. Lowered the bed rail near you if bed rails were used.	_____	_____	__________
12. Stood with your feet about 12 inches apart with one foot in front of the other. Flexed your knees.	_____	_____	__________
13. Crossed the person's arms over his or her chest.	_____	_____	__________
14. *Method 1:* Moving the person in segments:			
a. Placed your arm under the person's neck and shoulders. Grasped the far shoulder.	_____	_____	__________
b. Placed your other arm under the person's middle back.	_____	_____	__________
c. Moved the upper part of the person's body toward you. Rocked backward and shifted your weight to your rear leg.	_____	_____	__________
d. Placed one arm under the person's waist and one under his or her thighs.	_____	_____	__________
e. Rocked backward to move the lower part of the person toward you.	_____	_____	__________
f. Placed one arm under the person's thighs and the other under his or her calves.	_____	_____	__________
g. Rocked backward to move the legs and feet of the person toward you.	_____	_____	__________
15. *Method 2:* Moving the person with a lift sheet:			
a. Lowered both bed rails if bed rails were used.	_____	_____	__________
b. Rolled the lift sheet up close to the person.	_____	_____	__________

Procedure—cont'd

	S	U	Comments
c. Grasped the rolled up lift sheet near the person's shoulders and buttocks. Co-worker did the same. Supported the person's head.	____	____	____
d. Rocked backward on the count of "3," and moved the person toward you. Co-worker rocked backward slightly and then forward toward you, keeping arms straight.	____	____	____
e. Unrolled the lift sheet. Removed any wrinkles.	____	____	____

Post-Procedure

	S	U	Comments
16. Provided for comfort.	____	____	____
17. Positioned the person in good body alignment. Followed the nurse's direction and the plan of care.	____	____	____
18. Placed the call bell within reach.	____	____	____
19. Raised or lowered the bed rails. Followed the plan of care.	____	____	____
20. Lowered the bed to its lowest position.	____	____	____
21. Unscreened the person.	____	____	____
22. Decontaminated your hands.	____	____	____
23. Reported and recorded your observations.	____	____	____

Turning and Positioning a Person

QUALITY OF LIFE

Name: ______________________

Date: ______________________

Remembered to:
- ◆ **Knock before entering the person's room**
- ◆ **Address the person by name**
- ◆ **Introduce yourself by name and title**

Pre-Procedure	**S**	**U**	**Comments**
1. Followed Delegation Guidelines: Turning Person. Viewed Safety Alert: Turning Persons.	____	____	____________
2. Completed hand hygiene.	____	____	____________
3. Identified the person. Checked the identification bracelet against the assignment sheet. Called the person by name.	____	____	____________
4. Explained the procedure to the person.	____	____	____________
5. Provided for privacy.	____	____	____________
6. Locked the bed wheels.	____	____	____________
7. Raised the bed for body mechanics. Raised bed rails if used.	____	____	____________
Procedure			
8. Lowered the head of the bed to level appropriate for the person. It was as flat as possible.	____	____	____________
9. Stood on the opposite side of the bed to where you were turning the person. The far bed rail was up if used.	____	____	____________
10. Lowered the bed rail near you.	____	____	____________
11. Moved the person to the side near you.	____	____	____________
12. Crossed the person's arms over his or her chest. Crossed the leg near you over the far leg.	____	____	____________
13. Moved the person away from you:			
a. Stood with a wide base of support. Flexed your knees.	____	____	____________
b. Placed one hand on the person's shoulder. Placed the other on the person's buttock near you.	____	____	____________
c. Gently pushed the person toward the other side of the bed. Shifted your weight from your rear leg to your front leg.	____	____	____________
14. Moved the person toward you:			
a. Raised the bed rail.	____	____	____________
b. Went to the other side of the bed. Lowered the bed rail if used.	____	____	____________
c. Stood with a wide base of support. Flexed your knees.	____	____	____________
d. Placed one hand on the person's far shoulder. Placed your other hand on the person's far hip.	____	____	____________
e. Gently rolled the person toward you.	____	____	____________
15. Positioned the person. Followed the nurse's directions and the plan of care. Performed the following if appropriate for the person:	____	____	____________
a. Placed a pillow under the head and neck.	____	____	____________
b. Adjusted the shoulder. Person was not laying on his or her arm.	____	____	____________

Procedure—cont'd	S	U	Comments
c. Placed a small pillow under the person's upper hand and arm.	_____	_____	__________
d. Positioned a pillow against the back.	_____	_____	__________
e. Flexed the upper knee. Positioned the upper leg in front of the lower leg.	_____	_____	__________
f. Supported the upper leg and thigh on pillows.	_____	_____	__________

Post-Procedure

	S	U	Comments
16. Provided for comfort.	_____	_____	__________
17. Placed the call bell within reach.	_____	_____	__________
18. Raised or lowered bed rails. Followed the care plan.	_____	_____	__________
19. Lowered the bed to its lowest position.	_____	_____	__________
20. Unscreened the person.	_____	_____	__________
21. Decontaminated your hands.	_____	_____	__________
22. Reported and recorded your observations.	_____	_____	__________

Logrolling the Person

Quality of Life

Name: ____________________

Date: ____________________

Remembered to:
- **Knock before entering the person's room**
- **Address the person by name**
- **Introduce yourself by name and title**

Pre-Procedure	S	U	Comments
1. Followed Delegation Guidelines: Turning Persons. Viewed Safety Alerts: Turning Persons and Logrolling Persons.	____	____	____
2. Asked co-worker to assist you.	____	____	____
3. Completed hand hygiene.	____	____	____
4. Identified the person. Checked the identification bracelet against the assignment sheet. Called the person by name.	____	____	____
5. Explained the procedure to the person.	____	____	____
6. Provided for privacy.	____	____	____
7. Locked the bed wheels.	____	____	____
8. Raised the bed for body mechanics. Raised bed rails if used.	____	____	____
Procedure			
9. Made sure the bed was flat.	____	____	____
10. Stood on the opposite side to which you turned the person. Co-worker stood on the other side.	____	____	____
11. Lowered the bed rails if used.	____	____	____
12. Moved the person as a unit to the side of the bed near you. Used the turn sheet.	____	____	____
13. Placed the person's arms across his or her chest. Placed a pillow between the knees.	____	____	____
14. Raised the bed rail if used.	____	____	____
15. Went to the other side.	____	____	____
16. Stood near the shoulders and chest. Co-worker stood near the buttocks and thighs.	____	____	____
17. Stood with a broad base of support. Placed one foot in front of the other.	____	____	____
18. Asked the person to hold his or her body rigid.	____	____	____
19. Rolled the person toward you, or used a turn sheet. Turned the person as a unit.	____	____	____
Post-Procedure			
20. Provided for comfort. Positioned the person in good body alignment. Used pillows as directed by the nurse and care plan. Used the following if appropriate for the person (unless spinal cord involvement):	____	____	____
a. Placed one pillow against the back for support.	____	____	____
b. Placed one pillow under the head and neck if allowed.	____	____	____
c. Placed one pillow or folded bath blanket between the legs.	____	____	____
d. Placed a small pillow under the arm and hand.	____	____	____

Post-Procedure—cont'd

	S	U	Comments
21. Placed the call bell within reach.			
22. Raised or lowered bed rails. Followed care plan.			
23. Lowered the bed to its lowest position.			
24. Unscreened the person.			
25. Decontaminated your hands.			
26. Reported and recorded your observations.			

Helping the Person to Sit on the Side of the Bed (Dangle)

QUALITY OF LIFE

Name: ______________________

Date: ______________________

Remembered to:
- Knock before entering the person's room
- Address the person by name
- Introduce yourself by name and title

Pre-Procedure	S	U	Comments
1. Followed Delegation Guidelines: Dangling. Viewed Safety Alert: Dangling.			
2. Explained the procedure to the person.			
3. Completed hand hygiene.			
4. Identified the person. Checked the identification bracelet against the assignment sheet. Called the person by name.			
5. Decided what side of the bed to use.			
6. Moved furniture to provide moving space.			
7. Provided for privacy.			
8. Positioned the person in a side-lying position facing you. Lay the person on the strong side.			
9. Locked the bed wheels.			
10. Raised the bed for body mechanics. Raised bed rails if used.			

Procedure	S	U	Comments
11. Raised the head of the bed to a sitting position.			
12. Lowered the bed rail if up.			
13. Stood by the person's hips. Faced the foot of the bed.			
14. Stood with feet apart. The foot near the head of the bed was in front of the other foot.			
15. Slid one arm under the person's neck and shoulders. Grasped the person's far shoulder. Placed your other hand over his or her thighs near the knees.			
16. Pivoted toward the foot of the bed while moving the person's legs and feet over the side of the bed. As the legs went over the edge of the mattress, the person's truck became upright.			
17. Asked the person to hold onto the edge of the mattress. This supported the person in the sitting position.			
18. Made sure to never leave the person alone. Provided support if necessary.			
19. Checked the person's condition:			
a. Asked how the person felt. Asked if he or she was dizzy or lightheaded.			
b. Checked pulse and respirations.			
c. Checked for difficulty breathing.			
d. Noted whether the skin was pale or bluish in color (cyanosis).			
20. Helped the person lay down if necessary.			

Procedure—cont'd

	S	U	Comments
21. Reversed the procedure to return the person to bed:			
a. Stood at the side of the person nearest the headboard. Faced the foot of the bed.	_____	_____	__________
b. Placed one arm under the person's neck across the shoulders. Grasped the far shoulder. Slid your other arm under the thighs near the knees.	_____	_____	__________
c. Pivoted toward the head of the bed while moving the person's legs and feet up onto the mattress.	_____	_____	__________
22. Lowered the head of the bed after the person returned to bed. Helped the person move to center of the bed.	_____	_____	__________

Post-Procedure

	S	U	Comments
23. Provided for comfort. Positioned the person in good body alignment.	_____	_____	__________
24. Placed the call bell within reach.	_____	_____	__________
25. Lowered the bed to its lowest position.	_____	_____	__________
26. Raised or lowered bed rails. Followed the plan of care.	_____	_____	__________
27. Returned furniture to its proper place.	_____	_____	__________
28. Unscreened the person.	_____	_____	__________
29. Decontaminated your hands.	_____	_____	__________
30. Reported and recorded your observations.	_____	_____	__________

Applying a Transfer Belt

Quality of Life

Name: ______________________

Date: ______________________

Remembered to:
- **Knock before entering the person's room**
- **Address the person by name**
- **Introduce yourself by name and title**

Procedure	S	U	Comments
1. Viewed Safety Alert: Transfer Belts.	____	____	________
2. Completed hand hygiene.	____	____	________
3. Identified the person. Checked the identification bracelet against the assignment sheet. Called the person by name.	____	____	________
4. Explained the procedure to the person.	____	____	________
5. Provided for privacy.	____	____	________
6. Assisted the person into a sitting position.	____	____	________
7. Applied the belt around the person's waist over clothing. Did not apply it over bare skin.	____	____	________
8. Tightened the belt so that it was snug. Made sure that it did not cause discomfort or impair breathing. Slid your open flat hand under the belt.	____	____	________
9. Made sure that a woman's breast or folds of skin were not caught under the belt.	____	____	________
10. Placed the buckle off center in the front or in the back for the person's comfort. Make sure that the buckle was not over the spine.	____	____	________

Transferring the Person to a Chair

QUALITY OF LIFE

Name: ______________________

Date: ______________________

Remembered to:
- **Knock before entering the person's room**
- **Address the person by name**
- **Introduce yourself by name and title**

Pre-Procedure

	S	U	Comments
1. Followed Delegation Guidelines: Transferring Persons. Viewed Safety Alerts: Transferring Persons; Transfer Belts, and Chair or Wheelchair Transfers.			
2. Explained the procedure to the person.			
3. Collected:			
• Wheelchair or arm chair			
• Bath blanket			
• Lap blanket			
• Robe and nonskid footwear			
• Paper or sheet			
• Transfer belt if needed			
• Seat cushion if needed			
4. Completed hand hygiene.			
5. Identified the person. Checked the identification bracelet against the assignment sheet. Called the person by name.			
6. Provided for privacy.			
7. Decided which side of the bed to use. Moved furniture for moving space.			

Procedure

	S	U	Comments
8. Placed the chair at the head of the bed, even with the headboard.			
9. Placed a folded bath blanket or cushion on the seat if needed.			
10. Locked wheelchair wheels. Raised the footrests. Removed the footrests, or swung them out of the way.			
11. Lowered the bed to its lowest position. Locked the bed wheels.			
12. Fanfolded top linens to the foot of the bed.			
13. Placed the paper of the sheet under the person's feet. Put footwear on the person.			
14. Helped the person sit on the side of the bed. Made sure the person's feet touched the floor.			
15. Helped the person put on a robe.			
16. Applied the transfer belt if needed.			
17. *Method 1:* Transfer belt:			
a. Stood in front of the person.			
b. Had the person hold onto the mattress.			
c. Made sure the person's feet were flat on the floor.			

Procedure—cont'd	S	U	Comments
d. Had the person lean forward.	_____	_____	_____
e. Grasped the transfer belt at each side. Grasped the belt from underneath.	_____	_____	_____
f. Braced your knees against the person's knees. Blocked the person's feet with your feet, or used the knee and foot of one leg to block the person's weak foot. Placed your other foot slightly behind you for balance.	_____	_____	_____
g. Asked the person to push down on the mattress and to stand on the count of "3." Pulled the person into a standing position as you straightened your knees.	_____	_____	_____
18. *Method 2:* No transfer belt:			
a. Stood in front of the person.	_____	_____	_____
b. Had the person hold onto the mattress.	_____	_____	_____
c. Made sure the person's feet were on the floor.	_____	_____	_____
d. Slid your hands under the person's arms and placed them on the person's shoulder blades.	_____	_____	_____
e. Had the person lean forward.	_____	_____	_____
f. Braced your knees against the person's knees. Blocked the person's feet with your feet, or used the knee and foot of one leg to block the person's weak foot. Placed your other foot slightly behind you for balance.	_____	_____	_____
g. Asked the person to push down on the mattress and stand on the count of "3." Pulled the person up into a standing position as your knees straightened.	_____	_____	_____
19. Supported the person in the standing position. Held the transfer belt, or kept your hands around the person's shoulder blades. Continued to block the person's feet and knees with your feet and knees. Helped prevent the person from falling.	_____	_____	_____
20. Turned the person so he or she could grasp the far arm of the chair. The person's legs touched the edge of the chair.	_____	_____	_____
21. Continued to turn the person until the other armrest was grasped.	_____	_____	_____
22. Lowered the person into the chair as you bent your hips and knees. The person assisted by leaning forward and bending his or her elbows and knees.	_____	_____	_____
23. Made sure the buttocks are to the back of the seat. Positioned the person in good alignment.	_____	_____	_____
24. Attached the wheelchair footrests. Positioned the person's feet on the wheelchair footrests.	_____	_____	_____
25. Covered the person's lap and legs with a lap blanket. Kept the blanket off the floor and away from the wheels.	_____	_____	_____
26. Removed the transfer belt if used.	_____	_____	_____
27. Positioned the chair as the person preferred. Locked the wheelchair wheels.	_____	_____	_____

Post-Procedure	S	U	Comments
28. Placed the call bell and other needed items within reach.	_____	_____	____________________
29. Unscreened the person.	_____	_____	____________________
30. Decontaminated your hands.	_____	_____	____________________
31. Reported and recorded your observations.	_____	_____	____________________

Transferring the Person from a Chair or Wheelchair to the Bed

QUALITY OF LIFE

Name: ____________________

Date: ____________________

Remembered to:
- ◆ **Knock before entering the person's room**
- ◆ **Address the person by name**
- ◆ **Introduce yourself by name and title**

Pre-Procedure	S	U	Comments
1. Followed Delegation Guidelines: Transferring Persons. Viewed Safety Alerts: Transferring Persons; Safety Belts, and Chair or Wheelchair Transfers.	___	___	___
2. Explained the procedure to the person.	___	___	___
3. Collected paper or sheet and a transfer belt if needed.	___	___	___
4. Completed hand hygiene.	___	___	___
5. Identified the person. Checked the identification bracelet against the assignment sheet. Called the person by name.	___	___	___
6. Provided for privacy.	___	___	___

Procedure

	S	U	Comments
7. Moved furniture for moving space.	___	___	___
8. Raised the head of the bed to a sitting position. The bed was in the lowest position.	___	___	___
9. Moved the call bell so that it was on the strong side when the person was in bed.	___	___	___
10. Positioned the chair or wheelchair so that the person's strong side was next to the bed. Asked co-worker to help if necessary.	___	___	___
11. Locked the wheelchair and bed wheels.	___	___	___
12. Removed and folded the lap blanket.	___	___	___
13. Removed the person's feet from the footrests. Raised the footrests. Removed the footrests, or swung them out of the way.	___	___	___
14. Applied the transfer belt if needed.	___	___	___
15. Made sure the person's feet were flat on the floor.	___	___	___
16. Stood in front of the person.	___	___	___
17. Asked the person to hold on to the armrests, or slid your hands under the person's arms and placed them on the person's shoulder blades.	___	___	___
18. Had the person lean forward.	___	___	___
19. Grasped the transfer belt on each side if using it. Grasped the belt underhanded.	___	___	___
20. Braced your knees against the person's knees. Blocked the person's feet with your feet, or used your knee and foot of one leg to block the person's weak foot. Placed your other foot slightly behind you for balance.	___	___	___
21. Asked the person to push down on the armrests on the count of "3." Pulled the person into a standing position as you straightened your knees.	___	___	___

Procedure—cont'd	S	U	Comments
22. Supported the person in the standing position. Held the transfer belt, or kept your hands around the person's shoulder blades. Continued to block the person's knees and feet with your knees and feet.	_____	_____	_______________
23. Turned the person so he or she could reach the edge of the mattress. Make sure the person's legs touched the mattress.	_____	_____	_______________
24. Continued to turn the person until he or she reached the mattress with both hands.	_____	_____	_______________
25. Lowered the person onto the bed as you bent your hips and knees. The person assisted by leaning forward and by bending elbows and knees.	_____	_____	_______________
26. Removed the transfer belt.	_____	_____	_______________
27. Removed the robe and footwear.	_____	_____	_______________
28. Helped the person lay down.	_____	_____	_______________

Post-Procedure

29. Provided the comfort. Covered the person as needed.	_____	_____	_______________
30. Placed the call bell and other needed items within reach.	_____	_____	_______________
31. Arranged furniture to meet the person's needs.	_____	_____	_______________
32. Unscreened the person.	_____	_____	_______________
33. Decontaminated your hands.	_____	_____	_______________
34. Reported and recorded your observations.	_____	_____	_______________

Transferring the Person to a Wheelchair

QUALITY OF LIFE

Name: ______________________

Date: ______________________

Remembered to:
- ◆ **Knock before entering the person's room**
- ◆ **Address the person by name**
- ◆ **Introduce yourself by name and title**

Pre-Procedure	S	U	Comments
1. Followed Delegations Guidelines: Transferring Persons. Viewed Safety Alerts: Transferring Persons; Chair or Wheelchair Transfers, and Wheelchair Transfers With Assistance.	___	___	___
2. Asked a co-worker to assist.	___	___	___
3. Explained the procedure to the person.	___	___	___
4. Collected:			
• Wheelchair with removable armrests	___	___	___
• Bath blanket	___	___	___
• Lap blanket	___	___	___
• Nonskid footwear	___	___	___
• Seat cushion if used	___	___	___
5. Decontaminated your hands.	___	___	___
6. Identified the person. Checked the identification bracelet against the assignment sheet. Called the person by name.	___	___	___
7. Provided for privacy.	___	___	___
8. Decided which side of the bed to use. Moved furniture for moving space.	___	___	___

Procedure	S	U	Comments
9. Fanfolded tap linens to the foot of the bed.	___	___	___
10. Assisted the person to the side of the bed near you. Raised the head of the bed.	___	___	___
11. Placed the wheelchair at the side of the bed, even with the person's hips.	___	___	___
12. Removed the footrests.	___	___	___
13. Removed the armrest near the bed.	___	___	___
14. Placed the cushion or a folded bath blanket on the seat.	___	___	___
15. Locked wheelchair and bed wheels.	___	___	___
16. Stood behind the wheelchair. Slid your arms under the person's arms and grasped the person's forearms.	___	___	___
17. Co-worker grasped the person's thighs and calves.	___	___	___
18. Brought the person toward the chair on the count of "3." Lowered the person into the chair.	___	___	___
19. Made sure the person's buttocks were to the back of the seat. Positioned the person in good body alignment.	___	___	___
20. Replaced the armrest and footrests on the wheelchair.	___	___	___
21. Placed footwear on the person. Positioned the person's feet on the footrests.	___	___	___

Procedure—cont'd	S	U	Comments
22. Covered the person's lap and legs with a lap blanket. Kept the blanket off the floor and wheels.	____	____	____
23. Positioned the chair as the person preferred. Locked wheelchair wheels.	____	____	____

Post-Procedure

	S	U	Comments
24. Placed the call bell and other needed items within reach.	____	____	____
25. Unscreened the person.	____	____	____
26. Decontaminated your hands.	____	____	____
27. Reported and recorded your observations.	____	____	____
28. Reversed the procedure to return the person to bed:			
a. Placed the person in the wheelchair next to the side of the bed. Elevated the head of the bed.	____	____	____
b. Locked wheelchair and bed wheels.	____	____	____
c. Removed and folded the lap blanket.	____	____	____
d. Removed the person's feet from the footrests. Raised the footrests. Removed the footrests or swung them out of the way.	____	____	____
e. Removed armrest near the bed.	____	____	____
f. Stood behind the wheelchair. Slid your arms under the person's arms and grasped the person's forearms.	____	____	____
g. Co-worker grasped the person's thighs and calves.	____	____	____
h. Brought the person toward the bed on the count of "3."	____	____	____
i. Made sure that the person was positioned safely on the bed and in good body alignment.	____	____	____
j. Provided for comfort. Covered the person as needed.	____	____	____
k. Placed the call bell and other needed items within reach.	____	____	____
l. Arranged furniture to meet the person's needs.	____	____	____
m. Unscreened the person.	____	____	____
n. Decontaminated your hands.	____	____	____
o. Reported and recorded your observations.	____	____	____

Transferring a Person Using a Mechanical Lift

QUALITY OF LIFE

Name: ____________________

Date: ____________________

Remembered to:
- ◆ **Knock before entering the person's room**
- ◆ **Address the person by name**
- ◆ **Introduce yourself by name and title**

Pre-Procedure	**S**	**U**	**Comments**
1. Followed Delegation Guidelines: Transferring Persons. Viewed Safety Alerts: Transferring Persons and Mechanical Lifts.	____	____	____________
2. Asked co-worker to assist.	____	____	____________
3. Explained the procedure to the person.	____	____	____________
4. Collected:			
• Mechanical lift	____	____	____________
• Arm chair or wheelchair	____	____	____________
• Footwear	____	____	____________
• Bath blanket or cushion	____	____	____________
• Lap blanket	____	____	____________
5. Completed hand hygiene.	____	____	____________
6. Identified the person. Checked the identification bracelet against the assignment sheet. Called the person by name.	____	____	____________
7. Provided for privacy.	____	____	____________

Procedure

8. Centered the sling under the person. Positioned the sling according to the manufacturer's instructions.	____	____	____________
9. Placed the chair at the head of the bed, even with the head-board and about 1 foot away from the bedside. Placed a folded bath blanket or cushion in the chair.	____	____	____________
10. Locked the bed wheels. Lowered the bed to its lowest position.	____	____	____________
11. Raised the lift so that it was positioned over the person.	____	____	____________
12. Positioned the lift over the person.	____	____	____________
13. Locked the lift wheels in position.	____	____	____________
14. Attached the sling to the swivel bar.	____	____	____________
15. Raised the head of the bed to a sitting position.	____	____	____________
16. Crossed the person's arms over the chest, or made sure the person held on to the straps or chains and not the swivel bar.	____	____	____________
17. Raised the lift high enough until the person and sling were free of the bed.	____	____	____________
18. Had co-worker support the person's legs as you moved the lift and person away from the bed.	____	____	____________
19. Positioned the lift so that the person's back was toward the chair.	____	____	____________
20. Positioned the chair so that you could lower the person into it.	____	____	____________

Procedure—cont'd	S	U	Comments
21. Lowered and guided the person into the chair.	______	______	______________
22. Lowered the swivel bar to unhook the sling. Left the sling under the person unless otherwise indicated.	______	______	______________
23. Placed footwear on the person. Positioned the person's feet on the wheelchair footrests.	______	______	______________
24. Covered the person's lap and legs with a lap blanket. Kept it off the floor and wheels.	______	______	______________
25. Positioned the chair as the person preferred. Locked the wheelchair wheels.	______	______	______________

Post-Procedure

26. Placed the call bell and other needed items within reach.	______	______	______________
27. Unscreened the person.	______	______	______________
28. Decontaminated your hands.	______	______	______________
29. Reported and recorded your observations.	______	______	______________
30. Reversed the procedure to return the person to bed:			
a. Placed the wheelchair at the head of the bed, 1 foot away from the bed side.	______	______	______________
b. Locked wheelchair and bed wheels. Lowered bed to lowest position.	______	______	______________
c. Removed the person's footwear and lap blanket.	______	______	______________
d. Positioned the lift over the person.	______	______	______________
e. Locked the lift wheels in position.	______	______	______________
f. Attached the sling to the swivel bar.	______	______	______________
g. Crossed the person's arms over the chest, or made sure that the person hung on to the straps or chains but not the swivel bar.	______	______	______________
h. Raised the lift high enough until the person and sling were free of the chair.	______	______	______________
i. Had your co-worker support the person's legs as you moved the lift and person away from the chair.	______	______	______________
j. Positioned the lift so that the person was over the bed. The person's back was toward the head of the bed, and the person's legs were toward the foot of the bed.	______	______	______________
k. Lowered the person onto the bed. Guided the person into the center of the bed.	______	______	______________
l. Lowered the swivel bar to unhook the sling. Removed the sling according to manufacturer's instructions.	______	______	______________
m. Covered the person with appropriate linens.	______	______	______________
n. Placed the call bell and other needed items within reach.	______	______	______________
o. Unscreened the person.	______	______	______________
p. Decontaminated your hands.	______	______	______________
q. Reported and recorded your observations.	______	______	______________

Transferring a Person To and From the Toilet

QUALITY OF LIFE

Name: ______________________

Date: ______________________

Remembered to:
- ◆ Knock before entering the person's room
- ◆ Address the person by name
- ◆ Introduce yourself by name and title

Pre-Procedure	S	U	Comments
1. Followed Delegation Guidelines: Transferring Persons. Viewed Safety Alerts: Transfer Belts and Chair or Wheelchair Transfers.	______	______	______________
2. Completed hand hygiene.	______	______	______________
3. Made sure the person had an elevated toilet seat. The toilet seat and wheelchair were at the same level.	______	______	______________
4. Checked the grab bars by the toilet. Reported to the nurse if grab bars were loose and did not transfer the person to the toilet where the grab bars were not secure.	______	______	______________

Procedure

5. Had the person wear nonskid footwear.	______	______	______________
6. Positioned the wheelchair next to the toilet if enough room. If not, positioned the wheelchair at a right angle to the toilet with the person's stronger side nearest the toilet.	______	______	______________
7. Locked the wheelchair wheels.	______	______	______________
8. Raised the footrests. Removed or swung them out of the way.	______	______	______________
9. Applied the transfer belt.	______	______	______________
10. Helped the person unfasten clothing.	______	______	______________
11. Used the transfer belt to help the person stand and to turn to the toilet. Asked the person to use the grab bars to turn to the toilet.	______	______	______________
12. Supported the person with the transfer belt while he or she lowered clothing, or had the person hold on to the grab bars for support and you lowered the person's pants and undergarments.	______	______	______________
13. Used the transfer belt to lower the person onto the toilet seat.	______	______	______________
14. Removed the transfer belt.	______	______	______________
15. Told the person you will stay nearby. Reminded the person to use the call bell or call for you if help was needed.	______	______	______________
16. Closed the bathroom door to provide for privacy.	______	______	______________
17. Stayed near the bathroom. Completed other tasks in the person's room.	______	______	______________
18. Knocked on the bathroom door when the person called for you.	______	______	______________
19. Helped with wiping, perineal care, flushing, and hand-washing as needed.	______	______	______________
20. Applied transfer belt.	______	______	______________
21. Use the transfer belt to help the person stand.	______	______	______________

Procedure—cont'd	S	U	Comments
22. Helped the person rise and secured clothing.	______	______	______
23. Used the transfer belt to transfer the person to the wheelchair.	______	______	______
24. Made sure the person's buttocks were to the back of the seat. Positioned the person in good body alignment.	______	______	______
25. Positioned the person's feet on the footrests.	______	______	______
26. Covered the person's lap and legs with a lap blanket. Kept the blanket off the floor and away from the wheels.	______	______	______
27. Positioned the chair as the person preferred. Locked the wheelchair wheels.	______	______	______

Post-Procedure

28. Placed the call bell and other items within reach.	______	______	______
29. Unscreened the person.	______	______	______
30. Completed hand hygiene.	______	______	______
31. Reported and recorded your observations.	______	______	______

Transferring a Person to a Stretcher

QUALITY OF LIFE

Name: ______________________

Date: ______________________

Remembered to:
- ◆ Knock before entering the person's room
- ◆ Address the person by name
- ◆ Introduce yourself by name and title

Pre-Procedure	S	U	Comments
1. Followed Delegation Guidelines: Transferring Persons. Viewed Safety Alert: Stretcher Transfers.	_____	_____	__________
2. Asked two co-workers to help you.	_____	_____	__________
3. Explained the procedure to the person.	_____	_____	__________
4. Collected:			
• Stretcher covered with a sheet or bath blanket	_____	_____	__________
• Bath blanket	_____	_____	__________
• Pillow(s) if needed	_____	_____	__________
5. Completed hand hygiene.	_____	_____	__________
6. Identified the person. Checked the identification bracelet against the assignment sheet. Called the person by name.	_____	_____	__________
7. Provided privacy.	_____	_____	__________
8. Raised the bed to its highest level.	_____	_____	__________

Procedure	S	U	Comments
9. Positioned yourself and co-workers. Asked two co-workers to stand on the side of the bed where the stretcher would be and the third co-worker to stand on the other side of the bed.	_____	_____	__________
10. Covered the person with a bath blanket. Fanfolded top linens to the foot of the bed.	_____	_____	__________
11. Loosened the cotton drawsheet or lift sheet on each side if tucked in.	_____	_____	__________
12. Lowered the head of the bed as flat as possible.	_____	_____	__________
13. Lowered the bed rails if used.	_____	_____	__________
14. Moved the person to the side of the bed. Used drawsheet as a lift sheet.	_____	_____	__________
15. Protected the person from falling. Held his or her far arm and leg.	_____	_____	__________
16. Had your co-workers position the stretcher next to the bed. Asked them to stand behind the stretcher.	_____	_____	__________
17. Locked the bed and stretcher wheels.	_____	_____	__________
18. Rolled up and grasped the drawsheet. Provided support of the entire length of the person's body.	_____	_____	__________
19. Transferred the person to the stretcher on the count of "3." Lifted and pulled the person to the center of the stretcher.	_____	_____	__________
20. Placed one or more pillows under the person's head and shoulders if allowed. Raised the head of the stretcher if allowed.	_____	_____	__________

Procedure—cont'd	S	U	Comments
21. Covered the person. Provided for comfort.	____	____	________
22. Fastened safety straps. Raised the side rails.	____	____	________
23. Unlocked the stretcher's wheels. Transported the person.	____	____	________
Post-Procedure			
24. Decontaminated your hands.	____	____	________
25. Reported or recorded:			
• The time of the transport	____	____	________
• Where the person was transported	____	____	________
• Who went with the person	____	____	________
• How the transport was tolerated	____	____	________
26. Reversed the procedure to return the person to bed:			
a. Made sure top bed linens were fanfolded down and bed was raised to highest level with bed rails down if used.	____	____	________
b. Lowered side rail on stretcher that was next to the bed, and released safety strap.	____	____	________
c. Moved stretcher to side of bed.	____	____	________
d. Positioned yourself and two co-workers. Asked two co-workers to stand on the side of the bed where the stretcher was not. Ask the third worker to stand on the side with the stretcher.	____	____	________
e. Locked the bed and stretcher wheels.	____	____	________
f. Lowered the remaining stretcher side rail.	____	____	________
g. Removed pillows if used. Placed a pillow upright against headboard to protect person.	____	____	________
h. Rolled up the drawsheet or lift sheet next to the person. Provided support for the entire length of the person's body.	____	____	________
i. Transferred the person to the bed on the count of "3." Lifted and pulled the person to the center of the bed.	____	____	________
j. Placed pillow under person's head and shoulders. Covered the person with top linens and removed bath blanket. Provided comfort.	____	____	________
k. Raised bed rails if used. Lowered bed to the lowest level.	____	____	________
l. Unlocked the stretcher wheels and removed stretcher from bedside.	____	____	________
m. Decontaminated your hands.	____	____	________
n. Reported and recorded your observations.	____	____	________

Making a Closed Bed

QUALITY OF LIFE

Name: ______________________

Date: ______________________

Remembered to:
- ◆ **Knock before entering the person's room**
- ◆ **Address the person by name**
- ◆ **Introduce yourself by name and title**

Pre-Procedure

	S	U	Comments
1. Followed Delegation Guidelines: Making Beds. Viewed Safety Alert: Making Beds.	____	____	____________
2. Completed hand hygiene.	____	____	____________
3. Collected clean linen:			
• Mattress pad if needed	____	____	____________
• Bottom sheet (flat or fitted)	____	____	____________
• Plastic drawsheet or waterproof pad if needed	____	____	____________
• Cotton drawsheet if needed	____	____	____________
• Top sheet	____	____	____________
• Blanket	____	____	____________
• Bedspread	____	____	____________
• Two pillow cases	____	____	____________
• Bath towel(s)	____	____	____________
• Hand towel	____	____	____________
• Washcloth	____	____	____________
• Gown	____	____	____________
• Bath blanket	____	____	____________
• Gloves	____	____	____________
• Laundry bag	____	____	____________
4. Placed linen on a clean surface.	____	____	____________
5. Raised the bed for body mechanics.	____	____	____________

Procedure

	S	U	Comments
6. Put on gloves.	____	____	____________
7. Removed linen. Rolled each piece away from you. Placed each piece in a laundry bag. Discarded disposable bed protectors in the trash not in the laundry bag.	____	____	____________
8. Cleaned the bed frame and mattress if part of your job.	____	____	____________
9. Removed and discarded the gloves. Decontaminated your hands.	____	____	____________
10. Moved the mattress to the head of the bed.	____	____	____________
11. Placed the mattress pad on the mattress, even with the top of the mattress.	____	____	____________
12. Placed the bottom sheet on the mattress pad:			
a. Unfolded it lengthwise.	____	____	____________
b. Placed the center crease in the middle of the bed.	____	____	____________
c. Positioned the lower edge even with the bottom of the mattress.	____	____	____________

Procedure—cont'd	S	U	Comments
d. Placed the large hem at the top and the small hem at the bottom.	______	______	____________________
e. Faced hem-stitching downward, away from the person.	______	______	____________________
13. Opened the sheet. Fanfolded it to the other side of the bed.	______	______	____________________
14. Tucked the top of the sheet under the mattress. Made sure that the sheet was tight and smooth.	______	______	____________________
15. Made a mitered corner if using a flat sheet.	______	______	____________________
16. Placed the plastic drawsheet on the bed about 14 inches from the top of the mattress, or placed the waterproof pad on the bed.	______	______	____________________
17. Opened the plastic drawsheet. Fanfolded it to the other side of the bed.	______	______	____________________
18. Placed a cotton drawsheet over the plastic drawsheet, and covered the entire plastic drawsheet.	______	______	____________________
19. Opened the cotton drawsheet. Fanfolded it to the other side of the bed.	______	______	____________________
20. Tucked both drawsheets under the mattress one at a time or together.	______	______	____________________
21. Went to the other side of the bed.	______	______	____________________
22. Mitered the top corner of the flat bottom sheet.	______	______	____________________
23. Pulled the bottom sheet tight, allowing no wrinkles. Tucked in the sheet.	______	______	____________________
24. Pulled the drawsheets tight, allowing no wrinkles. Tucked both in together or separately.	______	______	____________________
25. Went to the other side of the bed.	______	______	____________________
26. Placed the top sheet on the bed:			
a. Unfolded it lengthwise.	______	______	____________________
b. Placed the center crease in the middle.	______	______	____________________
c. Placed the large hem even with the top of the mattress.	______	______	____________________
d. Opened the sheet. Fanfolded it to the other side.	______	______	____________________
e. Faced hem-stitching outward, away from the person.	______	______	____________________
f. Did not tuck the bottom in yet.	______	______	____________________
g. Never tucked top linens in on the sides.	______	______	____________________
27. Placed the blanket on the bed:			
a. Unfolded it lengthwise, placing the center crease in the middle.	______	______	____________________
b. Placed the upper hem about 6 to 8 inches from the top of the mattress.	______	______	____________________
c. Opened the blanket. Fanfolded it to the other side.	______	______	____________________
d. Made a cuff by turning top sheet down over the blanket with hem-stitching away from the person if performed in an agency.	______	______	____________________
28. Placed the bedspread on the bed:			
a. Unfolded it lengthwise, placing the center crease in the middle.	______	______	____________________
b. Placed the upper hem even with the top of the mattress.	______	______	____________________

Procedure—cont'd	S	U	Comments
c. Opened and fanfolded the spread to the other side.	______	______	____________
d. Made sure the spread that faced the door was even and covered all top linens.	______	______	____________
29. Tucked in top linens together at the foot of the bed. Made sure they were smooth and tight. Made a mitered corner.	______	______	____________
30. Went to the other side.	______	______	____________
31. Straightened all top linen. Worked from the head of the bed to the foot.	______	______	____________
32. Tucked in the top linens together. Made a mitered corner.	______	______	____________
33. Turned the top hem of the spread under the blanket to make a cuff, if cuff was not made yet.	______	______	____________
34. Turned the top sheet down over the spread. Hem-stitching was down (not done in all agencies in which the spread covers the pillow rather than tucked under the pillow).	______	______	____________
35. Placed the pillowcase on the pillow. Folded extra material under the pillow at the seam end of the pillowcase.	______	______	____________
36. Placed the pillow on the bed. Made sure the open end is away from the door and the seam of the pillowcase is toward the head of the bed.	______	______	____________

Post-Procedure

	S	U	Comments
37. Attached the call bell to the bed.	______	______	____________
38. Lowered the bed to its lowest position. Locked the bed wheels.	______	______	____________
39. Placed towels, washcloth, gown, and bath blanket in the bedside stand.	______	______	____________
40. Followed agency policy for dirty linen.	______	______	____________
41. Decontaminated your hands.	______	______	____________

Making an Open Bed

QUALITY OF LIFE

Name: ______________________

Date: ______________________

Remembered to:
- ◆ **Knock before entering the person's room**
- ◆ **Address the person by name**
- ◆ **Introduce yourself by name and title**

Procedure	S	U	Comments
1. Followed Delegation Guidelines: Making Beds. Viewed Safety Alert: Making Beds.	____	____	____________
2. Completed hand hygiene.	____	____	____________
3. Collected linen for a closed bed.	____	____	____________
4. Made a closed bed.	____	____	____________
5. Fanfolded linens to the foot of the bed.	____	____	____________
6. Attached the call bell to the bed.	____	____	____________
7. Lowered the bed to its lowest position.	____	____	____________
8. Placed towels, washcloth, gown, and bath blanket in the bedside stand.	____	____	____________
9. Followed agency policy for dirty linen.	____	____	____________
10. Decontaminated your hands.	____	____	____________

Making an Occupied Bed

QUALITY OF LIFE

Name: ______________________

Date: ______________________

Remembered to:
- ◆ **Knock before entering the person's room**
- ◆ **Address the person by name**
- ◆ **Introduce yourself by name and title**

Pre-Procedure

	S	U	Comments
1. Followed Delegation Guidelines: Making Beds. Viewed Safety Alerts: Making Beds and The Occupied Bed.			
2. Explained the procedure to the person.			
3. Completed hand hygiene.			
4. Collected the following:			
• Gloves			
• Laundry bag			
• Clean linen			
5. Placed linen on a clean surface.			
6. Identified the person. Checked the identification bracelet against the assignment sheet. Called the person by name.			
7. Provided for privacy.			
8. Removed the call bell.			
9. Raised the bed for body mechanics. Raised bed rails if used.			
10. Lowered the head of the bed with the head as flat as possible.			

Procedure

	S	U	Comments
11. Lowered the bed rail near you.			
12. Put on gloves.			
13. Loosened top linens at the foot of the bed.			
14. Removed the bedspread. Removed the blanket. Placed each over the chair.			
15. Covered the person with a bath blanket. Provided warmth and privacy.			
a. Unfolded a bath blanket over the top sheet.			
b. Asked the person to hold onto the bath blanket. If the person is unable, tucked the top part under the person's shoulders.			
c. Grasped the top sheet under the bath blanket at the shoulders. Brought the sheet down to the foot of the bed. Removed the sheet from under the blanket.			
16. Moved the mattress to the head of the bed.			
17. Positioned the person on the side of the bed away from you. Adjusted the pillow for comfort.			
18. Loosened bottom linens from the head of the bed to the foot.			
19. Fanfolded bottom linens one at a time toward the person. Started with the cotton drawsheet. If reusing the mattress pad, did not fanfold it.			

Procedure—cont'd	S	U	Comments
20. Placed a clean mattress pad on the bed if changed. Unfolded it lengthwise. Placed the center crease in the middle. Fanfolded the top part toward the person. If reusing the mattress pad, straightened and smoothed wrinkles.	_____	_____	____________
21. Placed the bottom sheet on the mattress pad. Placed hem-stitching away from the person. Unfolded the sheet so the crease was in the middle. The small hem was even with the bottom of the mattress. Fanfolded the top part toward the person.	_____	_____	____________
22. Made a mitered corner at the head of the bed. Tucked the sheet under the mattress from the lead to the foot.	_____	_____	____________
23. Pulled the plastic drawsheet toward you over the bottom sheet. Tucked excess material under the mattress. Performed the following for a clean plastic drawsheet:	_____	_____	____________
a. Placed the plastic drawsheet on the bed approximately 14 inches from the mattress top.	_____	_____	____________
b. Fanfolded the top part toward the person.	_____	_____	____________
c. Tucked in the excess fabric.	_____	_____	____________
24. Placed the cotton drawsheet over the plastic drawsheet. Covered the entire plastic drawsheet. Fanfolded the top part toward the person. Tucked in excess fabric.	_____	_____	____________
25. Raised the bed rail if used. Went to the other side and lowered the bed rail.	_____	_____	____________
26. Explained to the person that he or she would roll over a bump. Assured the person that he or she would not fall.	_____	_____	____________
27. Helped the person turn to the other side. Adjusted the pillow for comfort.	_____	_____	____________
28. Loosened bottom linens. Removed one piece at a time. Placed each piece in the laundry bag. Discarded disposable bed protectors in the trash. Did not put them in the laundry bag.	_____	_____	____________
29. Removed and discarded the gloves. Decontaminated your hands.	_____	_____	____________
30. Straightened and smoothed the mattress pad.	_____	_____	____________
31. Pulled the clean bottom sheet toward you. Made a mitered corner at the top. Tucked the sheet under the mattress from the head to the foot of the bed.	_____	_____	____________
32. Pulled the drawsheets tightly toward you. Tucked both under together or separately.	_____	_____	____________
33. Positioned the person supine in the center of the bed. Adjusted the pillow for comfort.	_____	_____	____________
34. Placed the top sheet on the bed. Unfolded it lengthwise. Placed the center crease in the middle. Made sure the large hem was even with the top of the mattress. Hem-stitching was on the outside.	_____	_____	____________
35. Asked the person to hold onto the top sheet as you removed the bath blanket, or tucked the top sheet under the person's shoulders. Removed the bath blanket.	_____	_____	____________

Procedure—cont'd	S	U	Comments
36. Placed the blanket on the bed. Unfolded it so that the center crease was in the middle and the blanket covered the person. Made sure that the upper hem was 6 to 8 inches from the top of the mattress.			
37. Placed the bedspread on the bed. Unfolded it so that the center crease was in the middle and the bedspread covered the person. Made sure that the top hem was even with the mattress top.			
38. Turned the top hem of the spread under the blanket to make a cuff.			
39. Brought the top sheet down over the spread to form a cuff.			
40. Went to the foot of the bed.			
41. Made a tow pleat. Made a 2-inch pleat across the foot of the bed and about 6 to 8 inches from the foot of the bed.			
42. Lifted the mattress corner with one arm. Tucked all top linens under the mattress together. Made a mitered corner.			
43. Raised the bed rail if used. Went to the other side and lowered the bed rail if used.			
44. Straightened and smoothed top linens.			
45. Tucked the top linens under the mattress. Made a mitered corner.			
46. Changed the pillowcase(s).			

Post-Procedure

	S	U	Comments
47. Placed the call bell within reach.			
48. Raised or lowered bed rails. Followed the care plan.			
49. Raised the head of the bed to the level appropriate for the person. Provided comfort.			
50. Lowered the bed to the lowest position. Locked the bed wheels.			
51. Placed towels, washcloth, gown, and bath blanket in the bedside stand.			
52. Unscreened the person. Thanked the person for cooperating.			
53. Followed agency policy for dirty linen.			
54. Decontaminated your hands.			

Making a Surgical Bed

QUALITY OF LIFE

Name: ______________________

Date: ______________________

Remembered to:
- ◆ **Knock before entering the person's room**
- ◆ **Address the person by name**
- ◆ **Introduce yourself by name and title**

Procedure	**S**	**U**	**Comments**
1. Followed Delegation Guidelines: Making Beds. Viewed Safety Alerts: Making Beds and Surgical Beds.	____	____	____________
2. Completed hand hygiene.	____	____	____________
3. Collected the following:			
• Clean linen	____	____	____________
• Gloves	____	____	____________
• Laundry bag	____	____	____________
• Equipment requested by the nurse	____	____	____________
4. Placed linen on a clean surface.	____	____	____________
5. Removed the call bell.	____	____	____________
6. Raised the bed for body mechanics.	____	____	____________
7. Removed all linen from the bed. Worn gloves.	____	____	____________
8. Made a closed bed. Did not tuck the top linens under the mattress.	____	____	____________
9. Folded all top linens at the foot of the bed back onto the bed. The fold was even with the edge of the mattress.	____	____	____________
10. Fanfolded linen lengthwise to the side of the bed farthest from the door.	____	____	____________
11. Placed the pillowcase(s) on the pillow(s).	____	____	____________
12. Placed the pillow(s) on a clean surface.	____	____	____________
13. Left the bed in its highest position.	____	____	____________
14. Left both bed rails down.	____	____	____________
15. Placed the towels, washcloth, gown, and bath blanket in the bedside stand.	____	____	____________
16. Moved furniture away from the bed. Allowed room for the stretcher and for the staff.	____	____	____________
17. Did not attach the call bell to the bed.	____	____	____________
18. Followed agency policy for soiled linen.	____	____	____________
19. Decontaminated your hands.	____	____	____________

Assisting the Person to Brush the Teeth

QUALITY OF LIFE

Name: ______________________

Date: ______________________

Remembered to:
- ◆ **Knock before entering the person's room**
- ◆ **Address the person by name**
- ◆ **Introduce yourself by name and title**

Pre-Procedure	S	U	Comments
1. Followed Delegation Guidelines: Oral Hygiene. Viewed Safety Alert: Oral Hygiene.	____	____	____________
2. Explained the procedure to the person.	____	____	____________
3. Completed hand hygiene.	____	____	____________
4. Collected the following:			
• Toothbrush	____	____	____________
• Toothpaste	____	____	____________
• Mouth wash, or solution noted on care plan	____	____	____________
• Dental floss if used	____	____	____________
• Water glass with cool water	____	____	____________
• Straw	____	____	____________
• Kidney basin	____	____	____________
• Hand towel	____	____	____________
• Paper towels	____	____	____________
5. Placed the paper towels on the overbed table. Arranged items on top of paper towels.	____	____	____________
6. Identified the person. Checked the identification bracelet against the assignment sheet. Called the person by name.	____	____	____________
7. Provided for privacy.	____	____	____________
8. Positioned the person so he or she could brush with ease.	____	____	____________
Procedure			
9. Lowered the bed rail if used.	____	____	____________
10. Placed the towel over the person's chest. Protected garments and linens from spills.	____	____	____________
11. Adjusted the overbed table in front of the person.	____	____	____________
12. Allowed the person to perform oral hygiene, including brushing the teeth, rinsing the mouth, flossing the teeth, and using mouthwash or other solution.	____	____	____________
13. Removed the towel when the person was done.	____	____	____________
14. Adjusted the overbed table next to the bed.	____	____	____________
Post-Procedure			
15. Provided for comfort.	____	____	____________
16. Placed the call bell within reach.	____	____	____________
17. Raised or lowered bed rails. Followed the care plan.	____	____	____________
18. Cleaned and returned items to their proper place. Wore gloves.	____	____	____________

Post-Procedure—cont'd	S	U	Comments
19. Wiped off the overbed table with the paper towels. Discarded the paper towels.			
20. Removed the gloves. Decontaminated your hands.			
21. Unscreened the person.			
22. Followed agency policy for dirty linen.			
23. Decontaminated your hands.			
24. Reported and recorded your observations.			

Brushing the Person's Teeth

QUALITY OF LIFE

Name: ____________________

Date: ____________________

Remembered to:
- ◆ Knock before entering the person's room
- ◆ Address the person by name
- ◆ Introduce yourself by name and title

Pre-Procedure	S	U	Comments
1. Followed Delegation Guidelines: Oral Hygiene. Viewed Safety Alert: Oral Hygiene.	____	____	____________
2. Explained the procedure to the person.	____	____	____________
3. Completed hand hygiene.	____	____	____________
4. Collected the following:			
• Gloves	____	____	____________
• Toothbrush	____	____	____________
• Tooth paste	____	____	____________
• Mouthwash or solution noted on care plan	____	____	____________
• Dental floss if used	____	____	____________
• Water glass with cool water	____	____	____________
• Straw	____	____	____________
• Kidney basin	____	____	____________
• Hand towel	____	____	____________
• Paper towels	____	____	____________
5. Placed the paper towels on the overbed table. Arranged items on top of paper towels.	____	____	____________
6. Identified the person. Checked the identification bracelet against the assignment sheet. Called the person by name.	____	____	____________
7. Provided for privacy.	____	____	____________
8. Raised the bed for body mechanics. Raised bed rails if used.	____	____	____________

Procedure	S	U	Comments
9. Lowered the bed rail nearest you if up.	____	____	____________
10. Assisted the person to a sitting position or to a side-lying position toward you.	____	____	____________
11. Placed the towel over the person's chest.	____	____	____________
12. Adjusted the overbed table so you could reach it with ease.	____	____	____________
13. Put on the gloves.	____	____	____________
14. Applied toothpaste to the toothbrush.	____	____	____________
15. Held the toothbrush over the kidney basin. Poured water over the brush.	____	____	____________
16. Gently brushed the teeth.	____	____	____________
17. Gently brushed the tongue.	____	____	____________

Procedure—cont'd	S	U	Comments
18. Allowed the person to rinse his or her mouth with water. Held the kidney basin under the person's chin. Repeated as needed.	_____	_____	_____
19. Flossed the person's teeth.	_____	_____	_____
20. Allowed the person to use mouthwash or other solution. Held the kidney basin under the person's chin.	_____	_____	_____
21. Removed the towel when done.	_____	_____	_____
22. Removed and discarded the gloves. Decontaminated your hands.	_____	_____	_____

Post-Procedure

23. Provided for comfort.	_____	_____	_____
24. Placed the call bell within reach.	_____	_____	_____
25. Lowered the bed to its lowest position.	_____	_____	_____
26. Raised or lowered bed rails. Followed care plan.	_____	_____	_____
27. Cleaned and returned equipment to its proper place. Wore gloves.	_____	_____	_____
28. Wiped off the overbed table with the paper towels. Discarded the paper towels.	_____	_____	_____
29. Removed the gloves. Decontaminated your hands.	_____	_____	_____
30. Adjusted the overbed table for the person.	_____	_____	_____
31. Unscreened the person.	_____	_____	_____
32. Followed agency policy for dirty linen.	_____	_____	_____
33. Decontaminated your hands.	_____	_____	_____
34. Reported and recorded your observations.	_____	_____	_____

Flossing the Person's Teeth

QUALITY OF LIFE

Name: ______________________

Date: ______________________

Remembered to:
- ◆ Knock before entering the person's room
- ◆ Address the person by name
- ◆ Introduce yourself by name and title

Pre-Procedure	S	U	Comments
1. Followed Delegation Guidelines: Oral Hygiene. Viewed Safety Alert: Oral Hygiene.	____	____	____________
2. Explained the procedure to the person.	____	____	____________
3. Completed hand hygiene.	____	____	____________
4. Collected the following:			
• Kidney basin	____	____	____________
• Water glass with cool water	____	____	____________
• Floss	____	____	____________
• Hand towel	____	____	____________
• Paper towels	____	____	____________
• Gloves	____	____	____________
5. Placed the paper towels on the overbed table. Arranged items on top of the paper towels.	____	____	____________
6. Identified the person. Checked the identification bracelet against the assignment sheet. Called the person by name.	____	____	____________
7. Provided for privacy.	____	____	____________
8. Raised the bed for body mechanics. Raised bed rails if used.	____	____	____________
Procedure			
9. Lowered the bed rail nearest you if up.	____	____	____________
10. Assisted the person to a sitting position or to a side-lying position facing you.	____	____	____________
11. Placed the towel over the person's chest.	____	____	____________
12. Adjusted the overbed table so you could reach it with ease.	____	____	____________
13. Put on gloves.	____	____	____________
14. Broke off an 18-inch piece of floss from the dispenser.	____	____	____________
15. Held the floss between the middle fingers of each hand.	____	____	____________
16. Stretched the floss with your thumbs.	____	____	____________
17. Started with the person's upper back tooth on the right side. Worked around to his or her left side.	____	____	____________
18. Moved the floss gently up and down between the teeth. Moved the floss up and down against the side of the tooth. Worked from the top of the crown to the gum line.	____	____	____________
19. Moved to a new section of floss after every second tooth.	____	____	____________
20. Flossed the lower teeth. Held the floss with your index fingers. Used up and down motions, and went under the gums the same as the upper teeth. Started on the right side. Worked around to the left side.	____	____	____________

Procedure—cont'd

	S	U	Comments
21. Allowed the person to rinse his or her mouth. Held the kidney basin under his or her chin. Repeated rinsing as necessary.	_____	_____	__________
22. Removed the towel when done.	_____	_____	__________
23. Removed and discarded the gloves. Decontaminated your hands.	_____	_____	__________

Post-Procedure

	S	U	Comments
24. Provided for comfort.	_____	_____	__________
25. Placed the call bell within reach.	_____	_____	__________
26. Lowered the bed to its lowest position.	_____	_____	__________
27. Raised or lowered bed rails. Followed the care plan.	_____	_____	__________
28. Cleaned and returned equipment to its proper place. Wore gloves.	_____	_____	__________
29. Wiped off the overbed table with the paper towels. Discarded the paper towels.	_____	_____	__________
30. Removed the gloves. Decontaminated your hands.	_____	_____	__________
31. Adjusted the overbed table for the person.	_____	_____	__________
32. Unscreened the person.	_____	_____	__________
33. Followed agency policy for dirty linen.	_____	_____	__________
34. Decontaminated your hands.	_____	_____	__________
35. Reported and recorded your observations.	_____	_____	__________

Providing Mouth Care for an Unconscious Person

QUALITY OF LIFE

Name: ______________________

Date: ______________________

Remembered to:
- ◆ Knock before entering the person's room
- ◆ Address the person by name
- ◆ Introduce yourself by name and title

Pre-Procedure

	S	U	Comments
1. Followed Delegation Guidelines: Oral Hygiene. Viewed Safety Alert: Oral Hygiene.	____	____	____________
2. Completed hand hygiene.	____	____	____________
3. Collected the following:			
• Cleaning agent (checked the care plan)	____	____	____________
• Sponge swabs	____	____	____________
• Padded tongue blade	____	____	____________
• Water glass with cool water	____	____	____________
• Hand towel	____	____	____________
• Kidney basin	____	____	____________
• Lip lubricant	____	____	____________
• Paper towels	____	____	____________
• Gloves	____	____	____________
4. Placed the paper towels on the overbed table. Arranged items on top of the paper towels.	____	____	____________
5. Identified the person. Checked the identification bracelet against the assignment sheet. Called the person by name.	____	____	____________
6. Explained the procedure to the person.	____	____	____________
7. Provided for privacy.	____	____	____________
8. Raised the bed for body mechanics. Raised bed rails if used.	____	____	____________

Procedure

	S	U	Comments
9. Lowered the bed rail nearest you if up.	____	____	____________
10. Put on the gloves.	____	____	____________
11. Positioned the person in a side-lying position toward you. Turned his or her head well to the side.	____	____	____________
12. Placed the towel under the person's face.	____	____	____________
13. Placed the kidney basin under his or her chin.	____	____	____________
14. Adjusted the overbed table so you could reach it with ease.	____	____	____________
15. Separated the upper and lower teeth. Gently used the padded tongue blade, never using force. If you had problems, asked the nurse for help.	____	____	____________
16. Cleaned the mouth using sponge swabs moistened with the cleaning agent.			
a. Cleaned the chewing and inner surfaces of the teeth.	____	____	____________
b. Cleaned the outer surfaces of the teeth.	____	____	____________
c. Swabbed the roof of the mouth, inside of the cheeks, and lips.	____	____	____________

Procedure—cont'd

	S	U	Comments
d. Swabbed the tongue.	____	____	____
e. Moistened a clean swab with water. Swabbed the mouth to rinse.	____	____	____
f. Placed used swabs in the kidney basin.	____	____	____
17. Applied lubricant to the lips.	____	____	____
18. Removed the towel.	____	____	____
19. Removed and discarded the gloves. Decontaminated your hands.	____	____	____
20. Explained that the procedure was done. Explained that you will reposition him or her.	____	____	____
21. Repositioned the person. Provided for comfort.	____	____	____
22. Raised or lowered bed rails. Followed the care plan.	____	____	____

Post-Procedure

	S	U	Comments
23. Placed the call bell within reach.	____	____	____
24. Lowered the bed to its lowest position.	____	____	____
25. Cleaned and returned equipment to its proper place. Discarded disposable items. Wore gloves.	____	____	____
26. Wiped off the overbed table with paper towels. Discarded the paper towels.	____	____	____
27. Removed the gloves. Decontaminated your hands.	____	____	____
28. Unscreened the person.	____	____	____
29. Told the person that you were leaving the room.	____	____	____
30. Followed agency policy for dirty linens.	____	____	____
31. Decontaminated your hands.	____	____	____
32. Reported and recorded observations.	____	____	____

Providing Denture Care

Quality of Life

Name: ______________________

Date: ______________________

Remembered to:
- ◆ Knock before entering the person's room
- ◆ Address the person by name
- ◆ Introduce yourself by name and title

Pre-Procedure	S	U	Comments
1. Followed Delegation Guidelines: Oral Hygiene. Viewed Safety Alerts: Oral Hygiene and Denture Care.	___	___	___
2. Explained the procedure to the person.	___	___	___
3. Completed hand hygiene.	___	___	___
4. Collected the following:			
• Denture brush or soft-bristled toothbrush	___	___	___
• Cleaning agent	___	___	___
• Water glass with cool water	___	___	___
• Straw	___	___	___
• Mouthwash or other noted solution	___	___	___
• Kidney basin	___	___	___
• Two hand towels	___	___	___
• Gauze squares	___	___	___
• Gloves	___	___	___
5. Identified the person. Checked the identification bracelet against the assignment sheet. Called the person by name.	___	___	___
6. Provided for privacy.	___	___	___

Procedure	S	U	Comments
7. Lowered the bed rail nearest you if used.	___	___	___
8. Placed a towel over the person's chest.	___	___	___
9. Put on the gloves.	___	___	___
10. Asked the person to remove the dentures. Carefully placed them in the kidney basin.	___	___	___
11. Removed the dentures if the person could not do so:			
a. Grasped the upper denture with your thumb and index finger. Moved it up and down slightly to break the seal. Gently removed the denture, and placed it in the kidney basin.	___	___	___
b. Grasped and removed the lower denture with your thumb and index finger. Turned it slightly, and lifted it out of the mouth. Placed it in the kidney basin.	___	___	___
c. Used gauze squares to get a good grip on the slippery dentures.	___	___	___
12. Followed the care plan for raising bed rails.	___	___	___
13. Took the kidney basin, denture cup, brush, and cleaning agent to the sink.	___	___	___
14. Lined the sink with a towel. Filled the sink with water.	___	___	___
15. Rinsed each denture under warm running water. (Some states require cool water.) Rinsed out the denture cup.	___	___	___

Procedure—cont'd	S	U	Comments
16. Returned dentures to the denture cup.			
17. Applied the cleaning agent to the brush.			
18. Brushed the dentures.			
19. Rinsed dentures under running water. Used warm or cool water as directed by the cleaning agent manufacturer. (Some states require cool water.)			
20. Placed dentures in the denture cup. Covered the dentures with cool water.			
21. Cleaned the kidney basin.			
22. Took the denture cup and kidney basin to the bedside table.			
23. Lowered the bed rail if up.			
24. Positioned the person for oral hygiene.			
25. Had the person use mouthwash or noted solution. Held the kidney basin under his or her chin.			
26. Asked the person to insert the dentures. Inserted them if the person could not.			
a. Held the upper denture firmly with your thumb and index finger. Raised the upper lip with the other hand. Inserted the denture. Gently pressed on the denture with your index fingers to make sure it was in place.			
b. Held the lower denture with your thumb and index finger. Pulled the lower lip down slightly. Inserted the denture. Gently pressed down on it to make sure it was in place.			
27. Placed the denture cup in the top drawer of the bedside stand if the dentures were not worn. Made sure the dentures were in water or in a denture-soaking solution.			
28. Removed the towel.			
29. Removed the gloves. Decontaminated your hands.			

Post-Procedure

	S	U	Comments
30. Provided for comfort.			
31. Placed the call bell within reach.			
32. Raised or lowered bed rails. Followed the care plan.			
33. Unscreened the person.			
34. Cleaned and returned equipment to its proper place. Discarded disposable items. Wore gloves.			
35. Removed gloves. Decontaminated your hands.			
36. Followed agency policy for dirty linen.			
37. Reported and recorded your observations.			

Giving a Complete Bed Bath

QUALITY OF LIFE

Name: ______________________

Date: ______________________

Remembered to:
- ◆ Knock before entering the person's room
- ◆ Address the person by name
- ◆ Introduce yourself by name and title

Pre-Procedure	S	U	Comments
1. Followed Delegation Guidelines: Bathing. Viewed Safety Alert: Bathing.			
2. Identified the person. Checked the identification bracelet against the assignment sheet. Called the person by name.			
3. Explained the procedure to the person.			
4. Offered the bedpan or urinal. Provided privacy.			
5. Completed hand hygiene.			
6. Collected clean linen for a closed bed. Placed linen on a clean surface.			
7. Collected the following:			
• Wash basin			
• Soap			
• Bath thermometer			
• Orange stick or nail file			
• Washcloth			
• Two bath towels and two hand towels			
• Bath blanket			
• Clothing, gown, or pajamas			
• Items for oral hygiene			
• Lotion			
• Powder			
• Deodorant or antiperspirant			
• Brush and comb			
• Other grooming items if requested			
• Paper towels			
• Gloves			
8. Arranged items on the overbed table. Adjusted the height as needed.			
9. Closed doors and windows to prevent drafts.			
10. Provided for privacy.			
11. Raised the bed for body mechanics. Raised bed rails if used.			

Procedure	S	U	Comments
12. Removed the call bell. Lowered the bed rail nearest you if up.			
13. Put on gloves.			
14. Provided oral hygiene.			

Procedure—cont'd

	S	U	Comments
15. Covered the person with a bath blanket. Removed top linens.	_____	_____	__________
16. Lowered the head of the bed as flat as possible. Made sure the person had at least one pillow.	_____	_____	__________
17. Covered the overbed table with paper towels.	_____	_____	__________
18. Raised the bed rail nearest you if used. Made sure both bed rails were up.	_____	_____	__________
19. Filled the wash basin half full of water. Made sure the water temperature was 110° to 115° F (43° to 46° C) for adults. Followed agency policy. Measured water temperature. Used a bath thermometer, or tested the water by dipping your elbow or inner wrist into the basin.	_____	_____	__________
20. Placed the basin on the overbed table.	_____	_____	__________
21. Lowered the bed rail if up.	_____	_____	__________
22. Placed a hand towel over the person's chest.	_____	_____	__________
23. Made a mitt with the washcloth. Used a mitt for the entire bath.	_____	_____	__________
24. Washed around the person's eyes with water. Did not use soap. Gently wiped from the inner to the outer aspect of the eye with a corner of the mitt. Cleaned the far eye first. Repeated for the nearest eye. Gently wiped from the inner to the outer aspect of the eye with a corner of the mitt. Used a clean part of the washcloth for each stroke.	_____	_____	__________
25. Asked the person if you should use soap to wash his or her face.	_____	_____	__________
26. Washed the face, ears, and neck. Rinsed and patted dry the person's face with the towel on the chest.	_____	_____	__________
27. Helped the person move to the side of the bed nearest you.	_____	_____	__________
28. Removed the gown. Avoided exposing the person. (Waited to remove the gown, helping the person feel less exposed and more comfortable with the bath.)	_____	_____	__________
29. Placed a bath towel lengthwise under the person's far arm.	_____	_____	__________
30. Supported the arm with your palm under the person's elbow. Made sure his or her forearm was resting on your forearm.	_____	_____	__________
31. Washed the arm, shoulder, and underarm. Used long, firm strokes. Rinsed and patted dry.	_____	_____	__________
32. Placed the basin on the towel. Placed the person's hand into the water. Washed the hand well. Cleaned under fingernails with an orange stick or nail file.	_____	_____	__________
33. Had the person exercise his or her hand and fingers.	_____	_____	__________
34. Removed the basin. Dried the hand well. Covered the arm with the bath blanket.	_____	_____	__________
35. Repeated for the nearest arm:			
a. Placed a bath towel lengthwise under the nearest arm.	_____	_____	__________
b. Supported the arm with your palm under the person's elbow. Made sure his or her forearm was resting on your forearm.	_____	_____	__________

Procedure—cont'd	S	U	Comments
c. Washed the arm, shoulder, and underarm. Used long strokes. Rinsed and patted dry.	_____	_____	_______________
d. Placed the basin on the towel. Placed the person's hand into the water. Washed the hand well. Cleaned under fingernails with an orange stick or nail file.	_____	_____	_______________
e. Had the person exercise his or her hand and fingers.	_____	_____	_______________
f. Removed the basin. Dried the hand well. Covered the arm with the bath blanket.	_____	_____	_______________
36. Placed a bath towel over the person's chest crosswise. Held the towel in place. Pulled the bath blanket from under the towel to the waist.	_____	_____	_______________
37. Lifted the towel slightly, and washed the chest. Avoided exposing the person. Rinsed and patted dry, especially under breasts.	_____	_____	_______________
38. Moved the towel lengthwise over the person's chest and abdomen. Avoided exposing the person. Pulled the bath blanket down to the pubic area.	_____	_____	_______________
39. Lifted the towel slightly, and washed the abdomen. Rinsed and patted dry.	_____	_____	_______________
40. Pulled the bath blanket up to the person's shoulders, covering both arms. Removed the towel.	_____	_____	_______________
41. Changed soapy or cool water. Measured bath water temperature. Used a bath thermometer or tested the water by dipping your elbow or inner wrist into the basin. Raised the bed rail nearest you if used before you left the bedside. Lowered bed rail if used when you returned.	_____	_____	_______________
42. Uncovered the far leg. Avoided exposing the genital area. Placed a towel lengthwise under the foot and leg.	_____	_____	_______________
43. Bent the knee, and supported the leg with your arm. Washed it with long, firm strokes. Rinsed and patted dry.	_____	_____	_______________
44. Placed the basin on the towel near the person's foot.	_____	_____	_______________
45. Lifted the leg slightly. Slid the basin under the foot.	_____	_____	_______________
46. Placed the foot in the basin. Used an orange stick or nail file to clean under toenails if necessary. If the person did not bend his or her knee:	_____	_____	_______________
a. Washed the foot. Carefully separated the toes. Rinsed and patted dry.	_____	_____	_______________
b. Cleaned under the toenails with an orange stick or nail file if needed.	_____	_____	_______________
47. Removed the basin. Dried the leg and foot. Covered the leg with the bath blanket. Removed the towel.	_____	_____	_______________
48. Repeated for the nearest leg:			
a. Uncovered the nearest leg. Avoided exposing the genital area. Placed a towel lengthwise under the foot and leg.	_____	_____	_______________
b. Bent the knee and supported the leg with your arm. Washed it with long, firm strokes. Rinsed and patted dry.	_____	_____	_______________
c. Placed the basin on the towel near the foot.	_____	_____	_______________
d. Lifted the leg slightly. Slid the basin under the foot.	_____	_____	_______________

Procedure—cont'd	S	U	Comments
e. Placed the foot in the basin. Used an orange stick or nail file to clean under toenails if needed. If person did not bend his or her knee:	____	____	________
• Washed the foot. Carefully separated the toes. Rinsed and patted dry.	____	____	________
• Cleaned under the toenails with an orange stick or nail file if needed.	____	____	________
f. Removed basin. Dried leg and foot. Covered the leg with the bath blanket. Removed the towel	____	____	________
49. Changed the water. Measured temperature of bath water. Used a bath thermometer, or tested the water by dipping your elbow or inner wrist into the basin. Raised the bed rail nearest you if used before you left the bedside. Lowered it when you returned.	____	____	________
50. Turned the person onto the side away from you. Made sure the person was covered with the bath blanket.	____	____	________
51. Uncovered the back and buttocks. Avoided exposing the person. Placed a towel lengthwise on the bed along the back.	____	____	________
52. Washed the person's back. Worked from the back of the neck to the lower end of the buttocks. Used long, firm, continuous strokes. Rinsed and dried well.	____	____	________
53. Gave back massage. The person may have wanted the back massage after the bath.	____	____	________
54. Turned the person on his or her back.	____	____	________
55. Changed the water for perineal care. Measured the temperature of the bath water. Used a bath thermometer, or tested the water by dipping your elbow or inner wrist into the basin. (Some states require changed gloves and hand hygiene.) Raised bed rail nearest you if used before leaving the bedside. Lowered it when you returned.	____	____	________
56. Allowed the person to wash his or her genital area. Adjusted the overbed table so he or she could reach the wash basin, soap, and towels with ease. Placed the call bell within reach. Asked the person to signal when finished. Made sure the person understood what to do.	____	____	________
57. Removed gloves. Decontaminated hands.	____	____	________
58. Promptly answered the call bell. Provided perineal care if person could not do so. (Wore gloves for perineal care, then removed and decontaminated hands.)	____	____	________
59. Gave a back massage if you had not already done so.	____	____	________
60. Applied deodorant or antiperspirant. Applied lotion and powder as requested. Viewed Safety Alert: Applying Powder.	____	____	________
61. Put clean garments on the person.	____	____	________
62. Combed and brushed his or her hair.	____	____	________
63. Made the bed. Attached the call bell.	____	____	________

Post-Procedure	S	U	Comments
64. Provided for comfort.			
65. Lowered the bed to its lowest position.			
66. Raised or lowered bed rails. Followed the care plan.			
67. Emptied and cleaned the wash basin. Returned it and other supplies to their proper place.			
68. Wiped off the overbed table with the paper towels. Discarded the paper towels.			
69. Unscreened the person.			
70. Followed agency policy for dirty linen.			
71. Decontaminated your hands.			
72. Reported and recorded your observations.			

Giving a Partial Bath

Quality of Life

Name: ____________________

Date: ____________________

Remembered to:
- Knock before entering the person's room
- Address the person by name
- Introduce yourself by name and title

Pre-Procedure	S	U	Comments
1. Followed Delegation Guidelines: Bathing. Viewed Safety Alert: Bathing.	_____	_____	____________
2. Identified the person. Checked the identification bracelet against the assignment sheet. Called the person by name.	_____	_____	____________
3. Explained the procedure to the person.	_____	_____	____________
4. Offered the bedpan or urinal. Provided privacy.	_____	_____	____________
5. Completed hand hygiene.	_____	_____	____________
6. Collected clean linen for a closed bed. Placed linen on a clean surface.	_____	_____	____________
7. Collected the following:			
a. Wash basin	_____	_____	____________
b. Soap	_____	_____	____________
c. Bath thermometer	_____	_____	____________
d. Orange stick or nail file	_____	_____	____________
e. Washcloth	_____	_____	____________
f. Two bath towels and two hand towels	_____	_____	____________
g. Bath blanket	_____	_____	____________
h. Clothing, gown, or pajamas	_____	_____	____________
i. Items for oral hygiene	_____	_____	____________
j. Lotion	_____	_____	____________
k. Powder	_____	_____	____________
l. Deodorant or antiperspirant	_____	_____	____________
m. Brush and comb	_____	_____	____________
n. Other grooming items if requested	_____	_____	____________
o. Paper towels	_____	_____	____________
p. Gloves	_____	_____	____________
8. Arranged items on the overbed table. Adjusted the height as needed.	_____	_____	____________
9. Closed doors and windows to prevent drafts.	_____	_____	____________
10. Provided for privacy.	_____	_____	____________
Procedure			
11. Made sure the bed was in the lowest position.	_____	_____	____________
12. Assisted with oral hygiene. Wore gloves. Adjusted the overbed table as needed.	_____	_____	____________
13. Removed top linens. Covered the person with a bath blanket.	_____	_____	____________
14. Covered the overbed table with paper towels.	_____	_____	____________

Procedure—cont'd	S	U	Comments
15. Filled the wash basin with water. Made sure water temperature was 110° to 115° F (43° to 46° C) for adults or as directed by the nurse and followed agency policy. Measured water temperature with the bath thermometer, or tested the bath water by dipping your elbow or inner wrist into the basin.	_____	_____	_____
16. Placed the basin on the overbed table.	_____	_____	_____
17. Positioned the person in the Fowler's position, or assisted him or her to sit at the bedside.	_____	_____	_____
18. Adjusted the overbed table so the person could reach the basin and supplies.	_____	_____	_____
19. Helped the person undress.	_____	_____	_____
20. Asked the person to wash easy-to-reach body parts. Explained that you would wash the back and areas the person could not reach.	_____	_____	_____
21. Placed the call bell within reach. Asked him or her to signal when help was needed or bathing was complete.	_____	_____	_____
22. Left the room after decontaminating your hands.	_____	_____	_____
23. Returned when the call light was on. Knocked before entering.	_____	_____	_____
24. Changed the bath water. Measured the water temperature with the bath thermometer, or tested the bath water by dipping your elbow or inner wrist into the basin.	_____	_____	_____
25. Raised the bed for body mechanics. Raised the far bed rail if used.	_____	_____	_____
26. Asked what was washed. Put on gloves. Washed and dried areas the person could not reach. The face, hands, underarms, back, buttocks, and perineal area should be washed during the partial bath.	_____	_____	_____
27. Removed the gloves. Decontaminated your hands.	_____	_____	_____
28. Gave a back massage.	_____	_____	_____
29. Applied lotion, powder, and deodorant or antiperspirant as requested.	_____	_____	_____
30. Helped the person put on clean garments.	_____	_____	_____
31. Assisted with hair care and other grooming needs.	_____	_____	_____
32. Assisted person to a chair, or turned the person on the side away from you. (Lowered the bed if person transferred to a chair.)	_____	_____	_____
33. Made the bed.	_____	_____	_____
34. Lowered the bed to its lowest position.	_____	_____	_____

Post-Procedure

35. Provided for comfort.	_____	_____	_____
36. Placed the call bell within reach	_____	_____	_____
37. Raised or lowered the bed rails. Followed the care plan.	_____	_____	_____
38. Emptied and cleaned the basin. Returned the basin and supplies to their proper place.	_____	_____	_____

Post-Procedure–cont'd	S	U	Comments
39. Wiped off the overbed table with the paper towels. Discarded the paper towels.	_____	_____	_____________
40. Unscreened the person.	_____	_____	_____________
41. Followed agency policy for dirty linen.	_____	_____	_____________
42. Decontaminated your hands.	_____	_____	_____________
43. Reported and recorded your observations.	_____	_____	_____________

Assisting With a Tub Bath or Shower

QUALITY OF LIFE

Name: ____________________

Date: ____________________

Remembered to:
- ◆ Knock before entering the person's room
- ◆ Address the person by name
- ◆ Introduce yourself by name and title

Pre-Procedure	S	U	Comments
1. Followed Delegation Guidelines: Tub Baths and Showers. Viewed Safety Alerts: Tub Baths and Showers.			
2. Reserved the bathtub or shower.			
3. Identified the person. Checked the identification bracelet against the assignment sheet. Called the person by name.			
4. Explained the procedure to the person.			
5. Completed hand hygiene.			
6. Collected the following:			
• Washcloth and two bath towels			
• Soap			
• Bath thermometer for a tub bath			
• Clothing, gown, or pajamas			
• Robe and nonskid footwear			
• Rubber bath mat if needed			
• Disposable bath mat			
• Gloves			
• Wheelchair or shower chair			

Procedure	S	U	Comments
7. Placed items in the tub shower room. Used the space provided or a chair.			
8. Cleaned the tub or shower.			
9. Placed a rubber bath mat in the tub or on the shower floor. Made sure that you did not block the drain.			
10. Placed the bath mat on the floor in front of the tub or shower.			
11. Placed the "Occupied" sign on the door.			
12. Returned to the person's room. Provided for privacy.			
13. Helped the person sit on the side of the bed.			
14. Helped the person put on a robe and nonskid footwear.			
15. Assisted or transported the person to the tub or shower room.			
16. *For a tub bath:*			
a. Had the person sit on a chair.			
b. Filled the tub halfway with warm water (105° F [41° C]). Measured water temperature with the bath thermometer, or checked the digital display.			

Procedure—cont'd	S	U	Comments
17. *For a shower:*			
a. Turned on the shower.			
b. Adjusted water temperature and pressure.			
18. Helped the person undress, and removed footwear.			
19. Helped the person into the tub or shower. Positioned the shower chair, and locked the wheels.			
20. Assisted with washing if necessary. Wore gloves.			
21. Asked the person to use the call bell when done or when help was needed. Reminded the person that a tub bath last no longer than 20 minutes.			
22. Placed a towel across the chair.			
23. Left the room if the person could bathe unattended. If not, stayed in the room or remained nearby. Removed the gloves and decontaminated your hands, if you left the room.			
24. Checked the person every 5 minutes.			
25. Returned when he or she signaled for you. Knocked before entering.			
26. Turned off the shower, or drained the tub. Covered the person while the tub drained.			
27. Helped the person out of the tub or shower and onto the chair.			
28. Helped the person dry off. Patted gently. Dried under breasts, between shin folds, in the perineal area, and between the toes.			
29. Assisted with lotion and other grooming items as needed.			
30. Helped the person dress and put on footwear.			
31. Helped the person return to the room. Provided for privacy.			
32. Assisted the person to a chair or into the bed.			
33. Provided a back massage if the person returned to bed.			
34. Assisted with hair care and other grooming needs.			

Post-Procedure

35. Made the bed. Provided for comfort.			
36. Raised or lowered bed rails. Followed the care plan.			
37. Placed the call bell within reach.			
38. Unscreened the person.			
39. Cleaned the tub or shower. Removed soiled linen. Wore gloves.			
40. Discarded disposable items. Placed the "Unoccupied" sign on the door. Returned supplies to their proper places.			
41. Followed agency policy for dirty linen.			
42. Decontaminated your hands.			
43. Reported or recorded your observations.			

Giving Back Massage

QUALITY OF LIFE

Name: ____________________

Date: ____________________

Remembered to:
- ◆ Knock before entering the person's room
- ◆ Address the person by name
- ◆ Introduce yourself by name and title

Pre-Procedure	S	U	Comments
1. Followed Delegation Guidelines: Back Massage. Viewed Safety Alert: Back Massage.	_____	_____	__________
2. Identified the person. Checked the identification bracelet against the assignment sheet. Called the person by name.	_____	_____	__________
3. Explained the procedure to the person.	_____	_____	__________
4. Completed hand hygiene.	_____	_____	__________
5. Collected the following:			
• Bath blanket	_____	_____	__________
• Bath towel	_____	_____	__________
• Lotion	_____	_____	__________
6. Provided for privacy.	_____	_____	__________
7. Raised the bed for body mechanics. Raised the bed rails if used.	_____	_____	__________

Procedure	S	U	Comments
8. Lowered the bed rail nearest you if used.	_____	_____	__________
9. Positioned the person in the prone or side-lying position. Made sure the person's back was toward you.	_____	_____	__________
10. Exposed the back, shoulders, upper arms, and buttocks. Covered the rest of the body with the bath blanket.	_____	_____	__________
11. Laid the towel on the bed along the back.	_____	_____	__________
12. Warmed the lotion.	_____	_____	__________
13. Explained that the lotion may feel cool and wet.	_____	_____	__________
14. Applied the lotion to the lower back area.	_____	_____	__________
15. Stroked up from the buttocks to the shoulders. Stroked down over the upper arms. Stroked up the upper arms, across the shoulders, and down the back to the buttocks. Used firm strokes. Kept your hands in contact with the person's skin.	_____	_____	__________
16. Continued for at least 3 minutes.	_____	_____	__________
17. Kneaded by grasping skin between your thumb and fingers. Kneaded half of the back. Started at the buttocks and moved up to the shoulder, then kneaded down from the shoulder to buttocks. Continued on the other half of the back.	_____	_____	__________
18. Applied lotion to bony areas. Used circular notions with the tips of your index and middle fingers. (Did not massage reddened bony areas.)	_____	_____	__________
19. Used fast movements to stimulate. Used slow movements to relax the person.	_____	_____	__________

Procedure—cont'd	S	U	Comments
20. Stroked with long, firm movements to end the massage. Told the person when finished.	______	______	____________________
21. Covered the person. Removed the towel and bath blanket.	______	______	____________________

Post-Procedure

	S	U	Comments
22. Provided for comfort.	______	______	____________________
23. Lowered the bed to its lowest position.	______	______	____________________
24. Raised or lowered bed rails. Followed the care plan.	______	______	____________________
25. Placed the call bell within reach.	______	______	____________________
26. Returned lotion to its proper place.	______	______	____________________
27. Unscreened the person.	______	______	____________________
28. Followed agency policy for dirty linen.	______	______	____________________
29. Decontaminated your hands.	______	______	____________________
30. Reported and recorded your observations.	______	______	____________________

Giving Female Perineal Care

QUALITY OF LIFE

Name: ______________________

Date: ______________________

Remembered to:
- ◆ **Knock before entering the person's room**
- ◆ **Address the person by name**
- ◆ **Introduce yourself by name and title**

Pre-Procedure

	S	U	Comments
1. Followed Delegation Guidelines: Perineal Care. Viewed Safety Alert: Perineal Care.	____	____	____________
2. Explained the procedure to the person.	____	____	____________
3. Completed hand hygiene.	____	____	____________
4. Collected the following:			
• Soap	____	____	____________
• At least four washcloths	____	____	____________
• Bath towel	____	____	____________
• Bath blanket	____	____	____________
• Bath thermometer	____	____	____________
• Washbasin	____	____	____________
• Waterproof pad	____	____	____________
• Gloves	____	____	____________
• Paper towels	____	____	____________
5. Covered the overbed table with paper towels. Arranged items on top of the paper towels.	____	____	____________
6. Identified the person. Checked the identification bracelet against the assignment sheet. Called her by name.	____	____	____________
7. Provided for privacy.	____	____	____________
8. Raised the bed for body mechanics. Raised bed rails if used.	____	____	____________

Procedure

	S	U	Comments
9. Lowered the bed rail nearest you if up.	____	____	____________
10. Covered the person with a bath blanket. Moved top linens to the foot of the bed.	____	____	____________
11. Positioned the person on her back.	____	____	____________
12. Draped her.	____	____	____________
13. Raised the bed rail if used.	____	____	____________
14. Filled the wash basin. Made sure water temperature was 105° to 109° F (41° to 43° C). Measured water temperature according to agency policy.	____	____	____________
15. Placed the basin on the overbed table.	____	____	____________
16. Lowered the bed rail if up.	____	____	____________
17. Put on the gloves.	____	____	____________
18. Helped the person flex her knees and spread her legs, or helped her spread her legs as much as possible with her knees straight.	____	____	____________
19. Placed a waterproof pad under her buttocks.	____	____	____________

Procedure—cont'd	S	U	Comments
20. Folded the corner of the bath blanket between her legs onto her abdomen.	____	____	____________
21. Wet the washcloth.	____	____	____________
22. Applied soap to a washcloth.	____	____	____________
23. Separated the labia. Cleaned downward from front to back with one stroke.	____	____	____________
24. Repeated until the area was clean:			
a. Applied soap to a washcloth.	____	____	____________
b. Separated the labia. Cleaned downward from front to back with one stroke.	____	____	____________
c. Used a clean part of the washcloth for each stroke.	____	____	____________
d. Used more than one washcloth if needed.	____	____	____________
25. Rinsed the perineum with a clean washcloth. Separated the labia. Stroke downward from front to back. Repeated as necessary. Used a clean part of the washcloth for each stroke. Used more than one washcloth if needed.	____	____	____________
26. Patted the area dry with the towel.	____	____	____________
27. Folded the blanket back between her legs.	____	____	____________
28. Helped the person lower her legs and turned her on her side away from you.	____	____	____________
29. Applied soap to a washcloth.	____	____	____________
30. Cleaned the rectal area. Cleaned from the vagina to the anus with one stroke.	____	____	____________
31. Repeated until the area was clean:			
a. Applied soap to a washcloth.	____	____	____________
b. Cleaned the rectal area. Cleaned from the vagina to the anus with one stroke.	____	____	____________
c. Used a clean part of the washcloth for each stroke.	____	____	____________
d. Used more than one washcloth if needed.	____	____	____________
32. Rinsed the rectal area with a washcloth. Stroked from the vagina to the anus. Repeated as necessary. Used a clean part of the washcloth for each stroke. Used more than one washcloth if needed.	____	____	____________
33. Patted the area dry with the towel.	____	____	____________
34. Removed the waterproof pad.	____	____	____________
35. Removed and discarded the gloves. Decontaminated your hands.	____	____	____________

Post-Procedure

36. Provided for comfort.	____	____	____________
37. Covered the person. Removed the bath blanket.	____	____	____________
38. Lowered the bed to its lowest position.	____	____	____________
39. Raised or lowered bed rails. Followed the care plan.	____	____	____________
40. Placed the call bell within reach.	____	____	____________
41. Emptied and cleaned the wash basin. Wore gloves.	____	____	____________
42. Returned the basin and supplies to their proper places.	____	____	____________

Post-Procedure—cont'd	S	U	Comments
43. Wiped off the overbed table with the paper towels. Discarded the paper towels.	_____	_____	__________________
44. Removed the gloves. Decontaminated your hands.	_____	_____	__________________
45. Unscreened the person.	_____	_____	__________________
46. Followed agency policy for dirty linen.	_____	_____	__________________
47. Decontaminated your hands.	_____	_____	__________________
48. Reported and recorded your observations.	_____	_____	__________________

Giving Male Perineal Care

Quality of Life

Name: ____________________

Date: ____________________

Remembered to:
- Knock before entering the person's room
- Address the person by name
- Introduce yourself by name and title

Pre-Procedure	S	U	Comments
1. Followed Delegation Guidelines: Perineal Care. Viewed Safety Alert: Perineal Care.			
2. Explained the procedure to the person.			
3. Completed hand hygiene.			
4. Collected the following:			
a. Soap			
b. At least four washcloths			
c. Bath towel			
d. Bath blanket			
e. Bath thermometer			
f. Washbasin			
g. Waterproof pad			
h. Gloves			
i. Paper towels			
5. Covered the overbed table with paper towels. Arranged items on top of them.			
6. Identified the person. Checked the identification bracelet against the assignment sheet. Called him by name.			
7. Provided for privacy.			
8. Raised the bed for body mechanics. Raised bed rails if used.			

Procedure

	S	U	Comments
9. Lowered the bed rail nearest you if up.			
10. Covered the person with a bath blanket. Moved top linens to the foot of the bed.			
11. Positioned the person on his back.			
12. Draped him.			
13. Raised the bed rail if used.			
14. Filled the wash basin. Made sure water temperature was 105° to 109° F (41° to 43° C). Measured water temperature according to agency policy.			
15. Placed the basin on the overbed table.			
16. Lowered the bed rail if up.			
17. Put on the gloves.			
18. Helped the person flex his knees and spread his legs, or helped him spread his legs as much as possible with his knees straight.			
19. Placed a waterproof pad under his buttocks.			

Procedure—cont'd	S	U	Comments
20. Folded the corner of the bath blanket between his legs onto his abdomen.			
21. Wet the washcloth.			
22. Applied soap to a washcloth.			
23. Retracted the foreskin if the person was not circumcised.			
24. Grasped the penis.			
25. Cleaned the tip. Used a circular motion. Started at the urethra and worked outward. Repeated as needed. Used a clean part of the washcloth each time.			
26. Rinsed the area with another washcloth.			
27. Returned the foreskin to its natural position.			
28. Cleaned the shaft of the penis. Used firm downward strokes. Rinsed the area.			
29. Helped the person flex his knees and spread his legs, or helped him spread his legs as much as possible with his knees straight.			
30. Cleaned the scrotum. Rinsed well. Observed for redness and irritation in the skin folds.			
31. Patted dry the penis and scrotum.			
32. Folded the bath blanket back between his legs.			
33. Helped him lower his legs, and turned him onto his side away from you.			
34. Cleaned the rectal area. Cleaned from the scrotum to the anus with one stroke. Repeated if necessary until the area was clean. Used more than one washcloth.			
35. Rinsed and dried well.			
36. Removed the waterproof pad.			
37. Removed and discarded the gloves. Decontaminated your hands.			

Post-Procedure

	S	U	Comments
38. Provided for comfort.			
39. Covered the person. Removed the bath blanket.			
40. Lowered the bed to its lowest position.			
41. Raised or lowered bed rails. Followed the care plan.			
42. Placed the call bell within reach.			
43. Emptied and cleaned the wash basin. Wore gloves.			
44. Returned the basin and supplies to their proper places.			
45. Wiped off the overbed table with the paper towels. Discarded the paper towels.			
46. Removed the gloves. Decontaminated your hands.			
47. Unscreened the person.			
48. Followed agency policy for dirty linen.			
49. Decontaminated your hands.			
50. Reported and recorded your observations.			

Brushing and Combing a Person's Hair

QUALITY OF LIFE

Name: ____________________

Date: ____________________

Remembered to:
- ◆ **Knock before entering the person's room**
- ◆ **Address the person by name**
- ◆ **Introduce yourself by name and title**

Pre-Procedure	S	U	Comments
1. Followed Delegation Guidelines: Brushing and Combing Hair. Viewed Safety Alert: Brushing and Combing Hair.	____	____	____________
2. Identified the person. Checked the ID bracelet against the assignment sheet. Called the person by name.	____	____	____________
3. Explained the procedure to the person. Asked the person about their style preference.	____	____	____________
4. Collected the following:			
• Comb and brush	____	____	____________
• Bath towel	____	____	____________
• Hair care items as requested	____	____	____________
5. Arranged items on the bedside stand.	____	____	____________
6. Completed hand hygiene.	____	____	____________
7. Provided for privacy.	____	____	____________

Procedure

8. Lowered the bed rail if used.	____	____	____________
9. Helped the person to the chair. The person put on a robe and nonskid footwear. (If the person was in bed, the bed was raised for body mechanics. Raised the bed rails if used. Lowered the near bed rail. Assisted the person to semi-Fowler's position, if allowed.)	____	____	____________
10. Placed a towel across the shoulders or across the pillow.	____	____	____________
11. Asked the person to remove eyeglasses. Placed them in the eyeglass case. Put the case inside the bedside stand.	____	____	____________
12. Parted hair into two sections. Divided one side into two sections.	____	____	____________
13. Brushed the hair. Started at the scalp and brushed toward the hair ends.	____	____	____________
14. Styled the hair as the person preferred.	____	____	____________
15. Removed the towel.	____	____	____________
16. Allowed the person to put on the eyeglasses.	____	____	____________

Post-Procedure

17. Provided for comfort.	____	____	____________
18. Lowered the bed to its lowest position.	____	____	____________
19. Raised or lowered bed rails. Followed the care plan.	____	____	____________
20. Placed the call bell within reach.	____	____	____________
21. Unscreened the person.	____	____	____________

Post-Procedure—cont'd	S	U	Comments
22. Cleaned and returned items to their proper place.	______	______	____________________
23. Followed agency policy for dirty linen.	______	______	____________________
24. Decontaminated your hands.	______	______	____________________

Shampooing the Person's Hair

QUALITY OF LIFE

Name: ______________

Date: ______________

Remembered to:
- ◆ Knock before entering the person's room
- ◆ Address the person by name
- ◆ Introduce yourself by name and title

Pre-Procedure	S	U	Comments
1. Followed Delegation Guidelines: Shampooing. Viewed Safety Alert: Shampooing.	____	____	________
2. Explained the procedure to the person.	____	____	________
3. Completed hand hygiene.	____	____	________
4. Collected the following:			
• Two bath towels	____	____	________
• Hand towel or washcloth	____	____	________
• Shampoo	____	____	________
• Hair conditioner if requested	____	____	________
• Bath thermometer	____	____	________
• Pitcher or nozzle if needed	____	____	________
• Shampoo tray if needed	____	____	________
• Basin or pan if needed	____	____	________
• Waterproof pad if needed	____	____	________
• Gloves if needed	____	____	________
• Comb and brush	____	____	________
• Hair dryer	____	____	________
5. Arranged items nearby.	____	____	________
6. Identified the person. Checked the identification bracelet against the assignment sheet. Called the person by name.	____	____	________
7. Provided for privacy.	____	____	________
8. Raised the bed for body mechanics for a shampoo in bed. Raised the far bed rail if bed rails were used.	____	____	________

Procedure	S	U	Comments
9. Positioned the person for the method you used. Placed the waterproof pad and shampoo tray under the head and shoulders if needed.	____	____	________
10. Placed a bath towel across the shoulders or pillow.	____	____	________
11. Brushed and combed the hair to remove snarls and tangles.	____	____	________
12. Raised the bed rail if used.	____	____	________
13. Obtained water. Made sure the water temperature was about 105° F (40.5° C). Tested temperature according to agency policy.	____	____	________
14. Lowered the bed rail if used.	____	____	________
15. Put on gloves if used.	____	____	________
16. Asked the person to hold a dampened hand towel or wash-cloth over the eyes. It did not cover the nose and mouth. (The dampened cloth was easier to hold and did not slip.)	____	____	________

Procedure—cont'd	S	U	Comments
17. Used the pitcher or nozzle to wet the hair.			
18. Applied a small amount of shampoo.			
19. Worked up a lather with both hands. Started at the hairline. Worked toward the back of the head.			
20. Massaged the scalp with your fingertips. Made sure you did not scratch the scalp.			
21. Rinsed the hair.			
22. Repeated:			
a. Asked the person to continue to hold the dampened cloth over the eyes only.			
b. Used the pitcher or nozzle to wet the hair.			
c. Applied a small amount of shampoo.			
d. Worked up a lather with both hands. Started at the hairline. Worked toward the back of the head.			
e. Massaged the scalp with your fingertips. Made sure you did not scratch the scalp.			
f. Rinsed the hair.			
23. Applied conditioner. Followed directions on the container.			
24. Squeezed water from the person's hair.			
25. Covered hair with a bath towel.			
26. Dried the person's face.			
27. Helped the person raise the head if appropriate.			
28. Rubbed the hair and scalp with the towel. Used the second towel if the first was wet.			
29. Combed the hair to remove snarls and tangles.			
30. Dried and styled hair as quickly as possible.			

Post-Procedure

31. Removed and discarded the gloves if used. Decontaminated your hands.			
32. Provided for comfort.			
33. Lowered the bed to its lowest position.			
34. Raised or lowered bed rails. Followed the care plan.			
35. Placed the call bell within reach.			
36. Unscreened the person.			
37. Cleaned and returned equipment to its proper place. Discarded disposable items.			
38. Followed agency policy for dirty linen.			
39. Decontaminated your hands.			

Shaving a Person

Quality of Life

Name: ______________________

Date: ______________________

Remembered to:
- ◆ Knock before entering the person's room
- ◆ Address the person by name
- ◆ Introduce yourself by name and title

Pre-Procedure	S	U	Comments
1. Followed Delegation Guidelines: Shaving. Viewed Safety Alert: Shaving.			
2. Explained the procedure to the person.			
3. Completed hand hygiene.			
4. Collected the following:			
• Wash basin			
• Bath towel			
• Hand towel			
• Washcloth			
• Safety razor			
• Mirror			
• Shaving cream, soap, or lotion			
• Shaving brush			
• After-shave lotion (men only)			
• Tissues or paper towels			
• Paper towels			
• Gloves			
5. Arranged paper towels and supplies on the overbed table.			
6. Identified the person. Checked the identification bracelet against the assignment sheet. Called the person by name.			
7. Provided for privacy.			
8. Raised the bed for body mechanics. Raised the bed rails if used.			

Procedure	S	U	Comments
9. Filled the basin with warm water.			
10. Placed the basin on the overbed table.			
11. Lowered the bed rail nearest you if up.			
12. Assisted the person to the semi-Fowler's or supine position if allowed.			
13. Adjusted lighting to see the person's face clearly.			
14. Placed the bath towel over the chest.			
15. Adjusted the overbed table for easy reach.			
16. Tightened the razor blade to the shaver.			
17. Washed the person's face. Did not dry.			
18. Soaked the washcloth or towel. Wrung it out.			
19. Applied the washcloth or towel to the face for a few minutes.			
20. Put on gloves.			

Procedure—cont'd	S	U	Comments
21. Applied shaving cream with your hands, or used a shaving brush to apply lather.	______	______	____________________
22. Held the skin taut with one hand.	______	______	____________________
23. Shaved in the direction of hair growth. Used shorter strokes around the chin and lips.	______	______	____________________
24. Raised the razor often. Wiped it with tissue or paper towels.	______	______	____________________
25. Applied direct pressure to any bleeding areas.	______	______	____________________
26. Washed off any remaining shaving cream or soap. Dried with a towel.	______	______	____________________
27. Applied after-shave lotion if requested.	______	______	____________________
28. Removed the towel and gloves. Decontaminated your hands.	______	______	____________________
29. Moved the overbed table to the side of the bed.	______	______	____________________

Post-Procedure

30. Provided for comfort.	______	______	____________________
31. Placed the call bell within reach.	______	______	____________________
32. Lowered the bed to its lowest position.	______	______	____________________
33. Raised or lowered the bed rails. Followed the care plan.	______	______	____________________
34. Cleaned and returned equipment and supplies to their proper place. Discarded disposable items. Worn gloves.	______	______	____________________
35. Wiped off the overbed table with the paper towels. Discarded the paper towels.	______	______	____________________
36. Removed the gloves. Decontaminated your hands.	______	______	____________________
37. Positioned the table for the person.	______	______	____________________
38. Unscreened the person.	______	______	____________________
39. Followed agency policy for dirty linen.	______	______	____________________
40. Decontaminated your hands.	______	______	____________________
41. Reported nicks or bleeding to the nurse.	______	______	____________________

Giving Nail and Foot Care

QUALITY OF LIFE

Name: ______________________

Date: ______________________

Remembered to:
- ◆ Knock before entering the person's room
- ◆ Address the person by name
- ◆ Introduce yourself by name and title

Pre-Procedure

	S	U	Comments
1. Followed Delegation Guidelines: Nail and Foot Care. Viewed Safety Alert: Nail and Foot Care.	____	____	____________
2. Explained the procedure to the person.	____	____	____________
3. Completed hand hygiene.	____	____	____________
4. Collected the following:			
• Wash basin or whirlpool footbath	____	____	____________
• Soap	____	____	____________
• Bath thermometer	____	____	____________
• Bath towel	____	____	____________
• Hand towel	____	____	____________
• Washcloth	____	____	____________
• Kidney basin	____	____	____________
• Nail clipper	____	____	____________
• Orange stick	____	____	____________
• Emery board or nail file	____	____	____________
• Lotion or petrolatum jelly	____	____	____________
• Paper towels	____	____	____________
• Disposable bath mat	____	____	____________
• Gloves	____	____	____________
5. Arranged paper towels and other items on the overbed table.	____	____	____________
6. Identified the person. Checked the identification bracelet against the assignment sheet. Called the person by name.	____	____	____________
7. Provided for privacy.	____	____	____________
8. Assisted the person to the bedside chair. Placed the call bell within reach.	____	____	____________

Procedure

	S	U	Comments
9. Placed the bath mat under the feet.	____	____	____________
10. Filled the wash basin or whirlpool footbath. The nurse told you what temperature to use. (Measured water temperature with a bath thermometer, or tested temperature according to agency policy.)	____	____	____________
11. Placed the basin of footbath on the bath mat.	____	____	____________
12. Helped the person put the feet into the basin or footbath.	____	____	____________
13. Adjusted the overbed table in front of the person.	____	____	____________
14. Filled the kidney basin. Used the bath thermometer to measure temperature, or followed agency policy.	____	____	____________
15. Placed the kidney basin on the overbed table.	____	____	____________

Procedure—cont'd

	S	U	Comments
16. Placed the person's fingers into the basin. Positioned the arms for comfort.			
17. Allowed the fingers to soak for 5 to 10 minutes. Allowed the feet to soak for 15 to 20 minutes. Warmed the water as needed.			
18. Put on gloves.			
19. Cleaned under the fingernails with an orange stick. Used a towel to wipe the orange stick after each nail.			
20. Removed the kidney basin. Thoroughly dried the hands and between the fingers.			
21. Clipped the fingernails straight across with the nail clippers.			
22. Shaped nails with an emery board or nail file.			
23. Pushed cuticles back with the orange stick or a washcloth.			
24. Moved the overbed table to the side.			
25. Washed the feet with soap and a washcloth. Washed between the toes.			
26. Removed the feet from the basin or footbath. Dried thoroughly, especially between the toes.			
27. Applied lotion or petrolatum jelly to the tops and soles of the feet. Did not apply between the toes. Warmed lotion before applying.			
28. Removed and discarded the gloves. Decontaminated your hands.			
29. Helped the person put on socks and nonskid footwear.			

Post-Procedure

	S	U	Comments
30. Provided for comfort.			
31. Placed the call bell within reach.			
32. Raised or lowered the bed rails. Followed the care plan.			
33. Cleaned and returned equipment and supplies to their proper place. Discarded disposable items. Wore gloves.			
34. Removed gloves. Decontaminated your hands.			
35. Unscreened the person.			
36. Followed agency policy for dirty linen.			
37. Decontaminated your hands.			
38. Reported and recorded your observations.			

Changing the Gown of a Person With an IV

QUALITY OF LIFE

Name: ____________________

Date: ____________________

Remembered to:
- Knock before entering the person's room
- Address the person by name
- Introduce yourself by name and title

Pre-Procedure

	S	U	Comments
1. Followed Delegation Guidelines: Changing Gowns. Viewed Safety Alert: Changing Gowns.			
2. Explained the procedure to the person.			
3. Completed hand hygiene.			
4. Collected a clean gown and bath blanket.			
5. Identified the person. Checked the identification bracelet against the assignment sheet. Called the person by name.			
6. Provided for privacy.			
7. Raised the bed for body mechanics. Raised the bed rails if used.			

Procedure

	S	U	Comments
8. Lowered the bed rail nearest you if up.			
9. Covered the person with a bath blanket. Fanfolded linens to the foot of the bed.			
10. Untied the gown. Freed parts that the person was lying on.			
11. Removed the gown from the arm with no IV.			
12. Gather up the sleeve of the arm with the IV. Slid it over the intravenous (IV) site and tubing. Removed the arm and hand from the sleeve.			
13. Kept the sleeve gathered. Slid your arm along the tubing to the bag.			
14. Removed the bag from the pole. Slid the bag and tubing through the sleeve. Did not pull on the tubing. Kept the bag above the person.			
15. Hung the IV bag on the pole.			
16. Gathered the sleeve of the clean gown that will go on the arm with the IV infusion.			
17. Removed the bag from the pole. Slipped the sleeve over the bag at the shoulder part of the gown. Hung the bag.			
18. Slid the gathered sleeve over the tubing, hand, arm, and IV site. Then slid it onto the shoulder.			
19. Put the other side of the gown on the person. Fastened the gown.			
20. Covered the person. Removed the bath blanket.			

Post-Procedure	S	U	Comments
21. Provided for comfort.	______	______	____________________
22. Placed the call bell within reach.	______	______	____________________
23. Lowered the bed to its lowest position.	______	______	____________________
24. Raised or lowered the bed rails. Followed the care plan.	______	______	____________________
25. Unscreened the person.	______	______	____________________
26. Followed agency policy for dirty linen.	______	______	____________________
27. Decontaminated your hands.	______	______	____________________
28. Checked the flow rate, or asked the nurse to check it.	______	______	____________________

Undressing a Person

Quality of Life

Name: ____________________

Date: ____________________

Remembered to:
- Knock before entering the person's room
- Address the person by name
- Introduce yourself by name and title

Pre-Procedure	S	U	Comments
1. Followed Delegation Guidelines: Dressing and Undressing.	______	______	______
2. Explained the procedure to the person.	______	______	______
3. Completed hand hygiene.	______	______	______
4. Got a bath blanket.	______	______	______
5. Identified the person. Checked the identification bracelet against the assignment sheet. Called the person by name.	______	______	______
6. Provided for privacy.	______	______	______
7. Raised the bed for body mechanics. Raised the bed rails if used.	______	______	______
8. Lowered the bed rail on the person's weak side.	______	______	______
9. Turned him or her to the supine position.	______	______	______
10. Covered the person with the bath blanket. Fanfolded linens to the foot of the bed.	______	______	______

Procedure

	S	U	Comments
11. Removed garments that open in the back:			
a. Raised the head and shoulders, or turned him or her onto the side away from you.	______	______	______
b. Undid buttons, zippers, ties, or snaps.	______	______	______
c. Brought the sides of the garment to the sides under the person. Folded the nearest side onto the chest.	______	______	______
d. Turned the person to the supine position.	______	______	______
e. Slid the garment off the shoulder on the strong side. Removed it from the arm.	______	______	______
f. Slid the garment off the shoulder on the weak side. Removed the garment from the arm.	______	______	______
12. Removed garments that open in the front:			
a. Undid buttons, zippers, ties, or snaps.	______	______	______
b. Slid the garment off the shoulder and arm on the strong side.	______	______	______
c. Raised the head and shoulders. Brought the garment over to the weak side. Lowered the head and shoulders.	______	______	______
d. Removed the garment from the weak side.	______	______	______
e. If unable to raise the head and shoulders:			
i. Turned the person toward you. Tucked the removed part under the person.	______	______	______
ii. Turned him or her on the side away from you.	______	______	______
iii. Pulled the side of the garment out from under the person. Made sure he or she was not lying on it when supine.	______	______	______

Procedure—cont'd	S	U	Comments
iv. Returned the person to the supine position.	_____	_____	_____
v. Removed the garment from the weak side.	_____	_____	_____
13. Removed pullover garments:			
a. Undid any buttons, zippers, ties, or snaps.	_____	_____	_____
b. Removed the garment from the strong side.	_____	_____	_____
c. Raised the head and shoulders, or turned the person on the side away from you. Brought the garment up to the person's neck.	_____	_____	_____
d. Removed the garment from the weak side.	_____	_____	_____
e. Brought the garment over the person's head.	_____	_____	_____
f. Turned him or her to the supine position.	_____	_____	_____
14. Removed pants or slacks:			
a. Removed footwear.	_____	_____	_____
b. Turned the person to the supine position.	_____	_____	_____
c. Undid buttons, zippers, ties, snaps, or buckles.	_____	_____	_____
d. Removed the belt.	_____	_____	_____
e. Asked the person to lift the buttocks off the bed. Slid the pants down over the hips and buttocks. Made sure the person lowered the hips and buttocks.	_____	_____	_____
f. If the person did not raise the hips off the bed:			
i. Turned the person toward you.	_____	_____	_____
ii. Slid the pants off the hips and buttocks on the strong side.	_____	_____	_____
iii. Turned the person away from you.	_____	_____	_____
iv. Slid the pants off the hips and buttocks on the weak side.	_____	_____	_____
g. Slid the pants down the legs and over the feet.	_____	_____	_____
15. Dressed the person.	_____	_____	_____
16. Helped the person get out of bed if he or she was allowed to be up. If the person stayed in bed:			
a. Covered the person, and removed the bath blanket.	_____	_____	_____
b. Provided for comfort.	_____	_____	_____
c. Lowered the bed to its lowest position.	_____	_____	_____
d. Raised or lowered the bed rails. Followed the care plan.	_____	_____	_____

Post-Procedure

	S	U	Comments
17. Placed the call bell within reach.	_____	_____	_____
18. Unscreened the person.	_____	_____	_____
19. Followed agency policy for soiled clothing.	_____	_____	_____
20. Decontaminated your hands.	_____	_____	_____
21. Reported and recorded your observations.	_____	_____	_____

Dressing the Person

Quality of Life

Name: ______________________

Date: ______________________

Remembered to:
- **Knock before entering the person's room**
- **Address the person by name**
- **Introduce yourself by name and title**

Pre-Procedure

	S	U	Comments
1. Followed Delegation Guidelines: Dressing and Undressing.			
2. Explained the procedure to the person.			
3. Completed hand hygiene.			
4. Collected a bath blanket and clothing requested by the person.			
5. Identified the person. Checked the identification bracelet against the assignment sheet. Called the person by name.			
6. Provided for privacy.			
7. Raised the bed for body mechanics. Raised the bed rails if used.			
8. Lowered the bed rail if up on the person's strong side.			
9. Undressed the person.			
10. Turned the person to the supine position.			

Procedure

	S	U	Comments
11. Covered the person with the bath blanket. Fanfolded linens to the foot of the bed.			
12. Put on garments that opened in the back.			
a. Slid the garment onto the arm and shoulder of the weak side.			
b. Slid the garment onto the arm and shoulder of the strong side.			
c. Raised the person's head and shoulders.			
d. Brought the sides to the back.			
e. If the person was in the side-lying position:			
i. Turned the person toward you.			
ii. Brought one side of the garment to the person's back.			
iii. Turned the person away from you.			
iv. Brought the other side to the person's back.			
f. Fastened buttons, snaps, ties, or zippers.			
g. Turned the person to the supine position.			
13. Put on garments opened in the front.			
a. Slid the garment onto the arm and shoulder on the weak side.			
b. Raised the head and shoulders. Brought the side of the garment around to the back. Lowered the person down. Slid the garment onto the arm and shoulder of the strong arm.			

Procedure—cont'd	S	U	Comments
c. If the person did not raise the head and shoulder:			
i. Turned the person toward you.	____	____	____
ii. Tucked the garment under the person.	____	____	____
iii. Turned the person away from you.	____	____	____
iv. Pulled the garment out from under the person.	____	____	____
v. Turned the person back to the supine position.	____	____	____
vi. Slid the garment over the arm and shoulder of the strong arm.	____	____	____
d. Fastened buttons, snaps, ties, or zippers.	____	____	____
14. Put on pullover garments:	____	____	____
a. Turned the person to the supine position.	____	____	____
b. Brought the neck of the garment over the head.	____	____	____
c. Slid the arm and shoulder of the garment onto the weak side.	____	____	____
d. Raised the person's head and shoulders.	____	____	____
e. Brought the garment down.	____	____	____
f. Slid the arm and shoulder of the garment onto the strong side.	____	____	____
g. If the person did not assume a semi-sitting position:			
i. Turned the person toward you.	____	____	____
ii. Tucked the garment under the person.	____	____	____
iii. Turned the person away from you.	____	____	____
iv. Pulled the garment out from under the person.	____	____	____
v. Turned the person to the supine position.	____	____	____
vi. Slid the arm and shoulder of the garment onto the strong side.	____	____	____
h. Fastened buttons, snaps, ties, or zippers.	____	____	____
15. Put on pants or slacks:			
a. Slid the pants over the feet and up the legs.	____	____	____
b. Asked the person to raise the hips and buttocks off the bed.	____	____	____
c. Brought the pants up over the buttocks and hips.	____	____	____
d. Asked the person to lower the hips and buttocks.	____	____	____
e. If the person did not raise the hips and buttocks:	____	____	____
i. Turned person onto strong side.	____	____	____
ii. Pulled the pants over the buttock and hip on the weak side.	____	____	____
iii. Turned the person onto the weak side.	____	____	____
iv. Pulled the pants over the buttock and hip on the strong side.	____	____	____
v. Turned the person to the supine position.	____	____	____
f. Fastened buttons, ties, snaps, the zipper, and the belt buckle.	____	____	____
16. Put socks and footwear on the person.	____	____	____

Procedure—cont'd	S	U	Comments
17. Helped the person get out of bed. If the person stayed in bed:			
a. Covered the person and removed the bath blanket.	____	____	____________
b. Provided for comfort.	____	____	____________
c. Lowered the bed to its lowest position.	____	____	____________
d. Raised or lowered bed rails. Followed the care plan.	____	____	____________

Post-Procedure

	S	U	Comments
18. Placed the call bell within reach.	____	____	____________
19. Unscreened the person.	____	____	____________
20. Followed agency policy for soiled clothing.	____	____	____________
21. Decontaminated your hands.	____	____	____________
22. Reported and recorded your observations.	____	____	____________

Giving the Bedpan

QUALITY OF LIFE

Name: ______________________

Date: ______________________

Remembered to:
- ◆ Knock before entering the person's room
- ◆ Address the person by name
- ◆ Introduce yourself by name and title

Pre-Procedure	**S**	**U**	**Comments**
1. Followed Delegation Guidelines: Bedpans. Viewed Safety Alert: Bedpan.	_____	_____	__________
2. Provided for privacy.	_____	_____	__________
3. Completed hand hygiene.	_____	_____	__________
4. Put on gloves.	_____	_____	__________
5. Collected the following:			
• Bedpan	_____	_____	__________
• Bedpan cover	_____	_____	__________
• Toilet tissue	_____	_____	__________
6. Arranged equipment on the chair or bed.	_____	_____	__________
7. Explained the procedure to the person.	_____	_____	__________

Procedure			
8. Warmed and dried the bedpan if necessary.	_____	_____	__________
9. Lowered the bed rail nearest to you if up.	_____	_____	__________
10. Turned the person to the supine position. Raised the head of the bed slightly.	_____	_____	__________
11. Folded the top linens and gown out of the way. Kept the lower body covered.	_____	_____	__________
12. Asked the person to flex the knees and raise the buttocks by pushing against the mattress with his or her feet.	_____	_____	__________
13. Slid your hand under the lower back. Helped raise the buttocks.	_____	_____	__________
14. Slid the bedpan under the person.	_____	_____	__________
15. If the person did not assist in getting on the bedpan:			
a. Turned the person onto the side away from you.	_____	_____	__________
b. Placed the bedpan firmly against the buttocks.	_____	_____	__________
c. Pushed the bedpan down and toward the person.	_____	_____	__________
d. Held the bedpan securely. Turned the person onto his or her back.	_____	_____	__________
e. Made sure the bedpan was centered under the person.	_____	_____	__________
16. Covered the person.	_____	_____	__________
17. Raised the head of the bed so the person was in a sitting position.	_____	_____	__________
18. Made sure the person was correctly positioned on the bedpan.	_____	_____	__________
19. Raised the bed rail if used.	_____	_____	__________
20. Placed the toilet tissue and call bell within reach.	_____	_____	__________

Procedure—cont'd

	S	U	Comments
21. Asked the person to signal when done or when help was needed.			
22. Removed the gloves. Decontaminated your hands.			
23. Left the room and closed the door.			
24. Returned when the person signaled. Knocked before entering,			
25. Decontaminated your hands. Put on gloves.			
26. Raised the bed for body mechanics. Lowered the bed rail if used and the head of the bed.			
27. Asked the person to raise his or her buttocks. Removed the bedpan, or held the bedpan and turned the person onto the side away from you.			
28. Cleaned the genital area if the person did not do so. Cleaned from front (urethra) to back (anus) with toilet tissue. Used fresh tissue for each wipe. Provided perineal care if needed.			
29. Covered the bedpan. Took it to the bathroom. Lowered the bed, and raised the bed rail, if used, before leaving the bedside.			
30. Noted the color, amount, and character of urine or feces.			
31. Emptied and rinsed the bedpan. Cleaned it with a disinfectant.			
32. Removed soiled gloves. Completed hand hygiene, and put on clean gloves.			
33. Returned the bedpan and clean cover to the bedside stand.			
34. Helped the person with handwashing.			
35. Removed the gloves. Decontaminated your hands.			

Post-Procedure

	S	U	Comments
36. Provided for comfort.			
37. Placed the call bell within reach.			
38. Raised or lowered the bed rails. Followed the care plan.			
39. Unscreened the person.			
40. Followed agency policy for soiled linen.			
41. Decontaminated your hands.			
42. Reported and recorded your observations.			

Giving the Urinal

QUALITY OF LIFE

Name: ______________________

Date: ______________________

Remembered to:
- Knock before entering the person's room
- Address the person by name
- Introduce yourself by name and title

Pre-Procedure	S	U	Comments
1. Followed Delegation Guidelines: Urinals. Viewed Safety Alert: Urinals.	____	____	____________
2. Provided for privacy.	____	____	____________
3. Determined whether the man will stand, sit, or lay in bed.	____	____	____________
4. Completed hand hygiene.	____	____	____________
5. Put on gloves.	____	____	____________

Procedure	S	U	Comments
6. Gave him the urinal if he was in bed. Reminded him to tilt the bottom down to prevent spills.	____	____	____________
7. If he stood:			
a. Helped him sit on the side of the bed.	____	____	____________
b. Put nonskid footwear on him.	____	____	____________
c. Helped him stand. Provided support if he was unsteady.	____	____	____________
d. Gave him the urinal.	____	____	____________
8. Positioned the urinal if necessary. Positioned his penis in the urinal if he did not do so.	____	____	____________
9. Provided for privacy.	____	____	____________
10. Placed the call bell within reach. Asked him to signal when done or when he needed help.	____	____	____________
11. Removed the gloves. Decontaminated your hands.	____	____	____________
12. Left the room, and closed the door.	____	____	____________
13. Returned when he signaled for you. Knocked before entering.	____	____	____________
14. Decontaminated your hands. Put on gloves.	____	____	____________
15. Closed the cap on the urinal. Took it to the bathroom.	____	____	____________
16. Noted the color, amount, and character of the urine.	____	____	____________
17. Emptied the urinal. Rinsed it with cold water. Cleaned it with a disinfectant.	____	____	____________
18. Returned the urinal to its proper place.	____	____	____________
19. Removed soiled gloves. Completed hand hygiene, and put on clean gloves.	____	____	____________
20. Assisted with handwashing.	____	____	____________
21. Removed the gloves. Decontaminated your hands.	____	____	____________

Post-Procedure	S	U	Comments
22. Provided for comfort.	_____	_____	__________________
23. Placed the call bell within reach.	_____	_____	__________________
24. Raised or lowered bed rails. Followed the care plan.	_____	_____	__________________
25. Unscreened him.	_____	_____	__________________
26. Followed agency policy for soiled linen.	_____	_____	__________________
27. Decontaminated your hands.	_____	_____	__________________
28. Reported and recorded your observations.	_____	_____	__________________

Helping the Person to the Commode

QUALITY OF LIFE

Name: ____________________

Date: ____________________

Remembered to:
- ◆ Knock before entering the person's room
- ◆ Address the person by name
- ◆ Introduce yourself by name and title

Pre-Procedure

	S	U	Comments
1. Followed Delegation Guidelines: Commodes. Viewed Safety Alert: Commodes.			
2. Explained the procedure to the person.			
3. Provided for privacy.			
4. Completed hand hygiene.			
5. Put on gloves.			
6. Collected the following:			
• Commode			
• Toilet tissue			
• Bath blanket			

Procedure

	S	U	Comments
7. Brought the commode next to the bed. Removed the chair seat and container lid.			
8. Helped the person sit on the side of the bed.			
9. Helped the person put on a robe and nonskid footwear.			
10. Assisted the person to the commode. Used the transfer belt.			
11. Covered the person with a bath blanket for warmth.			
12. Placed the toilet tissue and call bell within reach.			
13. Asked the person to signal when done or when help was needed. Stayed with the person if necessary. Was respectful. Provided as much privacy as possible.			
14. Removed the gloves. Decontaminated your hands.			
15. Left the room. Closed the door.			
16. Returned when the person signaled. Knocked before entering.			
17. Decontaminated your hands. Put on the gloves.			
18. Helped the person clean the genital area as needed. Removed the gloves and completed hand hygiene.			
19. Helped the person back to bed. Removed the robe and footwear. Raised the bed rail if used.			
20. Put on clean gloves. Removed and covered the commode container. Cleaned the commode.			
21. Took the container to the bathroom.			
22. Checked urine and feces for color, amount, and character.			
23. Cleaned and disinfected the container.			
24. Returned the container to the commode. Returned other supplies to their proper place.			
25. Returned the commode to its proper place.			

Procedure—cont'd	S	U	Comments
26. Removed soiled gloves. Completed hand hygiene, and put on clean gloves.			
27. Assisted with handwashing.			
28. Removed the gloves. Decontaminated your hands.			

Post-Procedure

	S	U	Comments
29. Provided for comfort.			
30. Placed the call bell within reach.			
31. Raised or lowered bed rails. Followed the care plan.			
32. Unscreened the person.			
33. Followed agency policy for soiled linen.			
34. Decontaminated your hands.			
35. Reported and recorded your observations.			

Giving Catheter Care

QUALITY OF LIFE

Name: ______________________

Date: ______________________

Remembered to:
- ◆ Knock before entering the person's room
- ◆ Address the person by name
- ◆ Introduce yourself by name and title

Pre-Procedure	S	U	Comments
1. Followed Delegation Guidelines: Catheters. Viewed Safety Alert: Catheters.	____	____	____________
2. Explained the procedure to the person.	____	____	____________
3. Completed hand hygiene.	____	____	____________
4. Collected the following:			
• Items for perineal care	____	____	____________
• Gloves	____	____	____________
• Bed protector	____	____	____________
• Bath blanket	____	____	____________
5. Identified the person. Checked the identification bracelet against the assignment sheet. Called the person by name.	____	____	____________
6. Provided for privacy.	____	____	____________
7. Raised the bed for body mechanics. Raised the bed rails if used.	____	____	____________

Procedure

Procedure	S	U	Comments
8. Lowered the nearest bed rail if up.	____	____	____________
9. Put on the gloves.	____	____	____________
10. Covered the person with a bath blanket. Fan-folded top linens to the foot of the bed.	____	____	____________
11. Draped the person for perineal care.	____	____	____________
12. Folded back the bath blanket to expose the genital area.	____	____	____________
13. Placed the bed protector under the buttocks. Asked the person to flex the knees and raise the buttocks off the bed.	____	____	____________
14. Gave perineal care.	____	____	____________
15. Applied soap to a clean, wet washcloth.	____	____	____________
16. Separated the labia (female). If an uncircumcised male, retracted the foreskin. Checked for crusts, abnormal drainage, or secretions.	____	____	____________
17. Held the catheter near the meatus.	____	____	____________
18. Cleaned the catheter from the meatus down the catheter about 4 inches. Cleaned downward, away from the meatus with one stroke. Made sure not to tug or pull on the catheter. With a clean area of the washcloth or a clean washcloth, repeated as needed:	____	____	____________
a. Cleaned the catheter from the meatus down the catheter about 4 inches.	____	____	____________
b. Cleaned downward, away from the meatus with one stroke.	____	____	____________
c. Made sure not to tug or pull on the catheter.	____	____	____________

Procedure—cont'd	S	U	Comments
19. Rinsed the catheter with a clean washcloth. Rinsed from the meatus down the catheter about 4 inches. Rinsed downward, away from the meatus with one stroke. Made sure not to tug or pull on the catheter. With a clean area of the washcloth or a clean washcloth, repeated as needed.	_____	_____	____________
20. Secured the catheter. Coiled and secured tubing.	_____	_____	____________
21. Removed the bed protector.	_____	_____	____________
22. Covered the person. Removed the bath blanket.	_____	_____	____________
23. Removed the gloves. Decontaminated your hands.	_____	_____	____________

Post-Procedure

24. Provided for comfort.	_____	_____	____________
25. Placed the call bell within reach.	_____	_____	____________
26. Raised or lowered bed rails. Followed the care plan.	_____	_____	____________
27. Lowered the bed to its lowest position.	_____	_____	____________
28. Cleaned and returned equipment to its proper place. Discarded disposable items. Wore gloves.	_____	_____	____________
29. Removed gloves. Decontaminated your hands.	_____	_____	____________
30. Unscreened the person.	_____	_____	____________
31. Followed agency policy for soiled linen.	_____	_____	____________
32. Decontaminated your hands.	_____	_____	____________
33. Reported and recorded your observations.	_____	_____	____________

Changing a Leg Bag to a Drainage Bag

QUALITY OF LIFE

Name: ______________________

Date: ______________________

Remembered to:
- ◆ Knock before entering the person's room
- ◆ Address the person by name
- ◆ Introduce yourself by name and title

Pre-Procedure	S	U	Comments
1. Followed Delegation Guidelines: Drainage Systems. Viewed Safety Alert: Drainage Systems.	____	____	____________
2. Explained the procedure to the person.	____	____	____________
3. Completed hand hygiene.	____	____	____________
4. Collected the following:			
• Gloves	____	____	____________
• Drainage bag and tubing	____	____	____________
• Antiseptic wipes	____	____	____________
• Bed protector	____	____	____________
• Sterile cap and plug	____	____	____________
• Catheter clamp	____	____	____________
• Paper towels	____	____	____________
• Bedpan	____	____	____________
• Bath blanket	____	____	____________
5. Arranged paper towels and equipment on the overbed table.	____	____	____________
6. Identified the person. Checked the identification bracelet against the assignment sheet. Called the person by name.	____	____	____________
7. Provided for privacy.	____	____	____________

Procedure

8. Had the person sit on the side of the bed.	____	____	____________
9. Put on the gloves.	____	____	____________
10. Exposed the catheter and leg bag.	____	____	____________
11. Clamped the catheter to prevent urine from draining from the catheter into the drainage tubing.	____	____	____________
12. Allowed urine to drain from below the clamped site into the drainage tubing to empty the lower end of the catheter.	____	____	____________
13. Helped the person lie down.	____	____	____________
14. Raised the bed rails if used. Raised the bed for body mechanics.	____	____	____________
15. Lowered the nearest bed rail if up.	____	____	____________
16. Covered the person with a bath blanket. Exposed the catheter and leg bag.	____	____	____________
17. Placed the bed protector under the person's leg.	____	____	____________
18. Opened the antiseptic wipes. Placed them on the paper towels.	____	____	____________
19. Opened the package with the sterile cap and plug.	____	____	____________
20. Opened the package with the drainage bag and tubing.	____	____	____________

Procedure—cont'd	S	U	Comments
21. Attached the drainage bag to the bed frame.	______	______	______
22. Disconnected the catheter from the drainage tubing. Made sure that nothing touched the ends.	______	______	______
23. Inserted the sterile plug unto the catheter end. Made sure that you touched only the end of the plug and that you did not touch the part that went inside the catheter. (If you contaminated the end of the catheter, wiped the end with an antiseptic. Did so before you inserted the sterile plug.)	______	______	______
24. Placed the sterile cap on the end of the leg bag drainage tube. (If you contaminated the tubing end, wiped the end with an antiseptic wipe. Did so before you put on the sterile cap.)	______	______	______
25. Removed the cap from the new drainage tubing.	______	______	______
26. Removed the sterile plug from the catheter.	______	______	______
27. Inserted the end for the drainage tubing into the catheter.	______	______	______
28. Removed the clamp from the catheter.	______	______	______
29. Looped drainage tubing on the bed. Secured tubing to the mattress.	______	______	______
30. Removed the leg bag. Placed it in the bedpan.	______	______	______
31. Removed and discarded the bed protector.	______	______	______
32. Covered the person. Removed the bath blanket.	______	______	______
33. Took the bedpan to the bathroom.	______	______	______
34. Removed the gloves. Completed hand hygiene.	______	______	______

Post-Procedure

	S	U	Comments
35. Provided for comfort.	______	______	______
36. Placed the call bell within reach.	______	______	______
37. Raised or lowered the bed rails. Followed the care plan.	______	______	______
38. Lowered the bed to its lowest position.	______	______	______
39. Unscreened the person.	______	______	______
40. Put on clean gloves. Discarded disposable supplies.	______	______	______
41. Emptied the drainage bag.	______	______	______
42. Discarded the drainage tubing and bag following agency policy, or cleaned the bag following agency policy.	______	______	______
43. Cleaned the bedpan. Placed it in a clean cover.	______	______	______
44. Returned the bedpan and other supplies to their proper places.	______	______	______
45. Removed the gloves. Decontaminated your hands.	______	______	______
46. Reported and recorded your observations.	______	______	______
47. Reversed the procedure to attach a leg bag:			
a. Clamped the catheter. This prevented urine from drainage during change over.	______	______	______
b. Opened the package with the leg bag.	______	______	______
c. Placed the leg bag next to the person's side.	______	______	______
d. Disconnected the catheter from the leg bag. Made sure nothing touch the ends.	______	______	______

Post-Procedure—cont'd	S	U	Comments
e. Inserted the sterile plug unto the catheter end. Made sure that you only touched the end of the plug and that the part that went inside the catheter was not touched. (If you contaminated the end of the catheter, wiped the end with an antiseptic. Did so before you inserted the sterile plug.)	______	______	______________________
f. Placed the sterile cap on the end of the drainage bag tubing. (If you contaminated the tubing end, wiped the end with an antiseptic wipe. Did so before you put on the sterile cap.)	______	______	______________________
g. Removed the cap from the new drainage tubing.	______	______	______________________
h. Removed the sterile plug from the catheter.	______	______	______________________
i. Inserted the end for the drainage tubing into the catheter.	______	______	______________________
j. Removed the clamp from the catheter.	______	______	______________________
k. Secured the leg bag around the person's leg. Followed manufacturer's instructions.	______	______	______________________
l. Removed the drainage bag and tubing. Followed agency policy for storage or disposal.	______	______	______________________
m. Removed and discarded the bed protector.	______	______	______________________
n. Covered the person. Removed the bath blanket.	______	______	______________________
o. Removed the gloves. Completed hand hygiene.	______	______	______________________

Emptying a Urinary Drainage Bag

QUALITY OF LIFE

Name: ______________________

Date: ______________________

Remembered to:
- ◆ Knock before entering the person's room
- ◆ Address the person by name
- ◆ Introduce yourself by name and title

Pre-Procedure	S	U	Comments
1. Followed Delegation Guidelines: Drainage Systems. Viewed Safety Alert: Drainage Systems.	_____	_____	__________
2. Collected equipment:			
• Graduate (measuring container)	_____	_____	__________
• Gloves	_____	_____	__________
• Paper towels	_____	_____	__________
3. Completed hand hygiene.	_____	_____	__________
4. Explained the procedure to the person.	_____	_____	__________
5. Identified the person. Checked the identification bracelet against the assignment sheet. Called the person by name.	_____	_____	__________
6. Provided for privacy.	_____	_____	__________

Procedure

7. Put on the gloves.	_____	_____	__________
8. Placed a paper towel on the floor. Placed the graduate on top of it.	_____	_____	__________
9. Positioned the graduate under the collection bag.	_____	_____	__________
10. Opened the clamp on the drain.	_____	_____	__________
11. Allowed all urine into the graduate. Did not let the drain touch the graduate.	_____	_____	__________
12. Closed and positioned the clamp.	_____	_____	__________
13. Measured urine.	_____	_____	__________
14. Removed and discarded the paper towel.	_____	_____	__________
15. Rinsed the graduate. Returned it to its proper place.	_____	_____	__________
16. Removed the gloves. Completed hand hygiene.	_____	_____	__________
17. Recorded the time and amount on the intake and output (I&O) record.	_____	_____	__________

Post-Procedure

18. Unscreened the person.	_____	_____	__________
19. Reported and recorded the amount and other observations.	_____	_____	__________

Applying a Condom Catheter

QUALITY OF LIFE

Name: ______________________

Date: ______________________

Remembered to:
- ◆ **Knock before entering the person's room**
- ◆ **Address the person by name**
- ◆ **Introduce yourself by name and title**

Pre-Procedure	S	U	Comments
1. Followed Delegation Guidelines: Condom Catheters. Viewed Safety Alert: Condom Catheters.	____	____	____________
2. Explained the procedure to the person.	____	____	____________
3. Completed hand hygiene.	____	____	____________
4. Collected the following:			
• Condom catheter	____	____	____________
• Elastic tape	____	____	____________
• Drainage bag or leg bag	____	____	____________
• Cap for the drainage bag	____	____	____________
• Basin of warm water	____	____	____________
• Soap	____	____	____________
• Towel and washcloths	____	____	____________
• Bath blanket	____	____	____________
• Gloves	____	____	____________
• Bed protector	____	____	____________
• Paper towels	____	____	____________
5. Arranged paper towels and equipment on the overbed table.	____	____	____________
6. Provided for privacy.	____	____	____________
7. Identified the person. Checked the identification bracelet against the assignment sheet. Called the person by name.	____	____	____________
8. Raised the bed for body mechanics. Raised the bed rails if used.	____	____	____________

Procedure

9. Lowered the nearest bed rail if up.	____	____	____________
10. Covered the person with a bath blanket. Lowered top linens to the knees.	____	____	____________
11. Asked the person to raise his buttocks off the bed, or turned him onto his side away from you.	____	____	____________
12. Slid the bed protector under his buttocks.	____	____	____________
13. Had the person lower his buttocks, or turned him onto his back.	____	____	____________
14. Secured the drainage bag to the bed frame, or had a leg bag ready. Closed the drain.	____	____	____________
15. Exposed the genital area.	____	____	____________
16. Put on the gloves.	____	____	____________

Procedure—cont'd	S	U	Comments
17. Removed the condom catheter:			
a. Removed the tape. Rolled the sheath off the penis.	_____	_____	______________
b. Disconnected the drainage tubing from the condom. Capped the drainage tube.	_____	_____	______________
c. Discarded the tape and condom.	_____	_____	______________
18. Provided perineal care. Observed the penis for reddened areas and skin breakdown or irritation.	_____	_____	______________
19. Removed the protective backing from the condom to expose the adhesive strip.	_____	_____	______________
20. Held the penis firmly. Rolled the condom onto the penis. Left a 1-inch space between the penis and the end of the catheter.	_____	_____	______________
21. Secured the condom with elastic tape. Applied tape in a spiral. Did not apply tape completely around penis.	_____	_____	______________
22. Connected the condom to the drainage tubing. Coiled excess tubing on the bed, or attached a leg bag.	_____	_____	______________
23. Removed the bed protector and gloves. Discarded them. Completed hand hygiene.	_____	_____	______________
24. Covered the person. Removed the bath blanket.	_____	_____	______________

Post-Procedure

25. Provided for comfort.	_____	_____	______________
26. Placed the call bell within reach.	_____	_____	______________
27. Raised or lowered bed rails. Followed the care plan.	_____	_____	______________
28. Lowered the bed to its lowest position.	_____	_____	______________
29. Unscreened the person.	_____	_____	______________
30. Decontaminated your hands. Put on clean gloves.	_____	_____	______________
31. Measured and recorded the amount of urine in the bag. Cleaned or discarded the collection bag.	_____	_____	______________
32. Cleaned and returned the wash basin and other equipment. Returned items to their proper places.	_____	_____	______________
33. Removed gloves. Decontaminated your hands.	_____	_____	______________
34. Reported and recorded your observations.	_____	_____	______________

Checking for a Fecal Impaction

Quality of Life

Name: ______________________

Date: ______________________

Remembered to:
- ◆ **Knock before entering the person's room**
- ◆ **Address the person by name**
- ◆ **Introduce yourself by name and title**

Pre-Procedure	S	U	Comments
1. Followed Delegation Guidelines: Fecal Impactions. Viewed Safety Alert: Fecal Impactions.	____	____	____________
2. Explained the procedure to the person.	____	____	____________
3. Completed hand hygiene.	____	____	____________
4. Collected the following:			
• Bedpan and cover	____	____	____________
• Bath blanket	____	____	____________
• Toilet tissue	____	____	____________
• Gloves	____	____	____________
• Lubricant	____	____	____________
• Waterproof pad	____	____	____________
• Basin of warm water	____	____	____________
• Soap	____	____	____________
• Washcloth	____	____	____________
• Bath towel	____	____	____________
5. Identified the person. Checked the identification bracelet against the assignment sheet. Called the person by name.	____	____	____________
6. Provided for privacy.	____	____	____________
7. Raised the bed for body mechanics. Raised the bed rails if used.	____	____	____________

Procedure			
8. Lowered the nearest bed rail if up.	____	____	____________
9. Covered the person with a bath blanket. Fan-folded top linens to the foot of the bed.	____	____	____________
10. Turned the person in the Sims' or left side-lying position.	____	____	____________
11. Put on gloves.	____	____	____________
12. Placed the waterproof pad under the buttocks.	____	____	____________
13. Exposed the anal area.	____	____	____________
14. Lubricated your gloved index finger.	____	____	____________
15. Asked the person to take a deep breath through his or her mouth.	____	____	____________
16. Inserted the gloved finger while the person was taking a deep breath.	____	____	____________
17. Checked for fecal mass.	____	____	____________
18. Removed your finger.	____	____	____________
19. Helped the person onto the bedpan or to the bathroom or commode if needed. Provided for privacy.	____	____	____________

Procedure—cont'd	S	U	Comments
20. Removed and discarded the gloves. Completed hand hygiene.	____	____	____
21. Put on clean gloves.	____	____	____
22. Washed the person's anal area with soap and water. Patted dry.	____	____	____
23. Removed the waterproof pad and your gloves. Decontaminated your hands.	____	____	____

Post-Procedure

	S	U	Comments
24. Provided for comfort.	____	____	____
25. Covered the person. Removed the bath blanket.	____	____	____
26. Placed the call bell within reach.	____	____	____
27. Lowered the bed to its lowest position.	____	____	____
28. Raised or lowered bed rails. Followed the care plan.	____	____	____
29. Unscreened the person.	____	____	____
30. Cleaned and returned equipment to its proper place. Discarded disposable items. Wore gloves.	____	____	____
31. Followed agency policy for soiled linen.	____	____	____
32. Removed your gloves. Decontaminated your hands.	____	____	____
33. Reported and recorded your observations.	____	____	____

Removing a Fecal Impaction

QUALITY OF LIFE

Name: ______________________

Date: ______________________

Remembered to:
- ◆ **Knock before entering the person's room**
- ◆ **Address the person by name**
- ◆ **Introduce yourself by name and title**

Procedure	S	U	Comments
1. Checked for a fecal impaction:			
a. Followed Delegation Guidelines: Fecal Impactions. Viewed Safety Alert: Fecal Impactions.	____	____	________
b. Explained the procedure to the person.	____	____	________
c. Completed hand hygiene.	____	____	________
d. Collected the following:			
• Bedpan and cover	____	____	________
• Bath blanket	____	____	________
• Toilet tissue	____	____	________
• Gloves	____	____	________
• Lubricant	____	____	________
• Waterproof pad	____	____	________
• Basin of warm water	____	____	________
• Soap	____	____	________
• Washcloth	____	____	________
• Bath towel	____	____	________
e. Identified the person. Checked the identification bracelet against the assignment sheet. Called the person by name.	____	____	________
f. Provided for privacy.	____	____	________
g. Raised the bed for body mechanics. Raised the bed rails if used.	____	____	________
h. Lowered the nearest bed rail if up.	____	____	________
i. Covered the person with a bath blanket. Fanfolded top linens to the foot of the bed.	____	____	________
j. Turned the person in the Sims' or left side-lying position.	____	____	________
k. Put on gloves.	____	____	________
l. Placed the waterproof pad under the buttocks.	____	____	________
2. Checked the person's pulse. Noted the rate and rhythm.	____	____	________
3. Exposed the anal area.	____	____	________
4. Lubricated your gloved index finger.	____	____	________
5. Asked the person to take a deep breath through the mouth.	____	____	________
6. Inserted your lubricated, gloved index finger.	____	____	________
7. Hooked your finger around a small piece of feces.	____	____	________
8. Removed your finger and the feces.	____	____	________
9. Dropped the stool into the bedpan.	____	____	________
10. Cleaned your finger with toilet tissue. Placed the toilet tissue in the bedpan.	____	____	________
11. Reapplied lubricant as needed.	____	____	________

Procedure—cont'd	S	U	Comments
12. Repeated until you no longer felt feces:			
a. Asked the person to take a deep breath through the mouth.	____	____	____________
b. Inserted your lubricated, gloved index finger.	____	____	____________
c. Hooked your index finger around a small piece of feces.	____	____	____________
d. Removed your finger and the feces.	____	____	____________
e. Dropped the stool into the bedpan.	____	____	____________
f. Cleaned your finger with toilet tissue. Placed the toilet tissue in the bedpan.	____	____	____________
13. Checked the person's pulse at intervals. Used your clean gloved hand. Noted the rate and rhythm. Stopped the procedure if the pulse rate had slowed or if the rhythm was irregular.	____	____	____________
14. Wiped the anal area with the toilet tissue.	____	____	____________
15. Covered the person with the bath blanket.	____	____	____________
16. Covered the bedpan.	____	____	____________
17. Removed and discarded the gloves. Completed hand hygiene, and put on clean gloves.	____	____	____________
18. Raised the bed rail if used. Took the bedpan to the bathroom.	____	____	____________
19. Emptied, cleaned, and disinfected the bedpan.	____	____	____________
20. Returned the bedpan to the bedside stand.	____	____	____________
21. Removed and discarded the gloves. Completed hand hygiene.	____	____	____________
22. Filled the wash basin with warm water.	____	____	____________
23. Lowered the nearest bed rail if up.	____	____	____________
24. Put on clean gloves.	____	____	____________
25. Washed the buttocks, and gave perineal care.	____	____	____________
26. Removed the waterproof pad and your gloves. Completed hand hygiene.	____	____	____________

Post-Procedure

	S	U	Comments
27. Provided for comfort.	____	____	____________
28. Covered the person, and removed the bath blanket.	____	____	____________
29. Placed the call bell within reach.	____	____	____________
30. Lowered the bed to its lowest position.	____	____	____________
31. Raised or lowered bed rails. Followed the care plan.	____	____	____________
32. Unscreened the person.	____	____	____________
33. Cleaned and returned equipment to its proper place. Discarded disposable items. Wore gloves.	____	____	____________
34. Followed agency policy for soiled linen.	____	____	____________
35. Removed the gloves. Completed hand hygiene.	____	____	____________
36. Reported and recorded your observations.	____	____	____________

Giving a Cleansing Enema

QUALITY OF LIFE

Name: ______________________

Date: ______________________

Remembered to:
- Knock before entering the person's room
- Address the person by name
- Introduce yourself by name and title

Pre-Procedure	S	U	Comments
1. Followed Delegation Guidelines: Enemas. Viewed Safety Alert: Enemas.	____	____	____________
2. Explained the procedure to the person.	____	____	____________
3. Completed hand hygiene.	____	____	____________
4. Collected the following:			
• Bedpan or commode	____	____	____________
• Disposable enema kit as directed by the nurse (enema bag, tube, clamp, and waterproof pad)	____	____	____________
• Bath thermometer	____	____	____________
• Waterproof pad	____	____	____________
• Gloves	____	____	____________
• 3 to 5 ml (1 teaspoon) castile soap or 1 to 2 teaspoons of salt	____	____	____________
• Toilet tissue	____	____	____________
• Bath blanket	____	____	____________
• IV pole	____	____	____________
• Robe and nonskid footwear	____	____	____________
• Paper towels	____	____	____________
5. Identified the person. Checked the identification bracelet with the assignment sheet. Called the person by name.	____	____	____________
6. Provided for privacy.	____	____	____________
7. Raised the bed for body mechanics. Raised the bed rails if used.	____	____	____________
Procedure			
8. Lowered the nearest bed rail if up.	____	____	____________
9. Covered the person with a bath blanket. Fan-folded top linens to the foot of the bed.	____	____	____________
10. Positioned the IV pole so the enema bag was 12 inches above the anus, or to the height directed by the nurse.	____	____	____________
11. Raised the bed rail if used.	____	____	____________
12. Prepared the enema:			
a. Closed the clamp on the tube.	____	____	____________
b. Adjusted water flow until it was lukewarm.	____	____	____________
c. Filled the enema bag for the amount ordered.	____	____	____________
d. Measured water temperature with the bath thermometer (usually 105° F [40.5° C] for adults and 100° F [37.5° C] for children).	____	____	____________

Procedure—cont'd	S	U	Comments
e. Prepared the enema solution as directed by the nurse:			
i. Saline enema: Added 1 to 2 teaspoons of salt	____	____	____________
ii. Soapsuds enema: Added 3 to 5 ml (1 teaspoon) of castile soap	____	____	____________
iii. Tap-water enema: Added nothing to the water	____	____	____________
f. Stirred the solution with the bath thermometer. Scooped off any suds (SSE).	____	____	____________
g. Sealed the bag.	____	____	____________
h. Hung the bag on the IV pole.	____	____	____________
13. Lowered the nearest bed rail.	____	____	____________
14. Turned the person in the Sims' left side-lying position.	____	____	____________
15. Put on the gloves.	____	____	____________
16. Placed a waterproof pad under the buttocks.	____	____	____________
17. Exposed the anal area.	____	____	____________
18. Placed the bedpan behind the person.	____	____	____________
19. Positioned the enema tube in the bedpan. Removed the cap from the tubing.	____	____	____________
20. Opened the clamp. Allowed solution to flow through the tube to remove air. Clamped the tube.	____	____	____________
21. Lubricated the tube 3 to 4 inches from the tip.	____	____	____________
22. Separated the buttocks to see the anus.	____	____	____________
23. Asked the person to take a deep breath through the mouth.	____	____	____________
24. Gently inserted the tube 3 to 4 inches into the adult's rectum as the person was exhaling. Stopped if the person complained of pain, if you felt resistance, or if bleeding occurred.	____	____	____________
25. Checked the amount of solution in the bag.	____	____	____________
26. Unclamped the tube. Gave the solution slowly.	____	____	____________
27. Asked the person to take slow deep breaths to help the person relax.	____	____	____________
28. Clamped the tube if the person needed to defecate, had cramping, or started to expel solution. Unclamped when symptoms subsided.	____	____	____________
29. Gave the amount of solution ordered. Stopped if the person did not tolerate the procedure.	____	____	____________
30. Clamped the tube before it was empty, which prevented air from entering the bowel.	____	____	____________
31. Held toilet tissue around the tube and against the anus. Removed the tube.	____	____	____________
32. Discarded the toilet tissue into the bedpan.	____	____	____________
33. Wrapped the tubing tip with paper towels. Placed it inside the enema bag.	____	____	____________
34. Helped the person onto the bedpan. Raised the head of the bed, and raised the bed rail if used, or assisted the person to the bathroom or commode. The person wore a robe and nonskid footwear when up. The bed was in the lowest position.	____	____	____________

Procedure—cont'd	S	U	Comments
35. Placed the call bell and toilet tissue within reach. Reminded the person not to flush the toilet.	_____	_____	____________________
36. Discarded disposable items.	_____	_____	____________________
37. Removed the gloves. Decontaminated your hands.	_____	_____	____________________
38. Left the room if the person could be left alone.	_____	_____	____________________
39. Returned when the person signaled. Knocked before entering.	_____	_____	____________________
40. Decontaminated your hands, and put on gloves. Lowered the bed rail if up.	_____	_____	____________________
41. Observed enema results for amount, color, consistency, and odor. Called for the nurse to observe the results.	_____	_____	____________________
42. Provided perineal care as needed.	_____	_____	____________________
43. Removed the bed protector.	_____	_____	____________________
44. Emptied, cleaned, and disinfected the bedpan or commode. Flushed the toilet after the nurse observed the results. Returned items to their proper place.	_____	_____	____________________
45. Removed the gloves. Completed hand hygiene.	_____	_____	____________________
46. Assisted with handwashing. Wore gloves if needed.	_____	_____	____________________
47. Covered the person. Removed the bath blanket.	_____	_____	____________________

Post-Procedure

48. Provided for comfort.	_____	_____	____________________
49. Placed the call bell within reach.	_____	_____	____________________
50. Lowered the bed to its lowest position.	_____	_____	____________________
51. Raised or lowered the bed rails. Followed the care plan.	_____	_____	____________________
52. Unscreened the person.	_____	_____	____________________
53. Followed agency policy for soiled linen and used supplies.	_____	_____	____________________
54. Decontaminated your hands.	_____	_____	____________________
55. Reported and recorded your observations.	_____	_____	____________________

Giving a Small Volume Enema

Quality of Life

Name: ______________________

Date: ______________________

Remembered to:
- ◆ **Knock before entering the person's room**
- ◆ **Address the person by name**
- ◆ **Introduce yourself by name and title**

Pre-Procedure	S	U	Comments
1. Followed Delegation Guidelines: Enemas. Viewed Safety Alert: Enemas.	____	____	____________
2. Explained the procedure to the person.	____	____	____________
3. Completed hand hygiene.	____	____	____________
4. Collected the following:			
• Small volume enema	____	____	____________
• Bedpan or commode	____	____	____________
• Waterproof pad	____	____	____________
• Toilet tissue	____	____	____________
• Gloves	____	____	____________
• Robe and nonskid footwear	____	____	____________
• Bath blanket	____	____	____________
5. Identified the person. Checked the identification bracelet against the treatment card. Called the person by name.	____	____	____________
6. Provided for privacy.	____	____	____________
7. Raised the bed for body mechanics. Raised the bed rails if used.	____	____	____________

Procedure			
8. Lowered the nearest bed rail if up.	____	____	____________
9. Covered the person with a bath blanket. Fan-folded top linens to the foot of the bed.	____	____	____________
10. Turned the person in the Sims' or left side-lying position.	____	____	____________
11. Put on the gloves.	____	____	____________
12. Placed the waterproof pad under the buttocks.	____	____	____________
13. Exposed the anal area.	____	____	____________
14. Positioned the bedpan near the person.	____	____	____________
15. Removed the cap from the enema.	____	____	____________
16. Separated the buttocks to see the anus.	____	____	____________
17. Asked the person to take a deep breath through the mouth.	____	____	____________
18. Inserted the enema tip 2 inches into the rectum as the person was exhaling. Inserted the tip gently. Stopped if the person complained of pain, if you felt resistance, or if bleeding occurred.	____	____	____________
19. Squeezed and rolled the bottle gently. Released pressure on the bottle after you removed the tip from the rectum.	____	____	____________
20. Put the bottle into the box, tip first.	____	____	____________

Procedure—cont'd	S	U	Comments
21. Helped the person onto the bedpan; raised the head of the bed. Raised or lowered bed rails according to the care plan, or assisted the person to the bathroom or commode. Made sure that the person wore a robe and nonskid footwear when up. Lowered the bed in the lowest position.			
22. Placed the call bell and toilet tissue within reach. Reminded the person not to flush the toilet.			
23. Discarded disposable items.			
24. Removed the gloves. Decontaminated your hands.			
25. Left the room if the person could be left alone.			
26. Returned when the person signaled. Knocked before entering.			
27. Decontaminated your hands. Lowered the bed rail if up.			
28. Put on the gloves.			
29. Observed enema results for amount, color, consistency, and odor.			
30. Helped the person with perineal care.			
31. Removed the bed protector.			
32. Emptied, cleaned, and disinfected the bedpan or commode. Flushed the toilet after the nurse observed the results.			
33. Returned equipment to its proper place.			
34. Removed the gloves. Completed hand hygiene.			
35. Assisted with handwashing. Wore gloves if necessary.			
36. Returned top linens. Removed the bath blanket.			

Post-Procedure

	S	U	Comments
37. Provided for comfort.			
38. Placed the call bell within reach.			
39. Lowered the bed to its lowest position.			
40. Raised or lowered bed rails. Followed the care plan.			
41. Unscreened the person.			
42. Followed agency policy for soiled linen and used supplies.			
43. Decontaminated your hands.			
44. Reported and recorded your observations.			

Giving an Oil-Retention Enema

QUALITY OF LIFE

Name: ______________________

Date: ______________________

Remembered to:
- ◆ Knock before entering the person's room
- ◆ Address the person by name
- ◆ Introduce yourself by name and title

Pre-Procedure

	S	U	Comments
1. Followed Delegation Guidelines: Enemas. Viewed Safety Alert: Enemas.	____	____	____________
2. Explained the procedure to the person.	____	____	____________
3. Completed hand hygiene.	____	____	____________
4. Collected the following:			
• Oil-retention enema	____	____	____________
• Waterproof pads	____	____	____________
• Gloves	____	____	____________
• Bath blanket	____	____	____________
5. Identified the person. Checked the identification bracelet against the assignment sheet. Called the person by name.	____	____	____________
6. Provided for privacy.	____	____	____________
7. Raised the bed for body mechanics. Raised the bed rails if used.	____	____	____________

Procedure

	S	U	Comments
8. Lowered the nearest bed rail if up.	____	____	____________
9. Covered the person with a bath blanket. Fan-folded top linens to the foot of the bed.	____	____	____________
10. Turned the person in the Sims' or left side-lying position.	____	____	____________
11. Put on the gloves.	____	____	____________
12. Placed the waterproof pad under the buttocks.	____	____	____________
13. Exposed the anal area.	____	____	____________
14. Positioned the bedpan near the person.	____	____	____________
15. Removed the cap from the enema.	____	____	____________
16. Separated the buttocks to see the anus.	____	____	____________
17. Asked the person to take a deep breath through the mouth.	____	____	____________
18. Inserted the enema tip 2 inches into the rectum as the person was exhaling. Gently inserted the tip. Stopped if the person complained of pain, if you felt resistance, or if bleeding occurred.	____	____	____________
19. Gently squeezed and rolled the bottle. Released pressure on the bottle after you removed the tip from the rectum.	____	____	____________
20. Put the bottle into the box, tip first.	____	____	____________
21. Covered the person. Turn him or her in the Sims' or side-lying position.	____	____	____________
22. Encourage him or her to retain the enema for the time ordered.	____	____	____________
23. Placed more waterproof pads on the bed if needed.	____	____	____________

Procedure—cont'd	S	U	Comments
24. Removed the gloves. Decontaminated your hands.			
25. Lowered the bed to its lowest position.			
26. Raised or lowered bed rails. Followed the care plan.			
27. Provided for comfort.			
28. Placed the call bell within reach.			
29. Unscreened the person.			
30. Decontaminated your hands.			
31. Checked the person often.			

Post-Procedure

	S	U	Comments
32. Provided for comfort.			
33. Placed the call bell within reach.			
34. Lowered the bed to its lowest position.			
35. Raised or lowered bed rails. Followed the care plan.			
36. Unscreened the person.			
37. Followed agency policy for soiled linen and used supplies.			
38. Decontaminated your hands.			
39. Reported and recorded your observations.			

Inserting a Rectal Tube

QUALITY OF LIFE

Name: ____________________

Date: ____________________

Remembered to:
- ◆ **Knock before entering the person's room**
- ◆ **Address the person by name**
- ◆ **Introduce yourself by name and title**

Pre-Procedure	**S**	**U**	**Comments**
1. Followed Delegation Guidelines: Rectal Tubes. Viewed Safety Alert: Rectal Tubes.	____	____	____________
2. Explained the procedure to the person.	____	____	____________
3. Completed hand hygiene.	____	____	____________
4. Collected the following:			
• Disposable rectal tube with flatus bag	____	____	____________
• Water-soluble lubricant	____	____	____________
• Tape	____	____	____________
• Gloves	____	____	____________
• Waterproof pad	____	____	____________
5. Identified the person. Checked the identification bracelet against the assignment sheet. Called the person by name.	____	____	____________
6. Provided for privacy.	____	____	____________
7. Raised the bed for body mechanics. Raised the bed rails if used.	____	____	____________

Procedure			
8. Lowered the nearest bed rail if up.	____	____	____________
9. Turned the person in the Sims' or left side-lying position.	____	____	____________
10. Put on the gloves.	____	____	____________
11. Placed the waterproof pad under the buttocks.	____	____	____________
12. Exposed the anal area.	____	____	____________
13. Lubricated 4 inches from the tube tip.	____	____	____________
14. Separated the buttocks to see the anus.	____	____	____________
15. Asked the person to take a deep breath through the mouth.	____	____	____________
16. Inserted the tube 4 inches into the rectum as the person was exhaling. Gently inserted the tube. Stopped if person complained of pain, if you felt resistance, or if bleeding occurred.	____	____	____________
17. Taped the rectal tube to the buttocks.	____	____	____________
18. Positioned the flatus bag so it rested on the bed protector.	____	____	____________
19. Covered the person.	____	____	____________
20. Left the tube in place for the time directed by the nurse (no longer than 30 minutes).	____	____	____________
21. Lowered the bed to its lowest position.	____	____	____________
22. Placed the call bell within reach.	____	____	____________
23. Raised or lowered bed rails. Followed the care plan.	____	____	____________
24. Removed the gloves. Decontaminated your hands.	____	____	____________

Procedure—cont'd	S	U	Comments
25. Left the room. Checked the person often. Knocked before entering the room.	______	______	____________________
26. Returned to the room when it was time to remove the tube. Knocked before entering the room.	______	______	____________________
27. Decontaminated your hands. Put on gloves.	______	______	____________________
28. Removed the tube. Wiped the rectal area.	______	______	____________________
29. Wrapped the rectal tube and flatus bag in the bed protector. Removed the bed protector and your gloves. Decontaminated your hands.	______	______	____________________
30. Asked the person about the amount of gas expelled.	______	______	____________________

Post-Procedure

31. Provided for comfort.	______	______	____________________
32. Placed the call bell within reach.	______	______	____________________
33. Unscreened the person.	______	______	____________________
34. Discarded disposable items. Followed agency policy for soiled linen. Wore gloves.	______	______	____________________
35. Removed the gloves. Decontaminated your hands.	______	______	____________________
36. Reported and recorded your observations.	______	______	____________________

Changing an Ostomy Pouch

QUALITY OF LIFE

Name: ______________________

Date: ______________________

Remembered to:
- ◆ Knock before entering the person's room
- ◆ Address the person by name
- ◆ Introduce yourself by name and title

Pre-Procedure	S	U	Comments
1. Followed Delegation Guidelines: Ostomy Pouches. Viewed Safety Alert: Ostomy Pouches.	____	____	____________
2. Explained the procedure to the person.	____	____	____________
3. Completed hand hygiene.	____	____	____________
4. Collected the following:			
• Clean pouch with skin barrier	____	____	____________
• Skin barrier (if not part of the pouch) as ordered	____	____	____________
• Pouch, clamp, and clip or wire closure	____	____	____________
• Clean ostomy belt if used	____	____	____________
• Gauze squares or wash cloths	____	____	____________
• Adhesive remover	____	____	____________
• Cotton balls	____	____	____________
• Bedpan with cover	____	____	____________
• Waterproof pad	____	____	____________
• Bath blanket	____	____	____________
• Toilet tissue	____	____	____________
• Wash basin	____	____	____________
• Bath thermometer	____	____	____________
• Prescribed soap or cleansing agent	____	____	____________
• Pouch deodorant	____	____	____________
• Paper towels	____	____	____________
• Gloves	____	____	____________
• Disposable bag	____	____	____________
5. Arranged your work area.	____	____	____________
6. Identified the person. Checked the identification bracelet against the assignment sheet. Called the person by name.	____	____	____________
7. Provided for privacy.	____	____	____________
8. Raised the bed for body mechanics. Raised the bed rails if used.	____	____	____________

Procedure			
9. Lowered the nearest bed rail if up.	____	____	____________
10. Covered the person with a bath blanket. Fan-folded the linens to the foot of the bed.	____	____	____________
11. Put on the gloves.	____	____	____________
12. Placed the waterproof pad under the buttocks.	____	____	____________
13. Disconnected the pouch from the belt if one was worn. Removed the belt.	____	____	____________

Procedure—cont'd	S	U	Comments
14. Gently removed the pouch. Gently pushed the skin down and away from the skin barrier. Placed the pouch in the bedpan.			
15. Wiped around the stoma with toilet tissue or gauze square, removing mucus and feces. Placed soiled tissue in the bedpan. Discarded gauze square in the bag.			
16. Moistened a cotton ball with adhesive remover. Cleaned around the stoma to remove any remaining skin barrier. Cleaned from the stoma outward.			
17. Covered the bedpan. Took it to the bathroom. (If the person used bed rails, raised them before you left the bedside.)			
18. Measured the amount of feces. Noted the color, amount, consistency, and odor of feces.			
19. Asked the nurse to observe abnormal feces. Then emptied the pouch and bedpan into the toilet. Put the pouch in the bag.			
20. Removed the gloves, and completed hand hygiene. Put on clean gloves.			
21. Filled the basin with warm water. Placed the basin on the overbed table on top of the paper towels. Lowered the nearest bed rail if up.			
22. Washed the skin around the stoma, using soap or other cleansing agent as directed by the nurse. Rinsed and patted dry.			
23. Applied the skin barrier if it was a separate device.			
24. Applied a clean ostomy belt on the person if worn.			
25. Added deodorant to the new pouch.			
26. Removed adhesive backing on the pouch.			
27. Centered the pouch over the stoma. Pointed the drain downward.			
28. Pressed around the skin barrier so that the pouch was sealed to the skin. Applied gentle pressure from the stoma outward.			
29. Maintained pressure for 1 to 2 minutes.			
30. Connected the belt to the pouch if worn.			
31. Removed the waterproof pad.			
32. Removed the gloves. Decontaminated your hands.			
33. Covered the person. Removed the bath blanket.			

Post-Procedure

	S	U	Comments
34. Provided for comfort.			
35. Raised or lowered bed rails. Followed the care plan.			
36. Lowered the bed to its lowest position.			
37. Placed the call bell within reach.			
38. Unscreened the person.			
39. Cleaned equipment. Wore gloves.			

Post-Procedure—cont'd	S	U	Comments
40. Returned equipment to its proper place.	_____	_____	__________________
41. Discarded the bag according to agency policy. Followed agency policy for soiled linen.	_____	_____	__________________
42. Removed the gloves. Completed hand hygiene.	_____	_____	__________________
43. Reported and recorded your observations.	_____	_____	__________________

Measuring Intake and Output

QUALITY OF LIFE

Name: ______________________

Date: ______________________

Remembered to:
- ◆ Knock before entering the person's room
- ◆ Address the person by name
- ◆ Introduce yourself by name and title

Pre-Procedure	S	U	Comments
1. Followed Delegation Guidelines: Intake and Output. Viewed Safety Alert: Intake and Output.	____	____	____________
2. Explained the procedure to the person.	____	____	____________
3. Completed hand hygiene.	____	____	____________
4. Collected the following:			
• Intake and output (I&O) record	____	____	____________
• Graduates	____	____	____________
• Gloves	____	____	____________
Procedure			
5. Put on the gloves.	____	____	____________
6. Measured intake as follows:			
a. Poured liquid remaining in a container into graduate.	____	____	____________
b. Measured the amount at eye level. Kept the container level.	____	____	____________
c. Checked the serving amount on the I&O record.			
d. Subtracted the remaining amount from the full serving amount. Recorded the amount.	____	____	____________
e. Repeated for each liquid:			
i. Measured the amount at eye level. Kept the container level.	____	____	____________
ii. Checked the serving amount on the I&O record.	____	____	____________
iii. Subtracted the remaining amount from the full serving amount. Recorded the amount.	____	____	____________
f. Added the amounts from each liquid together.	____	____	____________
g. Recorded the time and amount on the I&O record.	____	____	____________
7. Measured output as follows:			
a. Poured the fluid into the graduate used to measure output.	____	____	____________
b. Measured the amount at eye level. Kept the container level.	____	____	____________
8. Disposed of fluid in the toilet. Avoided splashes.	____	____	____________
9. Rinsed the graduate. Disposed of rinse into the toilet. Returned the graduate to its proper place.	____	____	____________
10. Cleaned and rinsed the bedpan, urinal, kidney basin, or other drainage container. Discarded the rinse into the toilet. Returned the item to its proper place.	____	____	____________
11. Removed the gloves. Decontaminated your hands.	____	____	____________
12. Recorded the amount on the I&O record.	____	____	____________
Post-Procedure			
13. Reported and recorded your observations.	____	____	____________

Preparing the Person for Meals

QUALITY OF LIFE

Name: ______________________

Date: ______________________

Remembered to:
- ◆ Knock before entering the person's room
- ◆ Address the person by name
- ◆ Introduce yourself by name and title

Pre-Procedure	S	U	Comments
1. Followed Delegation Guidelines: Preparing for Meals. Viewed Safety Alert: Preparing for Meals.	_____	_____	__________
2. Explained the procedure to the person.	_____	_____	__________
3. Completed hand hygiene.			
4. Collected the following:			
• Equipment for oral hygiene	_____	_____	__________
• Bedpan, urinal, or commode and toilet tissue	_____	_____	__________
• Wash basin	_____	_____	__________
• Soap	_____	_____	__________
• Washcloth	_____	_____	__________
• Towel	_____	_____	__________
• Gloves	_____	_____	__________
5. Provided for privacy.	_____	_____	__________

Procedure	S	U	Comments
6. Made sure eyeglasses and hearing aids were in place.	_____	_____	__________
7. Assisted with oral hygiene. Made sure dentures were in place.	_____	_____	__________
8. Assisted with elimination. Made sure the incontinent person was clean and dry.	_____	_____	__________
9. Assisted with handwashing.	_____	_____	__________
10. Performed the following if the person ate in bed:			
a. Raised the head of the bed to a comfortable position.	_____	_____	__________
b. Cleaned the overbed table. Adjusted it in front of the person.	_____	_____	__________
c. Placed the call bell within reach.	_____	_____	__________
d. Unscreened the person.	_____	_____	__________
11. Performed the following if the person sat in a chair:			
a. Positioned the person in a chair or wheelchair.	_____	_____	__________
b. Removed items from the overbed table. Cleaned the table.	_____	_____	__________
c. Adjusted the overbed table in front of the person.	_____	_____	__________
d. Placed the call bell within reach.	_____	_____	__________
e. Unscreened the person.	_____	_____	__________
12. Assisted the person to the dining area if he or she normally eats in the dining area.	_____	_____	__________

Post-Procedure	S	U	Comments
13. Returned to the room. Knocked before entering.	_____	_____	____________________
14. Cleaned and returned equipment to its proper place. Wore gloves for this step.	_____	_____	____________________
15. Straightened the room. Eliminated unpleasant noise, odors, or equipment.	_____	_____	____________________
16. Removed the gloves. Decontaminated your hands.	_____	_____	____________________

Serving Meal Trays

QUALITY OF LIFE

Name: ______________________

Date: ______________________

Remembered to:
- **Knock before entering the person's room**
- **Address the person by name**
- **Introduce yourself by name and title**

Pre-Procedure	**S**	**U**	**Comments**
1. Followed Delegation Guidelines: Serving Meal Trays. Viewed Safety Alert: Serving Meal Trays.	____	____	____________
2. Completed hand hygiene.	____	____	____________

Procedure			
3. Made sure the tray was complete. Checked items on the tray with the dietary card. Made sure adaptive equipment was included.	____	____	____________
4. Identified the person. Checked the identification bracelet with the dietary card. Called the person by name.	____	____	____________
5. Placed the tray within the person's reach. Adjusted the overbed table as needed.	____	____	____________
6. Removed food covers. Opened cartons, cut meat, and buttered bread as needed.	____	____	____________
7. Placed the napkin, clothes protector, adaptive equipment, and silverware within reach.	____	____	____________
8. Measured and recorded intake if ordered. Noted the amount and type of foods eaten.	____	____	____________
9. Checked for and removed any food in the mouth (pocketing). Wore gloves. Decontaminated your hands after you removed the gloves.	____	____	____________
10. Removed the tray.	____	____	____________
11. Cleaned spills. Changed soiled linen.	____	____	____________
12. Helped the person return to bed if indicated.	____	____	____________

Post-Procedure			
13. Assisted with oral hygiene and handwashing. Wore gloves.	____	____	____________
14. Removed the gloves. Decontaminated your hands.	____	____	____________
15. Provided for comfort.	____	____	____________
16. Placed the call bell within reach.	____	____	____________
17. Raised or lowered bed rails. Followed the care plan.	____	____	____________
18. Followed agency policy for soiled linen.	____	____	____________
19. Decontaminated your hands.	____	____	____________
20. Reported and recorded your observations.	____	____	____________

Feeding a Person

QUALITY OF LIFE

Name: ______________________

Date: ______________________

Remembered to:
- ◆ Knock before entering the person's room
- ◆ Address the person by name
- ◆ Introduce yourself by name and title

Pre-Procedure	S	U	Comments
1. Followed Delegation Guidelines: Feeding a Person. Viewed Safety Alert: Feeding a Person.	____	____	____________
2. Explained the procedure to the person.	____	____	____________
3. Completed hand hygiene.	____	____	____________
4. Positioned the person in a sitting position.	____	____	____________
5. Got the tray. Placed it on the overbed table or dining table.	____	____	____________

Procedure	S	U	Comments
6. Identified the person. Checked the identification bracelet with the dietary card. Called the person by name.	____	____	____________
7. Draped a napkin across the person's chest and underneath the chin.	____	____	____________
8. Told the person what foods and fluids were on the tray.	____	____	____________
9. Prepared food for eating. Seasoned food as the person preferred and was allowed on the care plan.	____	____	____________
10. Served foods in the order the person preferred. Alternated between solid and liquid foods. Used a spoon for safety. Allowed enough time for chewing. Avoided rushing the person.	____	____	____________
11. Used straws for liquids if the person did not drink out of a glass or cup. Had one straw for each liquid. Provided short straws for weak persons.	____	____	____________
12. Followed the care plan if the person had dysphagia. (Some persons with dysphagia do not use straws.) Gave thickened liquids with a spoon.	____	____	____________
13. Conversed with the person in a pleasant manner.	____	____	____________
14. Encouraged him or her to eat as much as possible.	____	____	____________
15. Wiped the person's mouth with a napkin.	____	____	____________
16. Noted how much and which foods were eaten.	____	____	____________
17. Measured and recorded intake if ordered.	____	____	____________
18. Removed the tray.	____	____	____________
19. Took the person back to his or her room.	____	____	____________
20. Assisted with oral hygiene and handwashing. Provided for privacy, and put on gloves. Decontaminated your hands after removing the gloves.	____	____	____________

Post-Procedure	S	U	Comments
21. Provided for comfort.	______	______	____________________
22. Placed the call bell within reach.	______	______	____________________
23. Raised or lowered bed rails. Followed the care plan.	______	______	____________________
24. Decontaminated your hands.	______	______	____________________
25. Reported and recorded your observations.	______	______	____________________

Taking a Temperature With a Glass Thermometer

QUALITY OF LIFE

Name: ______________________

Date: ______________________

Remembered to:
- Knock before entering the person's room
- Address the person by name
- Introduce yourself by name and title

Pre-Procedure	S	U	Comments
1. Followed Delegation Guidelines: Taking Temperatures. Viewed Safety Alerts: Taking Temperatures and Mercury-Glass Thermometers.	___	___	___
2. Explained the procedure to the person. For an oral temperature, asked the person not to eat, drink, smoke, or chew gum for at least 15 to 20 minutes or as required by agency policy.	___	___	___
3. Collected the following:			
• Oral or rectal thermometer and holder	___	___	___
• Tissues	___	___	___
• Plastic covers if used	___	___	___
• Gloves	___	___	___
• Toilet tissue (rectal temperature)	___	___	___
• Towel (axillary temperature)	___	___	___
4. Completed hand hygiene.	___	___	___
5. Identified the person. Checked the identification bracelet against the assignment sheet. Called the person by name.	___	___	___
6. Provided for privacy.	___	___	___

Procedure	S	U	Comments
7. Put on the gloves.	___	___	___
8. Rinsed the thermometer in cold water if it was soaked in a disinfectant. Dried it with tissues.	___	___	___
9. Checked for breaks, cracks, or chips.	___	___	___
10. Shook down the thermometer below the lowest number.	___	___	___
11. Inserted it into a plastic cover if used.	___	___	___
12. *For an oral temperature:*			
a. Asked the person to moisten his or her lips.	___	___	___
b. Placed the bulb end of the thermometer under the tongue.	___	___	___
c. Asked the person to close the lips around the thermometer to hold it in place.	___	___	___
d. Asked the person not to talk. Reminded the person not to bite down on the thermometer.	___	___	___
e. Left the thermometer in place for 2 to 3 minutes or as required by agency policy.	___	___	___

Procedure–cont'd	S	U	Comments
13. *For a rectal temperature:*			
a. Turned the person in the Sims' position.	_____	_____	__________
b. Put small amount of lubricant on a tissue. Lubricated the bulb end of the thermometer.	_____	_____	__________
c. Folded back top linens to expose the anal area.	_____	_____	__________
d. Raised the upper buttock, exposing the anus.	_____	_____	__________
e. Inserted the thermometer 1 inch into the rectum without forcing the thermometer. (Remember, glass thermometers can break.)	_____	_____	__________
f. Held the thermometer in place for 2 minutes or as required by agency policy without letting go of it while in the rectum.	_____	_____	__________
14. *For an axillary temperature:*			
a. Helped the person remove an arm from the gown. Did not expose the person.	_____	_____	__________
b. Dried the axilla with the towel.	_____	_____	__________
c. Placed the bulb end of the thermometer in the center of the axilla.	_____	_____	__________
d. Asked the person to place the arm over the chest to hold the thermometer in place. Held it and the arm in place if he or she could not help.	_____	_____	__________
e. Left the thermometer in place for 5 to 10 minutes or as required by agency policy.	_____	_____	__________
15. Removed the thermometer.	_____	_____	__________
16. Used tissues to remove the plastic cover. Wiped the thermometer with a tissue if no cover was used. Wiped from the stem to the bulb end.	_____	_____	__________
17. *For a rectal temperature:*			
a. Placed used toilet tissue on a paper towel or several thicknesses of toilet tissue.	_____	_____	__________
b. Placed the thermometer on clean toilet tissue.	_____	_____	__________
c. Wiped the anal area to remove excess lubricant and any feces.	_____	_____	__________
d. Covered the person.	_____	_____	__________
18. *For an axillary temperature:* Helped the person put the gown back on.	_____	_____	__________
19. Read the thermometer.	_____	_____	__________
20. Recorded the person's name and temperature on your note pad or assignment sheet. Wrote "R" for rectal temperature. Wrote "A" for axillary temperature.	_____	_____	__________
21. Shook down the thermometer.	_____	_____	__________
22. Cleaned it according to agency policy.	_____	_____	__________
23. Discarded tissue and the paper towel.	_____	_____	__________
24. Removed the gloves. Decontaminated your hands.	_____	_____	__________

Post-Procedure	S	U	Comments
25. Provided for comfort.	______	______	____________________
26. Placed the call bell within reach.	______	______	____________________
27. Unscreened the person.	______	______	____________________
28. Recorded the temperature in the proper place. Reported any abnormal temperature to the nurse. Noted the temperature site.	______	______	____________________

Taking a Temperature With an Electronic Thermometer

QUALITY OF LIFE

Name: ______________________

Date: ______________________

Remembered to:
- Knock before entering the person's room
- Address the person by name
- Introduce yourself by name and title

Pre-Procedure	S	U	Comments
1. Followed Delegation Guidelines: Taking Temperatures. Viewed Safety Alert: Temperature Sites.	____	____	________
2. Explained the procedure to the person. For an oral temperature, asked him or her not to eat, drink, smoke, or chew gum for at least 15 to 20 minutes.	____	____	________
3. Collected the following:			
• Thermometer—electronic or tympanic membrane	____	____	________
• Probe (blue for an oral or axillary temperature, red for a rectal temperature)	____	____	________
• Probe covers	____	____	________
• Toilet tissue (rectal temperature)	____	____	________
• Water-soluble lubricant (rectal temperature)	____	____	________
• Gloves	____	____	________
• Towels (axillary temperature)	____	____	________
4. Plugged the probe into the thermometer. (This was not done for a tympanic membrane thermometer.)	____	____	________
5. Completed hand hygiene.	____	____	________
6. Identified the person. Checked the identification bracelet against the assignment sheet. Called the person by name.	____	____	________
Procedure			
7. Provided for privacy. Positioned the person for an oral, rectal, axillary, or tympanic membrane temperature.	____	____	________
8. Put on gloves if contact with blood, body fluids, secretions, or excretions was likely.	____	____	________
9. Inserted the probe into a probe cover.	____	____	________
10. *For an oral temperature:*			
a. Asked the person to open the mouth and raise the tongue.	____	____	________
b. Placed the covered probe at the base of the tongue.	____	____	________
c. Asked the person to lower the tongue and close the mouth.	____	____	________
11. *For a rectal temperature:*			
a. Placed some lubricant on toilet tissue.	____	____	________
b. Lubricated the end of the covered probe.	____	____	________
c. Exposed the anal area.	____	____	________
d. Raised the upper buttock.	____	____	________
e. Inserted the probe 1/2 inch into the rectum.	____	____	________
f. Held the probe in place.	____	____	________

Procedure—cont'd

	S	U	Comments
12. *For an axillary temperature:*			
a. Helped the person remove an arm from the gown without exposing the person.	____	____	____
b. Dried the axilla with the towel.	____	____	____
c. Placed the covered probe in the axilla.	____	____	____
d. Placed the person's arm over the chest.	____	____	____
e. Held the probe in place.	____	____	____
13. *For a tympanic membrane temperature:*			
a. Asked the person to turn his or her head so the ear was in front of you.	____	____	____
b. Pulled back on the ear to straighten the ear canal.	____	____	____
c. Gently inserted the covered probe.	____	____	____
14. Started the thermometer.	____	____	____
15. Held the probe in place until you heard a tone or saw a flashing or steady light.	____	____	____
16. Read the temperature on the display.	____	____	____
17. Removed the probe. Pressed the eject button to discard the cover.	____	____	____
18. Recorded the person's name and temperature on your note pad or assignment sheet. Noted the temperature site.	____	____	____
19. Returned the probe to the holder.	____	____	____
20. Provided for comfort. Helped the person put the gown back on (axillary temperature). For a rectal temperature:	____	____	____
a. Wiped the anal area with tissue to remove lubricant.	____	____	____
b. Covered the person.	____	____	____
c. Discarded used toilet tissue.	____	____	____
d. Removed the gloves. Decontaminated your hands.	____	____	____

Post-Procedure

	S	U	Comments
21. Placed the call bell within reach.	____	____	____
22. Unscreened the person.	____	____	____
23. Returned the thermometer to the changing unit.	____	____	____
24. Decontaminated your hands.	____	____	____
25. Recorded the temperature in the proper place. Noted the temperature site. Reported any abnormal temperatures.	____	____	____

Taking a Radial Pulse

QUALITY OF LIFE

Name: ______________________

Date: ______________________

Remembered to:
- ◆ Knock before entering the person's room
- ◆ Address the person by name
- ◆ Introduce yourself by name and title

Pre-Procedure

	S	U	Comments
1. Followed Delegation Guidelines: Taking Pulses. Viewed Safety Alert: Taking Pulses.	____	____	____________
2. Completed hand hygiene.	____	____	____________
3. Identified the person. Checked the identification bracelet against the assignment sheet. Called the person by name.	____	____	____________
4. Explained the procedure to the person.	____	____	____________
5. Provided for privacy.	____	____	____________

Procedure

	S	U	Comments
6. Asked the person to sit or lie down.	____	____	____________
7. Located the radial pulse. Used your first two or three middle fingers.	____	____	____________
8. Noted if the pulse was strong or weak and regular or irregular.	____	____	____________
9. Counted the pulse for 30 seconds. Multiplied the number of beats by 2, or counted the pulse for 1 minute as directed by the nurse or as required by agency policy. (NNAAP skills evaluation required counting the pulse for 1 minute.)	____	____	____________
10. Counted the pulse for 1 minute if it was irregular.	____	____	____________
11. Recorded the person's name and pulse on your note pad or assignment sheet. Noted the strength of the pulse. Noted if it was regular or irregular.	____	____	____________

Post-Procedure

	S	U	Comments
12. Provided for comfort.	____	____	____________
13. Placed the call bell within reach.	____	____	____________
14. Unscreened the person.	____	____	____________
15. Decontaminated your hands.	____	____	____________
16. Reported and recorded the pulse rate and your observations.	____	____	____________

Taking an Apical Pulse

QUALITY OF LIFE

Name: ______________________

Date: ______________________

Remembered to:
- ◆ Knock before entering the person's room
- ◆ Address the person by name
- ◆ Introduce yourself by name and title

Pre-Procedure	S	U	Comments
1. Followed Delegation Guidelines: Taking Pulses. Viewed Safety Alert: Stethoscopes.			
2. Collected a stethoscope and antiseptic wipes.			
3. Completed hand hygiene.			
4. Identified the person. Checked the identification bracelet against the assignment sheet. Called the person by name.			
5. Explained the procedure to the person.			
6. Provided for privacy.			

Procedure

	S	U	Comments
7. Cleaned the earpieces and diaphragm with the wipes.			
8. Asked the person to sit or lie down.			
9. Exposed the nipple area of the left chest without exposing a woman's breasts.			
10. Warmed the diaphragm in your palm.			
11. Placed the earpieces in your ears.			
12. Found the apical pulse. Placed the diaphragm 2 to 3 inches to the left of the breastbone and below the left nipple.			
13. Counted the pulse for 1 minute. Noted if it was regular or irregular.			
14. Covered the person. Removed the earpieces.			
15. Recorded the person's name and pulse on your note pad or assignment sheet. Noted if the pulse was regular or irregular.			

Post-Procedure

	S	U	Comments
16. Provided for comfort.			
17. Placed the call bell within reach.			
18. Unscreened the person.			
19. Cleaned the earpieces and diaphragm with the wipes.			
20. Returned the stethoscope to its proper place.			
21. Decontaminated your hands.			
22. Reported and recorded your observations. Recorded the pulse rate with *Ap* for apical pulse.			

Taking an Apical-Radial Pulse

QUALITY OF LIFE

Name: ____________________

Date: ____________________

Remembered to:
- **Knock before entering the person's room**
- **Address the person by name**
- **Introduce yourself by name and title**

Pre-Procedure	**S**	**U**	**Comments**
1. Followed Delegation Guidelines: Taking Pulses. Viewed Safety Alerts: Stethoscopes and Taking Pulses.			
2. Asked a nurse or a nursing assistant to help you.			
3. Collected a stethoscope and antiseptic wipes.			
4. Completed hand hygiene.			
5. Identified the person. Checked the identification bracelet against the assignment sheet. Called the person by name.			
6. Explained the procedure to the person.			
7. Provided for privacy.			
Procedure			
8. Wiped the earpieces and diaphragm with the wipes.			
9. Asked the person to sit or lie down.			
10. Warmed the diaphragm in your palm.			
11. Exposed the left nipple area of the chest without exposing a woman's breasts.			
12. Placed the earpieces in your ears.			
13. Found the apical pulse while your co-worker found the radial pulse.			
14. Gave the signal to begin counting.			
15. Counted the pulse for 1 minute.			
16. Gave the signal to stop counting.			
17. Covered the person. Removed the earpieces.			
18. Recorded the person's name and the apical and radial pulses on your note pad or assignment sheet. Subtracted the radial pulse from the apical pulse for the pulse deficit. Noted whether the pulse was regular or irregular.			
Post-Procedure			
19. Provided for comfort.			
20. Placed the call bell within reach.			
21. Unscreened the person.			
22. Cleaned the earpieces and diaphragm with the wipes.			
23. Returned the stethoscope to its proper place.			
24. Decontaminated your hands.			
25. Reported and recorded your observations including:			
• Apical and radial pulse rates			
• Pulse deficit			

Counting Respirations

QUALITY OF LIFE

Name: ______________________

Date: ______________________

Remembered to:
- ◆ Knock before entering the person's room
- ◆ Address the person by name
- ◆ Introduce yourself by name and title

Pre-Procedure	S	U	Comments
1. Followed Delegation Guidelines: Respirations.	____	____	____________
2. Kept your fingers or the stethoscope over the pulse site.	____	____	____________
3. Did not tell the person you were counting respirations.	____	____	____________
4. Began counting when the chest rises. Counted each rise and fall or the chest as one respiration.	____	____	____________
5. Noted the following:			
• If respirations were regular	____	____	____________
• If both sides of the chest rose equally	____	____	____________
• Depth of the respirations	____	____	____________
• If the person had any pain or difficulty breathing	____	____	____________
6. Counted respirations for 30 seconds, and multiplied the number by 2. (The NNAAP skills evaluation requires counting respirations for 1 minute.)	____	____	____________
7. Counted respirations for 1 minute if they were abnormal or irregular.	____	____	____________
8. Recorded the person's name, respiratory rate, and other observations on your note pad or assignment sheet.	____	____	____________

Post-Procedure	S	U	Comments
9. Provided for comfort.	____	____	____________
10. Placed the call bell within reach.	____	____	____________
11. Decontaminated your hands.	____	____	____________
12. Reported and recorded your observations.	____	____	____________

Measuring Blood Pressure

QUALITY OF LIFE

Name: ______________________

Date: ______________________

Remembered to:
- ◆ Knock before entering the person's room
- ◆ Address the person by name
- ◆ Introduce yourself by name and title

Pre-Procedure

	S	U	Comments
1. Followed Delegation Guidelines: Measuring Blood Pressure. Viewed Safety Alerts: Stethoscopes and Equipment.	____	____	____________
2. Collected the following:			
• Sphygmomanometer	____	____	____________
• Stethoscope	____	____	____________
• Antiseptic wipes	____	____	____________
3. Completed hand hygiene.	____	____	____________
4. Identified the person. Checked the identification bracelet against the assignment sheet. Called the person by name.	____	____	____________
5. Explained the procedure to the person.	____	____	____________
6. Provided for privacy.	____	____	____________

Procedure

	S	U	Comments
7. Wiped the stethoscope earpieces and diaphragm with the wipes.	____	____	____________
8. Asked the person to sit or lie down.	____	____	____________
9. Positioned the person's arm level with the heart. The palm was up.	____	____	____________
10. Stood no more than 3 feet away from the sphygmomanometer. (Mercury model was vertical, on a flat surface, and at eye lever. Aneroid type was directly in front of you.)	____	____	____________
11. Exposed the upper arm.	____	____	____________
12. Squeezed the cuff to expel any remaining air. Closed the valve on the bulb.	____	____	____________
13. Found the brachial artery at the inner aspect of the elbow.	____	____	____________
14. Placed the arrow on the cuff over the brachial artery. Wrapped the cuff around the upper arm at least 1 inch above the elbow. It was even and snug.	____	____	____________
15. *Method 1:*			
a. Placed the stethoscope earpieces in your ears.	____	____	____________
b. Found the radial or brachial artery.	____	____	____________
c. Inflated the cuff until you could no longer feel the pulse. Noted this point.	____	____	____________
d. Inflated the cuff 30 mm Hg beyond the point where you last felt the pulse.	____	____	____________
Method 2:			
a. Found the radial or brachial artery.	____	____	____________
b. Inflated the cuff until you could no longer feel the pulse. Noted this point.	____	____	____________

Procedure—cont'd	S	U	Comments
c. Inflated the cuff 30 mm Hg beyond the point where you last felt the pulse.	______	______	______
d. Deflated the cuff slowly. Noted the point when you felt the pulse.	______	______	______
e. Waited 30 seconds.	______	______	______
f. Placed the stethoscope earpieces in your ears.	______	______	______
g. Inflated the cuff 30 mm Hg beyond the point where you felt the pulse return.	______	______	______
16. Placed the diaphragm over the brachial artery. Did not place it under the cuff.	______	______	______
17. Deflated the cuff at an even rate of 2 to 4 millimeters per second. Turned the valve counterclockwise to deflate the cuff.	______	______	______
18. Noted the point where you heard the first sound. This was the systolic reading. It is near the point where the radial pulse disappeared.	______	______	______
19. Continued to deflate the cuff. Noted the point where the sound disappeared. This was the diastolic reading.	______	______	______
20. Completely deflated the cuff. Removed it from the person's arm. Removed the stethoscope.	______	______	______
21. Recorded the person's name and blood pressure on your note pad or assignment sheet.	______	______	______
22. Returned the cuff to the case or wall holder.	______	______	______

Post-Procedure

23. Provided for comfort.	______	______	______
24. Placed the call bell within reach.	______	______	______
25. Unscreened the person.	______	______	______
26. Cleaned the earpieces and diaphragm with the wipes.	______	______	______
27. Returned the equipment to its proper place.	______	______	______
28. Decontaminated your hands.	______	______	______
29. Reported and recorded the blood pressure.	______	______	______

Performing Range-of-Motion Exercises

Quality of Life

Name: ____________________

Date: ____________________

Remembered to:
- **Knock before entering the person's room**
- **Address the person by name**
- **Introduce yourself by name and title**

Pre-Procedure

	S	U	Comments
1. Followed Delegation Guidelines: Range-of-Motion Exercises. Viewed Safety Alert: Range-of-Motion Exercises.			
2. Identified the person. Checked the identification bracelet against the assignment sheet. Called the person by name.			
3. Explained the procedure to the person.			
4. Completed hand hygiene.			
5. Obtained a bath blanket.			
6. Provided for privacy.			
7. Raised the bed for body mechanics. Raised bed rails if used.			

Procedure

	S	U	Comments
8. Lowered the nearest bed rail if up.			
9. Turned the person to the supine position.			
10. Covered the person with a bath blanket. Fanfolded top linens to the foot of the bed.			
11. Exercised the neck if allowed by your agency and if the nurse instructed you to do so:			
a. Placed your hands over the person's ears to support the head. Supported the jaws with your fingers.			
b. Flexion—Brought the head forward. The chin touched the chest.			
c. Extension—Straightened the head.			
d. Hyperextension—Brought the head backward until the chin pointed up.			
e. Rotation—Turned the head from side to side (chin to shoulder).			
f. Lateral flexion—Moved the head to the right and to the left (ear to shoulder).			
g. Repeated flexion, extension, hyperextension, rotation and lateral flexion five times or the number of times stated on the care plan.			
12. Exercised the shoulder:			
a. Grasped the wrist with one hand. Grasped the elbow with the other hand.			
b. Flexion—Raised the arm straight in front and over the head.			
c. Extension—Brought the arm down to the side.			
d. Hyperextension—Moved the arm behind the body if the person was sitting in a straight-backed chair or was standing.			

Procedure—cont'd	S	U	Comments
e. Abduction—Moved the straight arm away form the side of the body.	_____	_____	____________
f. Adduction—Moved the straight arm to the side of the body.	_____	_____	____________
g. Internal rotation—Bent the elbow. Placed the elbow at the same level as the shoulder. Moved the forearm down toward the body.	_____	_____	____________
h. External rotation—Moved the forearm toward the head.	_____	_____	____________
i. Repeated flexion, extension, hyperextension, abduction, adduction, and internal and external rotation five times or the number of times stated on the care plan.	_____	_____	____________
13. Exercised the elbow:			
a. Grasped the person's wrist with one hand. Grasped the elbow with your other hand.	_____	_____	____________
b. Flexion—Bent the arm so the same-side shoulder is touched.	_____	_____	____________
c. Extension—Straightened the arm.	_____	_____	____________
d. Repeated flexion and extension five times—or the number of times stated on the care plan.	_____	_____	____________
14. Exercised the forearm:			
a. Pronation—Turned the hand so the palm was down.	_____	_____	____________
b. Supination—Turned the hand so the palm was up.	_____	_____	____________
c. Repeated pronation and supination five times or the number of times stated on the care plan.	_____	_____	____________
15. Exercised the wrist:			
a. Held the wrist with both of your hands.	_____	_____	____________
b. Flexion—Bent the hand down.	_____	_____	____________
c. Extension—Straightened the hand.	_____	_____	____________
d. Hyperextension—Bent the hand back.	_____	_____	____________
e. Radial flexion—Turned the hand toward the thumb.	_____	_____	____________
f. Ulnar flexion—Turned the hand toward the little finger.	_____	_____	____________
g. Repeated flexion, extension, hyperextension, and radial and ulnar flexion five times or the number of times stated on the care plan.	_____	_____	____________
16. Exercised the thumb:			
a. Held the person's hand with one hand. Held the thumb with your other hand.	_____	_____	____________
b. Abduction—Moved the thumb out from the inner part of the index finger.	_____	_____	____________
c. Adduction—Moved the thumb back next to the index finger.	_____	_____	____________
d. Opposition—Touched each fingertip with the thumb.	_____	_____	____________
e. Flexion—Bent the thumb into the hand.	_____	_____	____________
f. Extension—Moved the thumb out to the side of the fingers.	_____	_____	____________
g. Repeated abduction, adduction, opposition, flexion, and extension five times or the number of times stated on the care plan.	_____	_____	____________

Procedure—cont'd	S	U	Comments
17. Exercised the fingers:			
a. Abduction—Spread apart the fingers and the thumb.	_____	_____	_______________
b. Adduction—Brought together the fingers and the thumb.	_____	_____	_______________
c. Extension—Straightened the fingers so the fingers, hand, and arm were straight.	_____	_____	_______________
d. Flexion—Made a fist.	_____	_____	_______________
e. Repeated abduction, adduction, extension, and flexion five times or the number of times stated on the care plan.	_____	_____	_______________
18. Exercised the hip:			
a. Supported the leg. Placed one hand under the knee. Placed your other hand under the ankle.	_____	_____	_______________
b. Flexion—Raised the leg.	_____	_____	_______________
c. Extension—Straightened the leg,	_____	_____	_______________
d. Abduction—Moved the leg away from the body.	_____	_____	_______________
e. Adduction—Moved the leg toward the other leg.	_____	_____	_______________
f. Internal rotation—Turned the leg inward.	_____	_____	_______________
g. External rotation—Turned the leg outward.	_____	_____	_______________
h. Repeated flexion, extension, abduction, adduction, and internal and external rotation five times or the number of times stated on the care plan.	_____	_____	_______________
19. Exercised the knee:			
a. Supported the knee. Placed one hand under the knee. Placed your hand under the ankle.	_____	_____	_______________
b. Flexion—Bent the leg.	_____	_____	_______________
c. Extension—Straightened the leg.	_____	_____	_______________
d. Repeated flexion and extension of the knee five times or the number of times stated on the care plan.	_____	_____	_______________
20. Exercised the ankle:			
a. Supported the foot and ankle. Placed one hand under the foot. Placed your other hand under the ankle.	_____	_____	_______________
b. Dorsiflexion—Pulled the foot forward. Pushed down on the heel at the same time, or pointed the toes up.	_____	_____	_______________
c. Plantar flexion—Turned the foot down, or pointed the toes down.	_____	_____	_______________
d. Repeated dorsiflexion and plantar flexion five times or the number of times stated on the care plan.	_____	_____	_______________
21. Exercised the foot:			
a. Continued to support the foot and ankle.	_____	_____	_______________
b. Pronation—Turned the outside of the foot up and the inside down.	_____	_____	_______________
c. Supination—Turned the inside of the foot up and the outside down.	_____	_____	_______________
d. Repeated pronation and supination five times or the number of times stated on the care plan.	_____	_____	_______________

Procedure—cont'd	S	U	Comments
22. Exercised the toes:			
a. Flexion—Curled the toes.	______	______	____________________
b. Extension—Straightened the toes.	______	______	____________________
c. Abduction—Spread the toes apart.	______	______	____________________
d. Adduction—Pulled the toes together.	______	______	____________________
e. Repeated flexion, extension, abduction, and adduction five times or the number of times stated on the care plan.	______	______	____________________
23. Covered the leg. Raised the bed rail if used.	______	______	____________________
24. Went to the other side. Lowered the nearest bed rail if used.	______	______	____________________
25. Repeated range-of-motion exercises on the person's other side:	______	______	____________________
a. Exercised the shoulder:			
i. Grasped the wrist with one hand. Grasped the elbow with the other hand.	______	______	____________________
ii. Flexion—Raised the arm straight in front and over the head.	______	______	____________________
iii. Extension—Brought the arm down to the side.	______	______	____________________
iv. Hyperextension—Moved the arm behind the body if the person was sitting in a straight-backed chair or was standing.	______	______	____________________
v. Abduction—Moved the straight arm away from the side of the body.	______	______	____________________
vi. Adduction—Moved the straight arm to the side of the body.	______	______	____________________
vii. Internal rotation—Bent the elbow. Placed the elbow at the same level as the shoulder. Moved the forearm down toward the body.	______	______	____________________
viii. External rotation—Moved the forearm toward the head.	______	______	____________________
ix. Repeated flexion, extension, hyperextension, abduction, adduction, and internal and external rotation five times or the number of times stated on the care plan.	______	______	____________________
b. Exercised the elbow:			
i. Grasped the person's wrist with one hand. Grasped the elbow with your other hand.	______	______	____________________
ii. Flexion—Bent the arm so the same-side shoulder is touched.	______	______	____________________
iii. Extension—Straightened the arm.	______	______	____________________
iv. Repeated flexion and extension five times or the number of times stated on the care plan.	______	______	____________________
c. Exercised the forearm:			
i. Pronation—Turned the hand so the palm was down.	______	______	____________________
ii. Supination—Turned the hand so the palm was up.	______	______	____________________
iii. Repeated pronation and supination five times or the number of times stated on the care plan.	______	______	____________________

Procedure—cont'd	S	U	Comments
d. Exercised the wrist:			
i. Held the wrist with both of your hands.	_____	_____	_____
ii. Flexion—Bent the hand down.	_____	_____	_____
iii. Extension—Straightened the hand.	_____	_____	_____
iv. Hyperextension—Bent the hand back.	_____	_____	_____
v. Radial flexion—Turned the hand toward the thumb.	_____	_____	_____
vi. Ulnar flexion—Turned the hand toward the little finger.	_____	_____	_____
vii. Repeated flexion, extension, hyperextension, and radial and ulnar flexion five times or the number of times stated on the care plan.	_____	_____	_____
e. Exercised the thumb:			
i. Held the person's hand with one hand. Held the thumb with your other hand.	_____	_____	_____
ii. Abduction—Moved the thumb out from the inner part of the index finger.	_____	_____	_____
iii. Adduction—Moved the thumb back next to the index finger.	_____	_____	_____
iv. Opposition—Touched each fingertip with the thumb.	_____	_____	_____
v. Flexion—Bent the thumb into the hand.	_____	_____	_____
vi. Extension—Moved the thumb out to the side of the fingers.	_____	_____	_____
vii. Repeated abduction, adduction, opposition, flexion, and extension five times—or the number of times stated on the care plan.	_____	_____	_____
f. Exercised the fingers.			
i. Abduction—Spread apart the fingers and thumb.	_____	_____	_____
ii. Adduction—Brought together the fingers and thumb.	_____	_____	_____
iii. Extension—Straightened the fingers so the fingers, hand, and arm were straight.	_____	_____	_____
iv. Flexion—Made a fist.	_____	_____	_____
v. Repeated abduction, adduction, extension, and flexion five times or the number of times stated on the care plan.	_____	_____	_____
g. Exercised the hip:			
i. Supported the leg. Placed one hand under the knee. Placed your other hand under the ankle.	_____	_____	_____
ii. Flexion—Raised the leg.	_____	_____	_____
iii. Extension—Straightened the leg.	_____	_____	_____
iv. Abduction—Moved the leg away from the body.	_____	_____	_____
v. Adduction—Moved the leg toward the other leg.	_____	_____	_____
vi. Internal rotation—Turned the leg inward.	_____	_____	_____
vii. External rotation—Turned the leg outward.	_____	_____	_____
viii. Repeated flexion, extension, abduction, adduction, and internal and external rotation five times or the number of times stated on the care plan.	_____	_____	_____

Procedure—cont'd	S	U	Comments
h. Exercised the knee:			
i. Supported the knee. Placed one hand under the knee. Placed your hand under the ankle.	_____	_____	__________
ii. Flexion—Bent the leg.	_____	_____	__________
iii. Extension—Straightened the leg.	_____	_____	__________
iv. Repeated flexion and extension of the knee five times or the number of times stated on the care plan.	_____	_____	__________
i. Exercised the ankle:			
i. Supported the foot and ankle. Placed one hand under the foot. Placed your other hand under the ankle.	_____	_____	__________
ii. Dorsiflexion—Pulled the foot forward. Pushed down on the heel at the same time, or pointed the toes up.	_____	_____	__________
iii. Plantar flexion—Turned the foot down, or pointed the toes down.	_____	_____	__________
iv. Repeated dorsiflexion and plantar flexion five times or the number of times stated on the care plan.	_____	_____	__________
j. Exercised the foot:			
i. Continued to support the foot and ankle.	_____	_____	__________
ii. Pronation—Turned the outside of the foot up and the inside down.	_____	_____	__________
iii. Supination—Turned the inside of the foot up and the outside down.	_____	_____	__________
iv. Repeated pronation and supination five times or the number of times stated on the care plan.	_____	_____	__________
k. Exercised the toes:			
i. Flexion—Curled the toes.	_____	_____	__________
ii. Extension—Straightened the toes.	_____	_____	__________
iii. Abduction—Spread the toes apart.	_____	_____	__________
iv. Adduction—Pulled the toes together.	_____	_____	__________
v. Repeated flexion, extension, abduction, and adduction five times or the number of times stated on the care plan.	_____	_____	__________

Post-Procedure

	S	U	Comments
26. Provided for comfort.	_____	_____	__________
27. Covered the person. Removed the bath blanket.	_____	_____	__________
28. Raised or lowered the bed rails. Followed the care plan.	_____	_____	__________
29. Lowered the bed to its lowest level.	_____	_____	__________
30. Placed the call bell within reach.	_____	_____	__________
31. Unscreened the person.	_____	_____	__________
32. Returned the bath blanket to its proper place.	_____	_____	__________
33. Decontaminated your hands.	_____	_____	__________
34. Reported and recorded your observations.	_____	_____	__________

Helping the Person to Walk

Quality of Life

Name: ______________________

Date: ______________________

Remembered to:
- ◆ Knock before entering the person's room
- ◆ Address the person by name
- ◆ Introduce yourself by name and title

Pre-Procedure	S	U	Comments
1. Followed Delegation Guidelines: Ambulation. Viewed Safety Alert: Ambulation.	_____	_____	__________
2. Explained the procedure to the person.	_____	_____	__________
3. Completed hand hygiene.	_____	_____	__________
4. Collected the following:			
• Robe and nonskid shoes	_____	_____	__________
• Paper or sheet to protect bottom linens	_____	_____	__________
• Gait (transfer) belt	_____	_____	__________
5. Identified the person. Checked the identification bracelet against the assignment sheet. Called the person by name.	_____	_____	__________
6. Provided for privacy.	_____	_____	__________

Procedure

	S	U	Comments
7. Lowered the bed to its lowest position. Locked the bed wheels. Lowered the bed rail if up.	_____	_____	__________
8. Fanfolded linens to the foot of the bed.	_____	_____	__________
9. Placed the paper or sheet under the person's feet. Put the shoes on the person.	_____	_____	__________
10. Helped the person to dangle.	_____	_____	__________
11. Helped the person put on the robe.	_____	_____	__________
12. Applied the gait belt.	_____	_____	__________
13. Helped the person stand. Grasped the gait belt at each side, or placed your arms under the person's arms around to the shoulder blades.	_____	_____	__________
14. Stood at the person's side while he or she gained balance. Held the belt at the side and back, or had one arm around the back to support the person.	_____	_____	__________
15. Encouraged the person to stand erect with the head up and back straight.	_____	_____	__________
16. Helped the person walk. Walked to the side and slightly behind the person. Provided support with the gait belt or had one arm around the back to support the person.	_____	_____	__________
17. Encouraged the person to walk normally (the heel struck the floor first). Discouraged shuffling, sliding, or walking on tiptoes.	_____	_____	__________
18. Walked the required distance if the person tolerated the activity. Did not rush the person.	_____	_____	__________
19. Helped the person return to bed.	_____	_____	__________

Procedure—cont'd	S	U	Comments
20. Lowered the head of the bed. Helped the person to the center of the bed.	_____	_____	_____________
21. Removed the shoes. Removed the paper or sheet over the bottom sheet.	_____	_____	_____________

Post-Procedure

	S	U	Comments
22. Provided for comfort. Covered the person.	_____	_____	_____________
23. Placed the call bell within reach.	_____	_____	_____________
24. Raised or lowered bed rails. Followed the care plan.	_____	_____	_____________
25. Returned the robe and shoes to their proper places.	_____	_____	_____________
26. Unscreened the person.	_____	_____	_____________
27. Decontaminated your hands.	_____	_____	_____________
28. Reported and recorded your observations.	_____	_____	_____________

Helping the Falling Person

QUALITY OF LIFE

Name: ______________________

Date: ______________________

Remembered to:
- ◆ Knock before entering the person's room
- ◆ Address the person by name
- ◆ Introduce yourself by name and title

Procedure	S	U	Comments
1. Stood with your feet apart. Kept your back straight.	____	____	____________
2. Brought the person close to your body as fast as possible. Used the gait belt, or wrapped your arms around the person's waist. (You could have held the person under the arms.)	____	____	____________
3. Moved your leg so the person's buttocks rested on it. Moved the leg near the person.	____	____	____________
4. Lowered the person to the floor. The person slid down your leg to the floor. Bent at your hips and knees as you lowered the person.	____	____	____________
5. Called the nurse to check the person. Stayed with the person.	____	____	____________
6. Helped the nurse return the person to bed. Got other staff to help if needed.	____	____	____________
7. Reported the following to the nurse:			
• How the fall occurred	____	____	____________
• How far the person walked	____	____	____________
• How activity was tolerated before the fall	____	____	____________
• Complaints before the fall	____	____	____________
• How much help the person needed while walking	____	____	____________
8. Completed an incident report.	____	____	____________

Preparing the Person's Room

QUALITY OF LIFE

Name: ______________________

Date: ______________________

Remembered to:
- Knock before entering the person's room
- Address the person by name
- Introduce yourself by name and title

Pre-Procedure

	S	U	Comments
1. Followed Delegation Guidelines: Admissions, Transfers, and Discharges.	___	___	___
2. Knew which room and bed to prepare. Found out if the person arrived by wheelchair or stretcher.	___	___	___
3. Completed hand hygiene.	___	___	___
4. Collected the following:			
• Admission kit—wash basin, soap, toothpaste, toothbrush, and water pitcher	___	___	___
• Bedpan and urinal (for a man)	___	___	___
• Admission form	___	___	___
• Urine specimen container if urine specimen was ordered	___	___	___
• Thermometer	___	___	___
• Sphygmomanometer	___	___	___
• Stethoscope	___	___	___
• Gown or pajamas if needed	___	___	___
• Towels and washcloths	___	___	___
• IV pole if needed	___	___	___
• Other items requested by the nurse	___	___	___

Procedure

	S	U	Comments
5. If the person was ambulatory or arrived by wheelchair:			
a. Opened the bed for a hospital patient. Left the bed closed for a nursing center resident.	___	___	___
b. Lowered the bed to its lowest position.	___	___	___
6. If the person arrived by stretcher:			
a. Made a surgical bed.	___	___	___
b. Raised the bed to its highest level.	___	___	___
7. Attached the call bell to the bed linen.	___	___	___
8. Placed the thermometer, sphygmomanometer, stethoscope, and admission checklist on the overbed table.	___	___	___
9. Placed the gown or pajamas on the bed.	___	___	___
10. Placed the wash basin, soap, toothpaste, and toothbrush in the bedside stand.	___	___	___
11. Placed the bedpan, urinal, towels, and washcloths in the bedside stand.	___	___	___
12. Placed the water pitcher, glass, and specimen container on the bedside stand or overbed table.	___	___	___
13. Decontaminated your hands.	___	___	___

Admitting the Person

QUALITY OF LIFE

Name: ______________________

Date: ______________________

Remembered to:
- Knock before entering the person's room
- Address the person by name
- Introduce yourself by name and title

Pre-Procedure

	S	U	Comments
1. Viewed Safety Alert: Admissions, Transfers, and Discharges.	____	____	____________
2. Completed hand hygiene.	____	____	____________
3. Prepared the room.	____	____	____________

Procedure

	S	U	Comments
4. Greeted the person by name. Asked if he or she preferred a certain name.	____	____	____________
5. Introduced yourself to the person and others present. Gave your name and title. Explained that you assisted the nurses in giving care.	____	____	____________
6. Introduced the roommate.	____	____	____________
7. Provided for privacy. Asked family members or friends to leave the room. Told them how much time you needed and where they could comfortably wait. Allowed a family member or friend stay if the person preferred.	____	____	____________
8. Had the person put on a gown or pajamas. Assisted as needed. (A nursing center resident could have stayed dressed if his or her condition permitted.)	____	____	____________
9. Provided for comfort. The person was in bed or in a chair as directed by the nurse.	____	____	____________
10. Completed the admission form. Measured vital signs and measured height and weight.	____	____	____________
11. Completed a list of clothing and personal belongings.	____	____	____________
12. Hung clothes in the closet. Put personal items in the drawers and bedside stand.	____	____	____________
13. Explained any ordered activity limits.	____	____	____________
14. Obtained a urine specimen if ordered. Took the specimen to the storage area or laboratory. Cleaned the equipment, and decontaminated your hands.	____	____	____________
15. Oriented the person to the area:			
a. Gave names of the nurses.	____	____	____________
b. Identified items in the bedside stand. Explained the purpose of each item.	____	____	____________
c. Showed how the call bell is used.	____	____	____________
d. Showed how to use the bed and television controls.	____	____	____________
e. Explained how to make phone calls. Placed the phone within reach.	____	____	____________
f. Explained visiting hours and policies.	____	____	____________
g. Explained where to find the nurses' station, lounge, chapel, dining room, gift shop, and other areas.	____	____	____________

Procedure—cont'd	S	U	Comments
h. Explained about newspapers, library, activities, education, religious, and other services.	____	____	____________
i. Identified staff—x-ray, laboratory, housekeeping, dietary, and physical therapy. In addition, identified students who were in the agency.	____	____	____________
j. Explained when meals and nourishments were served.	____	____	____________
16. Filled the water pitcher and glass if oral fluids were allowed.	____	____	____________
17. Placed the call bell within reach. Placed other controls and needed items within reach.	____	____	____________
18. Kept the bed in its lowest position.	____	____	____________
19. Raised or lowered bed rails. Followed the care plan.	____	____	____________
20. Unscreened the person.	____	____	____________
21. Cleaned used equipment. Discarded used disposable items. Decontaminated your hands.	____	____	____________
22. Provided a denture container if needed. Labeled it with the person's name and room number.	____	____	____________
23. Labeled personal property and personal care equipment for the nursing center resident. Items were labeled with the person's name.	____	____	____________

Post-Procedure

	S	U	Comments
24. Decontaminated your hands.	____	____	____________
25. Reported and recorded your observations.	____	____	____________

Measuring Height and Weight

QUALITY OF LIFE

Name: ______________________

Date: ______________________

Remembered to:
- Knock before entering the person's room
- Address the person by name
- Introduce yourself by name and title

Pre-Procedure

	S	U	Comments
1. Followed Delegation Guidelines: Measuring Height and Weight. Viewed Safety Alert: Measuring Height and Weight.			
2. Explained the procedure to the person.			
3. Asked the person to void.			
4. Completed hand hygiene.			
5. Brought the balance or lift scale and paper towels to the person's room.			
6. Identified the person. Checked the identification bracelet against the assignment sheet. Called the person by name.			
7. Provided for privacy.			

Procedure

	S	U	Comments
8. Balance scale:			
a. Placed the paper towels on the scale platform.			
b. Raised the height rod.			
c. Moved the weights to zero (0). The pointer was in the middle.			
d. Asked the person to remove the robe and footwear. Assisted as needed.			
e. Moved the weights until the balance pointer was in the middle.			
f. Recorded the weight on your note pad or assignment sheet.			
g. Asked the person to stand very straight.			
h. Lowered the height rod until it rested on the person's head.			
i. Recorded the height on your note pad or assignment sheet.			
9. Chair scale:			
a. Placed both weights on zero (0). Balanced the scale, following the manufacturer's instructions.			
b. Helped the person transfer from the wheelchair to the chair scale.			
c. Placed the person's feet on the foot platform.			
d. Moved the weights until the balance pointer was in the middle, or noted the digital display.			
e. Recorded the weight on your notepad or assignment sheet.			

Procedure—cont'd	S	U	Comments
10. Lift scale:			
a. Attached the sling to the lift.	_____	_____	_______________
b. Placed both weights on zero (0).	_____	_____	_______________
c. Leveled and balanced the scale. Followed the manufacturer's instructions.	_____	_____	_______________
d. Removed the sling from the scale.	_____	_____	_______________
e. Placed the person on the sling and attached it to the lift. Raised the person about 4 inches off the bed.	_____	_____	_______________
f. Moved the weights until the balance pointer was in the middle, or noted the digital display.	_____	_____	_______________
g. Recorded the weight on your notepad or assignment sheet.	_____	_____	_______________
h. Lowered the person to the bed.	_____	_____	_______________
i. Removed the sling.	_____	_____	_______________
11. Helped the person put on a robe and nonskid footwear if he or she remained up, or helped the person back to bed.	_____	_____	_______________

Post-Procedure

12. Provided for comfort.	_____	_____	_______________
13. Placed the call bell within reach.	_____	_____	_______________
14. Raised or lowered bed rails. Followed the care plan.	_____	_____	_______________
15. Unscreened the person.	_____	_____	_______________
16. Discarded the paper towels.	_____	_____	_______________
17. Returned the scale to its proper place.	_____	_____	_______________
18. Decontaminated your hands.	_____	_____	_______________
19. Reported and recorded the measurements.	_____	_____	_______________

Measuring Height: The Person Is in Bed

QUALITY OF LIFE

Name: ______________________

Date: ______________________

Remembered to:
- Knock before entering the person's room
- Address the person by name
- Introduce yourself by name and title

Pre-Procedure	S	U	Comments
1. Followed Delegation Guidelines: Measuring Height and Weight. Viewed Safety Alert: Measuring Height and Weight.			
2. Explained the procedure to the person.			
3. Completed hand hygiene.			
4. Collected a measuring tape and ruler.			
5. Asked a co-worker to help you.			
6. Identified the person. Checked the identification bracelet against the assignment sheet. Called the person by name.			
7. Provided for privacy.			

Procedure

	S	U	Comments
8. Positioned the person supine if allowed.			
9. Asked your co-worker to hold the end of the measuring tape at the person's heel.			
10. Pulled the measuring tape along the person's body until it extended past the head.			
11. Placed the ruler flat across the top of the person's head. Made sure that it extended from the person's head to the measuring tape and that the ruler was level.			
12. Recorded the height on your notepad or assignment sheet.			

Post-Procedure

	S	U	Comments
13. Provided for comfort.			
14. Raised or lowered bed rails. Followed the care plan.			
15. Placed the call bell within reach.			
16. Unscreened the person.			
17. Returned equipment to its proper location.			
18. Decontaminated your hands.			
19. Reported and recorded the height.			

Transferring the Person to Another Nursing Unit

QUALITY OF LIFE

Name: ______________________

Date: ______________________

Remembered to:
- ◆ Knock before entering the person's room
- ◆ Address the person by name
- ◆ Introduce yourself by name and title

	S	U	Comments
Pre-Procedure			
1. Followed Delegation Guidelines: Admissions, Transfers, and Discharges. Viewed Safety Alert: Admissions, Transfers, and Discharges.	_____	_____	__________
2. Found out where the person was going and if you needed to use the bed, wheelchair, or stretcher.	_____	_____	__________
3. Explained the procedure to the person.	_____	_____	__________
4. Got a stretcher or wheelchair, bath blanket, and utility cart if needed.	_____	_____	__________
5. Completed hand hygiene.	_____	_____	__________
6. Identified the person. Checked the identification bracelet against the transfer slip. Called the person by name.	_____	_____	__________
Procedure			
7. Collected the person's belongings and bedside equipment. Placed them on the utility cart.	_____	_____	__________
8. Assisted the person to the wheelchair or stretcher. Covered the person with a bath blanket.	_____	_____	__________
9. Transported the person to the new room.	_____	_____	__________
10. Introduced the person to the receiving nurse.	_____	_____	__________
11. Helped transfer the person to the bed or chair. Helped position the person.	_____	_____	__________
12. Brought personal belongings and equipment to the new room. Helped put them away.	_____	_____	__________
13. Reported the following to the receiving nurse:			
a. How the person tolerated the transfer	_____	_____	__________
b. That a nurse will bring the chart, care plan, Kardex, and medications.	_____	_____	__________
Post-Procedure			
14. Returned the wheelchair or stretcher and the utility cart to the storage area.	_____	_____	__________
15. Reported and recorded the following:			
• Time of the transfer	_____	_____	__________
• Where the person was taken	_____	_____	__________
• How the person was transferred (bed, wheelchair, or stretcher)	_____	_____	__________
• How the person tolerated the transfer	_____	_____	__________
• Who received the person	_____	_____	__________
• Any other observations	_____	_____	__________

Post-Procedure—cont'd	S	U	Comments
16. Stripped the bed and cleaned the unit. Wore gloves. (The housekeeping staff may have done this step.)	______	______	____________________
17. Decontaminated your hands.	______	______	____________________
18. Made a closed bed.	______	______	____________________
19. Decontaminated your hands.	______	______	____________________

Discharging the Person

QUALITY OF LIFE

Name: ______________________

Date: ______________________

Remembered to:
- Knock before entering the person's room
- Address the person by name
- Introduce yourself by name and title

Pre-Procedure	S	U	Comments
1. Followed Delegation Guidelines: Admissions, Transfers, and Discharges. Viewed Safety Alert: Admissions, Transfers, and Discharges.			
2. Made sure the person could leave. Found out if the person had transportation.			
3. Explained the procedure to the person.			
4. Completed hand hygiene.			
5. Identified the person. Checked the identification bracelet against the discharge slip. Called the person by name.			

Procedure	S	U	Comments
6. Provided for privacy.			
7. Helped the person dress as needed.			
8. Helped the person pack. Checked all drawers and closets. Made sure all items were collected.			
9. Checked off the clothing and personal belongings from the list. Gave the list to the nurse.			
10. Told the nurse that the person was ready for the final visit. The nurse:			
a. Gave prescriptions written by the doctor			
b. Provided discharge instructions			
c. Got valuables from the safe			
d. Had the person sign the lists of clothing and personal belongings			
11. Got a wheelchair and utility cart for the person's belongings. Asked a co-worker to help you.			
12. Assisted the person into the wheelchair.			
13. Took the person to the exit area. Locked the wheelchair wheels.			
14. Helped the person out of the wheelchair and into the car.			
15. Helped put the belongings into the car.			

Post-Procedure	S	U	Comments
16. Returned the wheelchair and cart to the storage area.			
17. Decontaminated your hands.			

Preparing the Person for an Examination

QUALITY OF LIFE

Name: ______________________

Date: ______________________

Remembered to:
- ◆ Knock before entering the person's room
- ◆ Address the person by name
- ◆ Introduce yourself by name and title

Pre-Procedure	S	U	Comments
1. Followed Delegation Guidelines: Preparing the Person. Viewed Safety Alert: Preparing the Person.	_____	_____	__________
2. Explained the procedure to the person.	_____	_____	__________
3. Completed hand hygiene.	_____	_____	__________
4. Collected the following:			
• Flashlight	_____	_____	__________
• Sphygmomanometer	_____	_____	__________
• Stethoscope	_____	_____	__________
• Thermometer	_____	_____	__________
• Tongue depressors (blades)	_____	_____	__________
• Laryngeal mirror	_____	_____	__________
• Ophthalmoscope	_____	_____	__________
• Otoscope	_____	_____	__________
• Nasal speculum	_____	_____	__________
• Percussion (reflex) hammer	_____	_____	__________
• Tuning fork	_____	_____	__________
• Tape measure	_____	_____	__________
• Gloves	_____	_____	__________
• Water-soluble lubricant	_____	_____	__________
• Vaginal speculum	_____	_____	__________
• Cotton-tipped applicators	_____	_____	__________
• Specimen containers and labels	_____	_____	__________
• Disposable bag	_____	_____	__________
• Kidney basin	_____	_____	__________
• Towel	_____	_____	__________
• Bath blanket	_____	_____	__________
• Tissues	_____	_____	__________
• Drape (sheet, bath blanket, drawsheet, or paper drape)	_____	_____	__________
• Paper towels	_____	_____	__________
• Cotton balls	_____	_____	__________
• Waterproof bed protector	_____	_____	__________
• Eye chart (Snellen chart)	_____	_____	__________
• Slides	_____	_____	__________
• Gown	_____	_____	__________
• Alcohol wipes	_____	_____	__________
• Wastebasket	_____	_____	__________
• Container for soiled instruments	_____	_____	__________
• Marking pencils or pens	_____	_____	__________

Pre-Procedure—cont'd	S	U	Comments
5. Identified the person. Checked the identification bracelet against the assignment sheet. Called the person by name.	____	____	____________
6. Provided for privacy.	____	____	____________

Procedure	S	U	Comments
7. Asked the person to put on the gown. Told him or her to remove all clothes. Assisted as needed.	____	____	____________
8. Asked the person to void. Offered the bedpan, commode, or urinal if necessary. Provided for privacy.	____	____	____________
9. Transported the person to the examination room if the examination was not performed in the person's room.	____	____	____________
10. Weighed and measured the person. Recorded the measurements on the examination form.	____	____	____________
11. Helped the person on to the examination table. Provided a step stool if necessary. (Omitted this step for an examination in the person's room.)	____	____	____________
12. Measured vital signs. Recorded them on the examination form.	____	____	____________
13. Raised the bed to its highest level. Raised the far bed rail if used. (This step was not performed if an examination table was used.)	____	____	____________
14. Positioned the person as directed.	____	____	____________
15. Draped the person.	____	____	____________
16. Placed a bed protector under the buttocks.	____	____	____________
17. Raised the nearest bed rail if used.	____	____	____________
18. Provided adequate lighting.	____	____	____________
19. Put the call bell on for the examiner. Did not leave the person alone.	____	____	____________

Collecting a Random Urine Specimen

Quality of Life

Name: ______________________

Date: ______________________

Remembered to:
- ◆ Knock before entering the person's room
- ◆ Address the person by name
- ◆ Introduce yourself by name and title

Pre-Procedure	S	U	Comments
1. Followed Delegation Guidelines: Urine Specimens. Viewed Safety Alert: Urine Specimens.	____	____	________
2. Explained the procedure to the person.	____	____	________
3. Completed hand hygiene.	____	____	________
4. Collected the following:			
• Voiding receptacle—bedpan and cover, urinal or specimen pan	____	____	________
• Specimen container and lid	____	____	________
• Label	____	____	________
• Gloves	____	____	________
• Plastic bag	____	____	________
Procedure			
5. Labeled the container.	____	____	________
6. Put the container and lid in the bathroom	____	____	________
7. Identified the person. Checked the identification bracelet against the requisition slip. Called the person by name.	____	____	________
8. Provided for privacy.	____	____	________
9. Put on the gloves.	____	____	________
10. Ask the person to void into the receptacle. Reminded him or her to put toilet tissue into the wastebasket or toilet. Toilet tissue was not put in the bedpan or specimen pan.	____	____	________
11. Took the receptacle to the bathroom.	____	____	________
12. Poured about 120 ml (4 oz) of urine into the specimen container. Disposed of excess urine.	____	____	________
13. Placed the lid on the specimen container. Placed the container in the plastic bag.	____	____	________
14. Cleaned and returned the receptacle to its proper place.	____	____	________
15. Assisted with handwashing.	____	____	________
16. Completed hand hygiene.	____	____	________
Post-Procedure			
17. Provided for comfort.	____	____	________
18. Placed the call bell within reach.	____	____	________
19. Raised or lowered bed rails. Followed the care plan.	____	____	________
20. Unscreened the person.	____	____	________
21. Decontaminated your hands.	____	____	________
22. Reported and recorded your observations.	____	____	________
23. Took the specimen and the requisition slip to the storage area or laboratory.	____	____	________

Collecting a Midstream Specimen

QUALITY OF LIFE

Name: ______________________

Date: ______________________

Remembered to:
- ◆ Knock before entering the person's room
- ◆ Address the person by name
- ◆ Introduce yourself by name and title

Pre-Procedure	S	U	Comments
1. Followed Delegation Guidelines: Urine Specimens. Viewed Safety Alert: Urine Specimens.	_____	_____	__________
2. Explained the procedure to the person.	_____	_____	__________
3. Completed hand hygiene.	_____	_____	__________
4. Collected the following:			
• Midstream specimen kit with antiseptic solution	_____	_____	__________
• Label	_____	_____	__________
• Disposable gloves	_____	_____	__________
• Sterile gloves if not part of the kit	_____	_____	__________
• Voiding receptacle—bedpan, urinal, or commode if needed	_____	_____	__________
• Plastic bag	_____	_____	__________
• Supplies for perineal care	_____	_____	__________
5. Labeled the container.	_____	_____	__________
6. Identified the person. Checked the identification bracelet against the requisition slip. Called the person by name.	_____	_____	__________
7. Provided for privacy.	_____	_____	__________

Procedure	S	U	Comments
8. Provided perineal care. Removed the gloves, and decontaminated your hands.	_____	_____	__________
9. Opened the sterile kit. Used sterile technique.	_____	_____	__________
10. Put on the sterile gloves.	_____	_____	__________
11. Poured the antiseptic solution over the cotton balls.	_____	_____	__________
12. Opened the sterile specimen container. Made sure that the inside of the container or lid was not touched. Set the lid down so the inside was up.	_____	_____	__________
13. *For a female:*			
a. Cleaned the perineum with cotton balls.	_____	_____	__________
b. Spread the labia with your thumb and index finger. Used your non-dominant hand. (This hand was now contaminated. It did not touch anything sterile.)	_____	_____	__________
c. Cleaned down the urethral area from front to back. Used a clean cotton ball for each stroke.	_____	_____	__________
d. Kept the labia separated until the urine specimen was collected.	_____	_____	__________

Procedure—cont'd	S	U	Comments
14. *For a male:*			
a. Cleaned the penis with cotton balls.	_____	_____	__________
b. Held the penis with your non-dominant hand.	_____	_____	__________
c. Cleaned the penis starting at the meatus. Used a cotton ball and cleaned in a circular motion. Started at the center and worked outward.	_____	_____	__________
d. Kept holding the penis until the specimen was collected.	_____	_____	__________
15. Asked the person to void into the receptacle.	_____	_____	__________
16. Passed the specimen container into the stream of urine.	_____	_____	__________
17. Collected about 30 to 60 ml of urine (1 to 2 oz)	_____	_____	__________
18. Removed the specimen container before the person stopped voiding.	_____	_____	__________
19. Released the labia or penis.	_____	_____	__________
20. Allowed the person to finish voiding into the receptacle.	_____	_____	__________
21. Placed the lid on the specimen container. Touched only the outside of the container or lid.	_____	_____	__________
22. Wiped the outside of the container.	_____	_____	__________
23. Placed the container in a plastic bag.	_____	_____	__________
24. Provided toilet tissue after the person was done voiding.	_____	_____	__________
25. Took the receptacle to the bathroom.	_____	_____	__________
26. Measured urine if I&O was ordered. Included the amount in the specimen container.	_____	_____	__________
27. Cleaned the receptacle and other items. Returned equipment to its proper place.	_____	_____	__________
28. Removed soiled gloves. Completed hand hygiene.	_____	_____	__________
29. Put on clean gloves.	_____	_____	__________
30. Assisted with handwashing.	_____	_____	__________
31. Removed the gloves. Decontaminated your hands.	_____	_____	__________

Post-Procedure

32. Provided for comfort.	_____	_____	__________
33. Placed the call bell within reach.	_____	_____	__________
34. Raised or lowered bed rails. Followed the care plan.	_____	_____	__________
35. Unscreened the person.	_____	_____	__________
36. Decontaminated your hands.	_____	_____	__________
37. Reported and recorded your observations.	_____	_____	__________
38. Took the specimen and the requisition slip to the storage area or laboratory.	_____	_____	__________

Collecting a 24-Hour Urine Specimen

QUALITY OF LIFE

Name: ____________________

Date: ____________________

Remembered to:
- ◆ Knock before entering the person's room
- ◆ Address the person by name
- ◆ Introduce yourself by name and title

Pre-Procedure	S	U	Comments
1. Followed Delegation Guidelines: Urine Specimens. Viewed Safety Alert: Urine Specimens.	___	___	___
2. Reviewed the procedure with the nurse.	___	___	___
3. Explained the procedure to the person.	___	___	___
4. Completed hand hygiene.	___	___	___
5. Collected the following:			
• Urine container for a 24-hour collection	___	___	___
• Preservative if needed	___	___	___
• Bucket with ice if needed	___	___	___
• Two 24-hour urine specimen labels	___	___	___
• Funnel	___	___	___
• Voiding receptacle—bedpan, urinal, commode, or specimen pan	___	___	___
• Gloves	___	___	___
• Graduate	___	___	___
6. Labeled the urine container.	___	___	___
7. Identified the person. Checked the identification bracelet against the requisition slip. Called the person by name.	___	___	___
8. Arranged equipment in the person's bathroom.	___	___	___
9. Placed one label in the bathroom. Placed the other near the bed.	___	___	___

Procedure	S	U	Comments
10. Put on the gloves.	___	___	___
11. Offered the bedpan or urinal, or assisted the person to the bathroom or commode.	___	___	___
12. Asked the person to void.	___	___	___
13. Discarded the urine, and noted the time, starting the 24-hour collection period.	___	___	___
14. Cleaned the bedpan, urinal, commode, or specimen pan.	___	___	___
15. Removed the gloves. Practiced hand hygiene.	___	___	___
16. Marked the time the test began and the time it ended on the room and bathroom labels. In addition, marked the urine container.	___	___	___
17. Asked the person to use the bedpan, urinal, commode, or specimen pan when voiding during the next 24 hours. Asked the person to signal after voiding. Reminded him or her not to have a bowel movement at the same time and not to put toilet tissue in the receptacle.	___	___	___

Procedure—cont'd	S	U	Comments
18. Put on the gloves.	____	____	____________
19. Measured all urine if I&O was ordered.	____	____	____________
20. Poured urine into the urine container using the funnel to avoid spilling any urine. Restarted the test if you spilled or discarded urine.	____	____	____________
21. Cleaned the receptacle. Removed the gloves, and completed hand hygiene.	____	____	____________
22. Added ice to the bucket as needed.	____	____	____________
23. Asked the person to void at the end of the 24-hour period. Poured the urine into the urine container. Wore gloves for this step.	____	____	____________

Post-Procedure

24. Provided for comfort.	____	____	____________
25. Placed the call bell within reach.	____	____	____________
26. Raised or lowered bed rails. Followed the care plan.	____	____	____________
27. Removed the labels from the room and bathroom.	____	____	____________
28. Cleaned and returned equipment to its proper place. Discarded disposable items. Wore gloves for this step.	____	____	____________
29. Removed the gloves, and completed hand hygiene.	____	____	____________
30. Reported and recorded your observations.	____	____	____________
31. Took the specimen and requisition slip to the laboratory.	____	____	____________

Collecting a Double-Voided Specimen

QUALITY OF LIFE

Name: ______________________

Date: ______________________

Remembered to:
- ◆ Knock before entering the person's room
- ◆ Address the person by name
- ◆ Introduce yourself by name and title

Pre-Procedure	S	U	Comments
1. Followed Delegation Guidelines: Urine Specimens. Viewed Safety Alert: Urine Specimens.	____	____	____________
2. Explained the procedure to the person.	____	____	____________
3. Completed hand hygiene.	____	____	____________
4. Collected the following:			
• Voiding receptacle—bedpan, urinal, commode, or specimen pan	____	____	____________
• Two specimen containers	____	____	____________
• Urine testing equipment	____	____	____________
• Gloves	____	____	____________
5. Identified the person. Checked the identification bracelet against the assignment sheet. Called the person by name.	____	____	____________
6. Provided for privacy.	____	____	____________

Procedure

Procedure	S	U	Comments
7. Put on the gloves.	____	____	____________
8. Asked the person to void into the receptacle. Reminded the person not to put toilet tissue in the receptacle.	____	____	____________
9. Took the receptacle to the bathroom.	____	____	____________
10. Poured some urine into the specimen container.	____	____	____________
11. Tested the specimen in case you could not obtain a second specimen. Discarded the urine.	____	____	____________
12. Cleaned the receptacle, and returned it to its proper place.	____	____	____________
13. Removed the gloves. Completed hand hygiene.	____	____	____________
14. Assisted with handwashing. Wore gloves if needed. Decontaminated your hands after gloves were removed.	____	____	____________
15. Asked the person to drink an 8-ounce glass of water.	____	____	____________
16. Provided for comfort. Raised the bed rails if used. Placed the call bell within reach.	____	____	____________
17. Unscreened the person.	____	____	____________
18. Decontaminated your hands.	____	____	____________
19. Returned to the room in 20 to 30 minutes.	____	____	____________
20. Repeated procedure for the second specimen:			
a. Provided privacy.	____	____	____________
b. Put on the gloves.	____	____	____________
c. Asked the person to void into the receptacle. Reminded the person not to put toilet tissue in the receptacle.	____	____	____________
d. Took the receptacle to the bathroom.	____	____	____________
e. Poured some urine into the specimen container.	____	____	____________

Procedure—cont'd	S	U	Comments
f. Tested the specimen. Discarded the urine.	_____	_____	____________
g. Cleaned the receptacle, and returned it to its proper place.	_____	_____	____________
h. Removed the gloves. Completed hand hygiene.	_____	_____	____________
i. Assisted with handwashing. Wore gloves, if needed. Decontaminated your hands after removing gloves.	_____	_____	____________

Post-Procedure

	S	U	Comments
21. Provided for comfort.	_____	_____	____________
22. Raised the bed rails if used. Followed the care plan.	_____	_____	____________
23. Placed the call bell within reach.	_____	_____	____________
24. Unscreened the person.	_____	_____	____________
25. Decontaminated your hands.	_____	_____	____________
26. Reported the results of the second test and any other observations.	_____	_____	____________

Collecting a Urine Specimen From an Infant or Child

QUALITY OF LIFE

Name: ____________

Date: ____________

Remembered to:
- Knock before entering the person's room
- Address the person by name
- Introduce yourself by name and title

Pre-Procedure	S	U	Comments
1. Followed Delegation Guidelines: Urine Specimens. Viewed Safety Alert: Urine Specimens.	____	____	____
2. Explained the procedure to the child and parents.	____	____	____
3. Completed hand hygiene.	____	____	____
4. Collected the following:			
• Collection bag	____	____	____
• Wash basin	____	____	____
• Cotton balls	____	____	____
• Bath towel	____	____	____
• Two diapers	____	____	____
• Specimen container	____	____	____
• Gloves	____	____	____
• Plastic bag	____	____	____
• Scissors	____	____	____
5. Identified the child. Checked the identification bracelet against the requisition slip. Called the child by name.	____	____	____
6. Provided for privacy.	____	____	____

Procedure

	S	U	Comments
7. Put on the gloves.	____	____	____
8. Removed and disposed of the diaper.	____	____	____
9. Cleaned the perineal area. Used a new cotton ball for each stroke. Rinsed and dried the area.	____	____	____
10. Removed the gloves, and completed hand hygiene. Bed rails were up before leaving the bedside.	____	____	____
11. Put on clean gloves.	____	____	____
12. Positioned the child on the back. Flexed the child's knees and separated the legs.	____	____	____
13. Removed the adhesive backing from the collection bag.	____	____	____
14. Applied the bag to the perineum. Did not cover the anus.	____	____	____
15. Cut a slit in the bottom of the new diaper.	____	____	____
16. Diapered the child.	____	____	____
17. Pulled the collection bag through the slit in the diaper.	____	____	____
18. Removed the gloves. Decontaminated your hands.	____	____	____
19. Raised the head of the crib if allowed, which helped urine to collect in the bottom of the bag.	____	____	____
20. Unscreened the child.	____	____	____
21. Decontaminated your hands.	____	____	____

Procedure—cont'd

	S	U	Comments
22. Checked the child often. Checked the bag for urine. Wore gloves and provided for privacy.	____	____	____
23. Provided privacy when the child voided.	____	____	____
24. Removed the diaper.	____	____	____
25. Gently removed the collection bag.	____	____	____
26. Pressed the adhesive surfaces of the bag together, or transferred urine to the specimen container using the drainage tab.	____	____	____
27. Cleaned the perineal area. Rinsed and dried well.	____	____	____
28. Diapered the child.	____	____	____
29. Removed the gloves. Completed hand hygiene.	____	____	____

Post-Procedure

	S	U	Comments
30. Provided for comfort. Raised the bed rail.	____	____	____
31. Unscreened the child.	____	____	____
32. Labeled the specimen container. Placed it in the plastic bag.	____	____	____
33. Cleaned and returned equipment to its proper place. Discarded disposable items. Wore gloves for this step.	____	____	____
34. Completed hand hygiene.	____	____	____
35. Reported and recorded your observations.	____	____	____
36. Took the requisition slip and the specimen to the storage area or laboratory.	____	____	____

Testing Urine With Reagent Strips

QUALITY OF LIFE

Name: ______________________

Date: ______________________

Remembered to:
- ◆ Knock before entering the person's room
- ◆ Address the person by name
- ◆ Introduce yourself by name and title

Pre-Procedure	S	U	Comments
1. Followed Delegation Guidelines: Testing Urine. Viewed Safety Alerts: Testing Urine and Using Reagent Strips.	_____	_____	__________
2. Explained the procedure to the person.	_____	_____	__________
3. Completed hand hygiene.	_____	_____	__________
4. Identified the person. Checked the identification bracelet against the assignment sheet. Called the person by name.	_____	_____	__________
Procedure			
5. Put on the gloves.	_____	_____	__________
6. Collected the following:			
• Urine specimen (routine specimen for pH and occult blood; double-voided specimen for sugar and ketones)	_____	_____	__________
• Reagent strip as ordered	_____	_____	__________
• Gloves	_____	_____	__________
7. Removed a strip from the bottle. Tightly put the cap on the bottle at once.	_____	_____	__________
8. Dipped the strip test areas into the urine.	_____	_____	__________
9. Removed the strip after the correct amount of time. Followed the manufacturer's instructions.	_____	_____	__________
10. Gently tapped the strip against the container, which removed excess urine.	_____	_____	__________
11. Waited the required amount of time. Followed the manufacturer's instructions.	_____	_____	__________
12. Compared the strip with the color chart on the bottle. Read the results.	_____	_____	__________
13. Discarded disposable items and the specimen.	_____	_____	__________
Post-Procedure			
14. Cleaned and returned equipment to its proper place.	_____	_____	__________
15. Removed the gloves. Completed hand hygiene.	_____	_____	__________
16. Reported and recorded the results and other observations.	_____	_____	__________

Straining Urine

QUALITY OF LIFE

Name: ______________________

Date: ______________________

Remembered to:
- ◆ Knock before entering the person's room
- ◆ Address the person by name
- ◆ Introduce yourself by name and title

Pre-Procedure	S	U	Comments
1. Followed Delegation Guidelines: Testing Urine. Viewed Safety Alert: Testing Urine.	____	____	____________
2. Explained the procedure to the person. In addition, explained that the urinal, bedpan, commode, or specimen pan is used for voiding.	____	____	____________
3. Completed hand hygiene.	____	____	____________
4. Collected the following:			
• Strainer or 4 × 4 gauze	____	____	____________
• Specimen container	____	____	____________
• Bedpan, urinal, commode, or specimen pan	____	____	____________
• Two labels stating that all urine is strained	____	____	____________
• Gloves	____	____	____________
• Plastic bag	____	____	____________
5. Identified the person. Checked the identification bracelet against the assignment sheet. Called the person by name.	____	____	____________
6. Arranged items in the person's bathroom. Placed the specimen pan in the toilet.	____	____	____________
7. Placed one label in the bathroom. Placed the other near the bed.	____	____	____________

Procedure	S	U	Comments
8. Put on the gloves.	____	____	____________
9. Offered the bedpan or urinal, or assisted the person to the commode or bathroom.	____	____	____________
10. Provided for privacy.	____	____	____________
11. Told the person to signal after voiding.	____	____	____________
12. Removed the gloves. Decontaminated your hands.	____	____	____________
13. Returned when the person signaled for you. Knocked before entering the room.	____	____	____________
14. Decontaminated your hands. Put on gloves.	____	____	____________
15. Placed the strainer or gauze into the specimen container.	____	____	____________
16. Poured urine into the specimen container. Made sure urine passed through the strainer or gauze.	____	____	____________
17. Discarded the urine.	____	____	____________
18. Placed the strainer or gauze in the specimen container if any crystals, stones, or particles appeared.	____	____	____________
19. Provided perineal care if needed.	____	____	____________
20. Cleaned and returned equipment to its proper place.	____	____	____________

Procedure—cont'd	S	U	Comments
21. Removed soiled gloves. Completed hand hygiene, and put on clean gloves.	______	______	______________________
22. Assisted with handwashing.	______	______	______________________
23. Removed the gloves. Decontaminated your hands.	______	______	______________________

Post-Procedure

	S	U	Comments
24. Provided for comfort.	______	______	______________________
25. Placed the call bell within reach.	______	______	______________________
26. Raised or lowered bed rails. Followed the care plan.	______	______	______________________
27. Unscreened the person.	______	______	______________________
28. Labeled the specimen container. Put it in the plastic bag. Wore gloves for this step.	______	______	______________________
29. Removed gloves. Decontaminated your hands.	______	______	______________________
30. Reported and recorded your observations.	______	______	______________________
31. Took the specimen and requisition slip to the laboratory or storage area.	______	______	______________________

Collecting a Stool Specimen

QUALITY OF LIFE

Name: ______________________

Date: ______________________

Remembered to:
- ◆ **Knock before entering the person's room**
- ◆ **Address the person by name**
- ◆ **Introduce yourself by name and title**

Pre-Procedure	**S**	**U**	**Comments**
1. Followed Delegation Guidelines: Stool Specimens. Viewed Safety Alert: Stool Specimens.	_____	_____	_____________
2. Explained the procedure to the person.	_____	_____	_____________
3. Completed hand hygiene.	_____	_____	_____________
4. Collected the following:			
• Bedpan and cover or commode	_____	_____	_____________
• Urinal for voiding	_____	_____	_____________
• Specimen pan for the toilet or commode	_____	_____	_____________
• Specimen container and lid	_____	_____	_____________
• Tongue blade	_____	_____	_____________
• Disposable bag	_____	_____	_____________
• Gloves	_____	_____	_____________
• Toilet tissue	_____	_____	_____________
• Laboratory requisition slip	_____	_____	_____________
• Plastic bag	_____	_____	_____________

Procedure			
5. Labeled the container.	_____	_____	_____________
6. Identified the person. Checked the identification bracelet against the requisition slip. Called the person by name.	_____	_____	_____________
7. Provided for privacy.	_____	_____	_____________
8. Asked the person to void. Provided the bedpan, commode, or urinal for voiding if the person did not use the bathroom. Emptied and cleaned the device.	_____	_____	_____________
9. Put the specimen pan on the toilet if the person used the bathroom.	_____	_____	_____________
10. Assisted the person onto the bedpan, toilet, or commode. Made sure the person wore a robe and nonskid footwear while up.	_____	_____	_____________
11. Asked the person not to put toilet tissue in the bedpan, commode, or specimen pan. Provided a bag for toilet tissue.	_____	_____	_____________
12. Placed the call bell and toilet tissue within reach. Raised or lowered bed rails. Followed the care plan.	_____	_____	_____________
13. Decontaminated your hands. Left the room.	_____	_____	_____________
14. Returned when the person signaled. Knocked before entering. Decontaminated your hands.	_____	_____	_____________
15. Lowered the nearest bed rail if up.	_____	_____	_____________
16. Put on the gloves. Provided perineal care if needed.	_____	_____	_____________

Procedure—cont'd	S	U	Comments
17. Used a tongue blade to take about 2 tablespoons of stool to the specimen container. Took the sample from the middle of a formed stool. If required by agency policy, took stool from two different places on the specimen.	____	____	________
18. Put the lid on the specimen container without touching the inside of the lid or container. Placed the container in the plastic bag.	____	____	________
19. Wrapped the tongue blade in toilet tissue.	____	____	________
20. Discarded the tongue blade into the bag.	____	____	________
21. Emptied, cleaned, and disinfected equipment.	____	____	________
22. Removed the gloves. Decontaminated your hands.	____	____	________
23. Returned equipment to its proper place.	____	____	________
24. Helped the person with handwashing. Wore gloves if necessary.	____	____	________

Post-Procedure

	S	U	Comments
25. Provided for comfort.	____	____	________
26. Placed the call bell within reach.	____	____	________
27. Lowered the bed to its lowest position.	____	____	________
28. Raised or lowered bed rails. Followed the care plan.	____	____	________
29. Unscreened the person.	____	____	________
30. Took the specimen and requisition slip to the laboratory.	____	____	________
31. Decontaminated your hands.	____	____	________
32. Reported and recorded your observations.	____	____	________

Testing a Stool Specimen for Blood

QUALITY OF LIFE

Name: ______________________

Date: ______________________

Remembered to:
- ◆ Knock before entering the person's room
- ◆ Address the person by name
- ◆ Introduce yourself by name and title

Pre-Procedure	S	U	Comments
1. Followed Delegation Guidelines: Testing Stool Specimens. Viewed Safety Alert: Testing Stool Specimens.	_____	_____	____________
2. Explained the procedure to the person.	_____	_____	____________
3. Decontaminated your hand.	_____	_____	____________

Procedure	S	U	Comments
4. Collected a stool specimen.	_____	_____	____________
5. Collected the following:			
• Paper towels	_____	_____	____________
• Hemoccult test kit	_____	_____	____________
• Tongue blades	_____	_____	____________
• Gloves	_____	_____	____________
6. Put on the gloves.	_____	_____	____________
7. Opened the test kit.	_____	_____	____________
8. Used the tongue blade to obtain a small amount of stool.	_____	_____	____________
9. Applied a thin smear of stool on box A on the test paper.	_____	_____	____________
10. Used another tongue blade to obtain stool from another part of the specimen.	_____	_____	____________
11. Applied a thin smear of stool on box B on the test paper.	_____	_____	____________
12. Closed the test packet.	_____	_____	____________
13. Turned the test packet to the other side. Opened the flap. Applied developer from the kit to boxes A and B. Followed the manufacturer's instructions.	_____	_____	____________
14. Waited the amount of time noted in the manufacturer's instructions. Time varies from 10 to 60 seconds.	_____	_____	____________
15. Noted and recorded the color changes.	_____	_____	____________
16. Disposed of the test packet.	_____	_____	____________
17. Wrapped the tongue blades with toilet tissue. Discarded them.	_____	_____	____________
18. Disposed of the specimen.	_____	_____	____________
19. Removed the gloves. Decontaminated your hands.	_____	_____	____________
20. Reported and recorded the test results and your observations.	_____	_____	____________

Collecting a Sputum Specimen

QUALITY OF LIFE

Name: ______________________

Date: ______________________

Remembered to:
- ◆ **Knock before entering the person's room**
- ◆ **Address the person by name**
- ◆ **Introduce yourself by name and title**

Pre-Procedure

	S	U	Comments
1. Followed Delegation Guidelines: Sputum Specimens. Viewed Safety Alert: Sputum Specimens.	______	______	______________________
2. Explained the procedure to the person.	______	______	______________________
3. Completed hand hygiene.	______	______	______________________
4. Collected the following:			
• Sputum specimen container and label	______	______	______________________
• Laboratory requisition	______	______	______________________
• Disposable bag	______	______	______________________
• Gloves	______	______	______________________
• Tissues	______	______	______________________
5. Labeled the container.	______	______	______________________
6. Identified the person. Checked the identification bracelet against the requisition slip. Called the person by name.	______	______	______________________
7. Provided for privacy. Allowed the person to go into the bathroom for the procedure if able.	______	______	______________________

Procedure

	S	U	Comments
8. Asked the person to rinse the mouth out with clear water.	______	______	______________________
9. Put on gloves.	______	______	______________________
10. Had the person hold the container. Touched the outside of the container only.	______	______	______________________
11. Asked the person to cover the mouth and nose with a tissue when coughing.	______	______	______________________
12. Asked him or her to take two or three deep breaths, and cough up sputum.	______	______	______________________
13. Had the person expectorate directly into the container. Sputum did not touch the outside of the container.	______	______	______________________
14. Collected 1 to 2 tablespoons of sputum unless was told to collect more.	______	______	______________________
15. Placed the lid on the container.	______	______	______________________
16. Placed the container in the bag. Attached the requisition to the bag.	______	______	______________________
17. Removed the gloves.	______	______	______________________

Post-Procedure	S	U	Comments
18. Provided for comfort.			
19. Placed the call bell within reach.			
20. Unscreened the person.			
21. Decontaminated your hands.			
22. Took the bag to the laboratory or storage area.			
23. Decontaminated your hands.			
24. Reported and recorded your observations.			

The Surgical Skin Preparation

QUALITY OF LIFE

Name: ____________________

Date: ____________________

Remembered to:
- ◆ **Knock before entering the person's room**
- ◆ **Address the person by name**
- ◆ **Introduce yourself by name and title**

Pre-Procedure

	S	U	Comments
1. Followed Delegation Guidelines: Skin Preparation. Viewed Safety Alert: Skin Preparation.	___	___	___
2. Explained the procedure to the person.	___	___	___
3. Completed hand hygiene.	___	___	___
4. Collected the following:			
• Skin preparation kit (with drape)	___	___	___
• Bath blanket	___	___	___
• Warm water	___	___	___
• Gloves	___	___	___
• Waterproof pad	___	___	___
• Bath towel	___	___	___
5. Identified the person. Checked the identification bracelet against the assignment sheet. Called the person by name.	___	___	___
6. Provided for privacy.	___	___	___

Procedure

	S	U	Comments
7. Made sure you had good lighting.	___	___	___
8. Raised the bed for body mechanics. Lowered the nearest bed rail if up.	___	___	___
9. Covered the person with a bath blanket. Fanfolded top linens to the foot of the bed.	___	___	___
10. Placed the waterproof pad under the area you will shave.	___	___	___
11. Opened the skin preparation kit.	___	___	___
12. Positioned the person for the skin preparation.	___	___	___
13. Draped him or her with the drape.	___	___	___
14. Added warm water to the basin. Raised bed rails, if used, before you left the bedside.	___	___	___
15. Put on gloves.	___	___	___
16. Lathered the skin with the sponge.	___	___	___
17. Held the skin taut. Shaved in the direction of hair growth.	___	___	___
18. Shaved outward from the center using short strokes.	___	___	___
19. Rinsed the razor often.	___	___	___
20. Made sure the entire area was free of hair. Checked for cuts, scratches, or nicks.	___	___	___
21. Rinsed the skin thoroughly. Patted dry.	___	___	___
22. Removed the drape and waterproof pad.	___	___	___
23. Removed the gloves. Decontaminated your hands.	___	___	___
24. Returned top linens. Removed the bath blanket.	___	___	___

Post-Procedure	S	U	Comments
25. Provided for comfort.	_____	_____	____________
26. Raised or lowered bed rails. Followed the care plan.	_____	_____	____________
27. Lowered the bed to its lowest position.	_____	_____	____________
28. Placed the call bell within reach.	_____	_____	____________
29. Unscreened the person.	_____	_____	____________
30. Returned equipment to its proper place.	_____	_____	____________
31. Discarded supplies. Followed agency policy for soiled linen.	_____	_____	____________
32. Decontaminated your hands.	_____	_____	____________
33. Reported and recorded your observations.	_____	_____	____________

Giving a Douche

QUALITY OF LIFE

Name: ______________________

Date: ______________________

Remembered to:
- ◆ Knock before entering the person's room
- ◆ Address the person by name
- ◆ Introduce yourself by name and title

Pre-Procedure

	S	U	Comments
1. Followed Delegation Guidelines: Giving a Douche. Viewed Safety Alert: Giving a Douche.	____	____	____________
2. Explained the procedure to the person.	____	____	____________
3. Completed hand hygiene.	____	____	____________
4. Collected the following:			
• Douche kit	____	____	____________
• 1000 ml of solution	____	____	____________
• Bath thermometer	____	____	____________
• Bath blanket	____	____	____________
• Bedpan	____	____	____________
• Toilet tissue	____	____	____________
• Waterproof pad	____	____	____________
• Gloves	____	____	____________
• IV pole	____	____	____________
• Water pitcher	____	____	____________
• Equipment for perineal care	____	____	____________
5. Identified the person. Checked the identification bracelet against the assignment sheet. Called the person by name.	____	____	____________
6. Provided for privacy.	____	____	____________
7. Asked the woman to void. Assisted her to the bathroom or commode, or provided the bedpan. Wore gloves for this step.	____	____	____________
8. Removed the gloves. Completed hand hygiene.	____	____	____________
9. Raised the bed for body mechanics. Raised bed rails if used.	____	____	____________

Procedure

	S	U	Comments
10. Warmed the solution to the temperature directed by the nurse. Followed agency policy for warming the solution and measuring its temperature.	____	____	____________
11. Clamped the tubing. Poured the solution into the douche bag.	____	____	____________
12. Hung the bag from the IV pole, 12 to 18 inches above the vagina.	____	____	____________
13. Covered the person with a bath blanket. Fanfolded top linens to the foot of the bed.	____	____	____________
14. Turned the person in the supine position. Draped her with the bath blanket for perineal care.	____	____	____________
15. Put on gloves.	____	____	____________
16. Placed the waterproof pad under her buttocks.	____	____	____________

Procedure—cont'd	S	U	Comments
17. Gave perineal care.			
18. Positioned her on the bedpan.			
19. Unclamped the tubing. Allowed some solution to run over the vulva and perineal area.			
20. Inserted the nozzle 2 to 3 inches into the vagina. Gently turned the nozzle back and forth during the procedure.			
21. Clamped the tubing when the bag was empty. Removed the nozzle.			
22. Placed the tubing in the douche bag.			
23. Raised the head of the bed to allow the solution to drain from the vagina into the bedpan.			
24. Lowered the head of the bed.			
25. Removed the bedpan. Dried the perineal area with toilet tissue.			
26. Removed the waterproof pad.			
27. Took the bedpan into the bathroom. Raised the bed rails if used.			
28. Cleaned and returned equipment to its proper place.			
29. Discarded used disposable items.			
30. Changed damp linen.			
31. Removed the gloves. Completed hand hygiene.			

Post-Procedure

32. Provided for comfort.			
33. Returned top linens. Removed the bath blanket.			
34. Lowered the bed to its lowest position.			
35. Raised or lowered bed rails. Followed the care plan.			
36. Placed the call bell within reach.			
37. Unscreened the person.			
38. Decontaminated your hands.			
39. Reported and recorded your observations.			

Applying Elastic Stockings

QUALITY OF LIFE

Name: ______________________

Date: ______________________

Remembered to:
- ◆ Knock before entering the person's room
- ◆ Address the person by name
- ◆ Introduce yourself by name and title

Pre-Procedure	**S**	**U**	**Comments**
1. Followed Delegation Guidelines: Elastic Stockings. Viewed Safety Alert: Elastic Stockings.	_____	_____	__________
2. Explained the procedure to the person.	_____	_____	__________
3. Completed hand hygiene.	_____	_____	__________
4. Obtained elastic stockings in the correct size and length.	_____	_____	__________
5. Identified the person. Checked the identification bracelet against the assignment sheet. Called the person by name.	_____	_____	__________
6. Provided for privacy.	_____	_____	__________
7. Raised the bed for body mechanics. Raised the bed rails if used.	_____	_____	__________
Procedure			
8. Lowered the nearest bed rail if up.	_____	_____	__________
9. Turned the person in the supine position.	_____	_____	__________
10. Exposed the legs. Fanfolded top linens toward the thighs.	_____	_____	__________
11. Turned the stocking inside out down to the heel.	_____	_____	__________
12. Slipped the foot of the stocking over the toes, foot, and heel.	_____	_____	__________
13. Grasped the stocking top. Slipped it over the foot and heel. Pulled it up the leg, turning it right side out as it was pulled up. Made sure the stocking was even and snug.	_____	_____	__________
14. Removed twists, creases, or wrinkles.	_____	_____	__________
15. Repeated steps for other leg:			
a. Turned the stocking inside out down to the heel.	_____	_____	__________
b. Slipped the foot of the stocking over the toes, foot and heel.	_____	_____	__________
c. Grasped the stocking top. Slipped it over the foot and heel. Pulled it up the leg, turning it right side out as it was pulled up. Made sure the stocking was even and snug.	_____	_____	__________
d. Removed twists, creases, or wrinkles.	_____	_____	__________
Post-Procedure			
16. Provided for comfort.	_____	_____	__________
17. Covered the person.	_____	_____	__________
18. Lowered the bed.	_____	_____	__________
19. Raised or lowered the bed rails. Followed the care plan.	_____	_____	__________
20. Placed the call bell within reach.	_____	_____	__________
21. Unscreened the person.	_____	_____	__________
22. Decontaminated your hands.	_____	_____	__________
23. Reported and recorded your observations.	_____	_____	__________

Applying Elastic Bandages

QUALITY OF LIFE

Name: ______________________

Date: ______________________

Remembered to:
- ◆ Knock before entering the person's room
- ◆ Address the person by name
- ◆ Introduce yourself by name and title

Pre-Procedure

	S	U	Comments
1. Followed Delegation Guidelines: Elastic Bandages. Viewed Safety Alert: Elastic Bandages.			
2. Explained the procedure to the person.			
3. Completed hand hygiene.			
4. Collected the following:			
• Elastic bandage as directed by the nurse			
• Tape or metal clips unless the bandage has Velcro			
5. Identified the person. Checked the identification bracelet against the assignment sheet. Called the person by name.			
6. Provided for privacy.			
7. Raised the bed for body mechanics. Raised the bed rails if used.			

Procedure

	S	U	Comments
8. Lowered the nearest bed rail if up.			
9. Helped the person to a comfortable position. Exposed the part you needed to bandage.			
10. Made sure the area was clean and dry.			
11. Held the bandage so the roll was up and the loose end was on the bottom.			
12. Applied the bandage to the smallest part of the wrist, foot, ankle, or knee.			
13. Made two circular turns around the part.			
14. Made overlapping spiral turns in an upward direction. Each turn overlapped about two thirds of the previous turn.			
15. Applied the bandage smoothly with firm, even pressure. Made sure it was not too tight.			
16. Secured the bandage in place with Velcro, tape, or clips. Made sure the clips were not under the body part.			
17. Checked the fingers or toes for coldness or cyanosis (bluish color). Asked about pain, itching, numbness, or tingling. Removed the bandage if any was noted. Reported your observations to the nurse.			

Post-Procedure	S	U	Comments
18. Provided for comfort.	______	______	______
19. Placed the call bell within reach.	______	______	______
20. Lowered the bed.	______	______	______
21. Raised or lowered bed rails. Followed the care plan.	______	______	______
22. Unscreened the person.	______	______	______
23. Decontaminated your hands.	______	______	______
24. Reported and recorded your observations.	______	______	______

Applying a Dry Nonsterile Dressing

QUALITY OF LIFE

Name: ______________________

Date: ______________________

Remembered to:
- ◆ Knock before entering the person's room
- ◆ Address the person by name
- ◆ Introduce yourself by name and title

Pre-Procedure	S	U	Comments
1. Followed Delegation Guidelines: Applying Dressings. Viewed Safety Alert: Applying Dressings.	_____	_____	____________
2. Explained the procedure to the person.	_____	_____	____________
3. Allowed time for pain relief medications to take effect.	_____	_____	____________
4. Provided for fluid and elimination needs.	_____	_____	____________
5. Completed hand hygiene.	_____	_____	____________
6. Collected the following:			
• Gloves	_____	_____	____________
• Personal protective equipment as needed.	_____	_____	____________
• Tape or Montgomery ties.	_____	_____	____________
• Adhesive remover	_____	_____	____________
• Scissors	_____	_____	____________
• Plastic bag	_____	_____	____________
• Bath blanket	_____	_____	____________
7. Identified the person. Checked the identification bracelet against the assignment sheet. Called the person by name.	_____	_____	____________
8. Provided for privacy.	_____	_____	____________
9. Arranged your work area. Made sure that you would not have to reach over or turn your back on the work area.	_____	_____	____________
10. Raised the bed for body mechanics. Raised the bed rails if used.	_____	_____	____________

Procedure	S	U	Comments
11. Lowered the nearest bed rail if up.	_____	_____	____________
12. Helped the person to a comfortable position.	_____	_____	____________
13. Covered the person with a bath blanket. Fanfolded top linens to the foot of the bed.	_____	_____	____________
14. Exposed the affected body part.	_____	_____	____________
15. Made a cuff on the plastic bag. Placed it within reach.	_____	_____	____________
16. Put on a gown and mask if needed.	_____	_____	____________
17. Put on the gloves.	_____	_____	____________
18. Undid Montgomery ties or removed tape:			
a. Montgomery ties: Folded ties away from the wound.	_____	_____	____________
b. Tape: Held the skin down. Gently pulled the tape toward the wound.	_____	_____	____________
19. Removed adhesive from the skin if necessary. Moistened a 4 × 4 gauze dressing with the adhesive remover. Cleaned away from the wound.	_____	_____	____________

Procedure—cont'd	S	U	Comments
20. Removed gauze dressings. Started with the top dressing. Made sure the soiled side was away from the person's sight. Put dressings in the bag, and avoided touching the outside of the bag with the dressings.	______	______	____________________
21. Very gently removed the dressing directly over the wound. Made sure it does not stick to the wound or drain.	______	______	____________________
22. Observed the wound, drain site, and wound drainage.	______	______	____________________
23. Removed the gloves, and put them into the bag. Decontaminated your hands.	______	______	____________________
24. Put on clean gloves.	______	______	____________________
25. Opened the dressings.	______	______	____________________
26. Cut the length of tape needed.	______	______	____________________
27. Applied dressings as directed by the nurse.	______	______	____________________
28. Secured the dressings in place. Used tape or Montgomery ties.	______	______	____________________
29. Removed your gloves, and put them in the bag. Decontaminated your hands.	______	______	____________________

Post-Procedure

	S	U	Comments
30. Provided for comfort.	______	______	____________________
31. Covered the person. Removed the bath blanket.	______	______	____________________
32. Placed the call bell within reach.	______	______	____________________
33. Lowered the bed to its lowest position.	______	______	____________________
34. Raised or lowered bed rails. Followed the care plan.	______	______	____________________
35. Unscreened the person.	______	______	____________________
36. Discarded supplies into the bag. Tied the bag closed. Discarded the bag according to agency policy.	______	______	____________________
37. Cleaned your work surface. Followed the Bloodborne Pathogen Standard.	______	______	____________________
38. Decontaminated your hands.	______	______	____________________
39. Reported and recorded your observations.	______	______	____________________

Applying Hot Compresses

QUALITY OF LIFE

Name: ______________________

Date: ______________________

Remembered to:
- ◆ Knock before entering the person's room
- ◆ Address the person by name
- ◆ Introduce yourself by name and title

Pre-Procedure	**S**	**U**	**Comments**
1. Followed Delegation Guidelines: Applying Heat and Cold. Viewed Safety Alert: Applying Heat and Cold.	_____	_____	__________
2. Explained the procedure to the person.	_____	_____	__________
3. Completed hand hygiene.	_____	_____	__________
4. Collected the following:			
• Basin	_____	_____	__________
• Bath thermometer	_____	_____	__________
• Small towel, washcloth, or gauze squares	_____	_____	__________
• Plastic wrap or aquathermia pad	_____	_____	__________
• Ties, tape, or rolled gauze	_____	_____	__________
• Bath towel	_____	_____	__________
• Waterproof pad	_____	_____	__________
5. Identified the person. Checked the identification bracelet against the assignment sheet. Called the person by name.	_____	_____	__________
6. Provided for privacy.	_____	_____	__________

Procedure

7. Placed the waterproof pad under the body part.	_____	_____	__________
8. Filled the basin one-half to two-thirds full with hot water as directed by the nurse. Measured water temperature. Followed agency policy.	_____	_____	__________
9. Placed the compress in the water.	_____	_____	__________
10. Wrung out the compress.	_____	_____	__________
11. Applied the compress to the area. Noted the time.	_____	_____	__________
12. Quickly covered the compress. Used one of the following as directed by the nurse:	_____	_____	__________
a. Applied plastic wrap and then a bath towel. Secured the towel in place with ties, tape, or rolled gauze.	_____	_____	__________
b. Applied an aquathermia pad.	_____	_____	__________
13. Placed the call bell within reach.	_____	_____	__________
14. Raised or lowered bed rails. Followed the care plan.	_____	_____	__________
15. Checked the area every 5 minutes. Checked for redness and complaints of pain, discomfort, or numbness. Removed the compress if any had occurred. Told the nurse at once.	_____	_____	__________
16. Changed the compress if cooling had occurred.	_____	_____	__________
17. Removed the compress after 20 minutes or as directed by the nurse. Patted dry the area. Lowered the bed rail for this step if it was up.	_____	_____	__________

Post-Procedure	S	U	Comments
18. Provided for comfort.	_____	_____	__________
19. Unscreened the person.	_____	_____	__________
20. Raised or lowered bed rails. Followed the care plan.	_____	_____	__________
21. Placed the call bell within reach.	_____	_____	__________
22. Cleaned equipment. Discarded disposable items. Wore gloves for this step.	_____	_____	__________
23. Followed agency policy for soiled linen.	_____	_____	__________
24. Decontaminated your hands.	_____	_____	__________
25. Reported and recorded your observations.	_____	_____	__________

The Hot Soak

Quality of Life

Name: ______________________

Date: ______________________

Remembered to:
- ◆ **Knock before entering the person's room**
- ◆ **Address the person by name**
- ◆ **Introduce yourself by name and title**

Pre-Procedure	**S**	**U**	**Comments**
1. Followed Delegation Guidelines: Applying Heat and Cold. Viewed Safety Alert: Applying Heat and Cold.	_____	_____	_____________
2. Explained the procedure to the person.	_____	_____	_____________
3. Completed hand hygiene.	_____	_____	_____________
4. Collected the following:			
• Water basin or an arm or foot bath	_____	_____	_____________
• Bath thermometer	_____	_____	_____________
• Bath blanket	_____	_____	_____________
• Waterproof pad	_____	_____	_____________
5. Identified the person. Checked the identification bracelet against the assignment sheet. Called the person by name.	_____	_____	_____________
6. Provided for privacy.	_____	_____	_____________
Procedure			
7. Positioned the person for the procedure. Placed the call bell within reach.	_____	_____	_____________
8. Placed a waterproof pad under the area.	_____	_____	_____________
9. Filled the container one-half full with hot water as directed by the nurse. Measured water temperature. Followed agency policy.	_____	_____	_____________
10. Exposed the area. Avoided unnecessary exposure.	_____	_____	_____________
11. Placed the part into the water. Padded the edge of the container with a towel. Noted the time.	_____	_____	_____________
12. Covered the person with a bath blanket for extra warmth.	_____	_____	_____________
13. Checked every 5 minutes. Checked for redness and complaints of pain, numbness, or discomfort. Discontinued the soak if any of these occurred. Wrapped the part in a towel, and told the nurse at once.	_____	_____	_____________
14. Checked water temperature every 5 minutes. Changed water as necessary. Wrapped the part in a towel while changing the water.	_____	_____	_____________
15. Removed the part from the water in 15 to 20 minutes. Patted dry.	_____	_____	_____________

Post-Procedure	S	U	Comments
16. Provided for comfort.	______	______	______________________
17. Unscreened the person.	______	______	______________________
18. Raised or lowered bed rails. Followed the care plan.	______	______	______________________
19. Placed the call bell within reach.	______	______	______________________
20. Cleaned equipment. Discarded disposable items. Wore gloves for this step.	______	______	______________________
21. Followed agency policy for soiled linen.	______	______	______________________
22. Decontaminated your hands.	______	______	______________________
23. Reported and recorded your observations.	______	______	______________________

Assisting the Person to Take a Sitz Bath

Quality of Life

Name: ____________________

Date: ____________________

Remembered to:
- ◆ Knock before entering the person's room
- ◆ Address the person by name
- ◆ Introduce yourself by name and title

Pre-Procedure	S	U	Comments
1. Followed Delegation Guidelines: Applying Heat and Cold. Viewed Safety Alert: Applying Heat and Cold.	_____	_____	__________
2. Explained the procedure to the person.	_____	_____	__________
3. Completed hand hygiene.	_____	_____	__________
4. Collected the following:			
• Disposable sitz bath if used	_____	_____	__________
• Wheelchair if the built-in sitz bath is used	_____	_____	__________
• Bath thermometer	_____	_____	__________
• Two bath blankets, bath towels, and clean gown	_____	_____	__________
• Footstool if the person is short	_____	_____	__________
• Disinfectant solution	_____	_____	__________
• Utility gloves	_____	_____	__________
5. Identified the person. Checked the identification bracelet against the assignment sheet. Called the person by name.	_____	_____	__________
6. Provided for privacy.	_____	_____	__________

Procedure

7. Performed one of the following:			
a. Placed the disposable sitz bath on the toilet seat.	_____	_____	__________
b. Transported the person by wheelchair to the sitz bath room.	_____	_____	__________
8. Filled the sitz bath two-thirds full with water as directed by the nurse. Measured water temperature. Followed agency policy.	_____	_____	__________
9. Padded the metal part of the sitz bath with towels. Padded the part in contact with the person.	_____	_____	__________
10. Secured the gown above the waist.	_____	_____	__________
11. Helped the person sit in the sitz bath.	_____	_____	__________
12. Placed a bath blanket around the shoulders. Placed another over the legs for warmth.	_____	_____	__________
13. Provided a footstool if the edge of the sitz bath causes pressure under the knees.	_____	_____	__________
14. Placed the call bell within reach. Provided for comfort.	_____	_____	__________
15. Stayed with the person who is weak or unsteady.	_____	_____	__________
16. Checked the person every 5 minutes for complaints of weakness, faintness, and drowsiness. Checked for a rapid pulse. If any occurred, called the nurse. Assisted the person back to bed.	_____	_____	__________

Procedure—cont'd	S	U	Comments
17. Helped the person out of the sitz bath after 20 minutes or as directed by the nurse.	_____	_____	__________
18. Assisted the person with drying and dressing.	_____	_____	__________
19. Assisted the person back to bed.	_____	_____	__________

Post-Procedure

	S	U	Comments
20. Provided for comfort.	_____	_____	__________
21. Unscreened the person.	_____	_____	__________
22. Placed the call bell within reach.	_____	_____	__________
23. Raised or lowered bed rails. Followed the care plan.	_____	_____	__________
24. Cleaned the sitz bath with disinfectant solution. Wore utility gloves.	_____	_____	__________
25. Cleaned and returned reusable items to their proper place. Followed agency policy for soiled linen. Wore gloves for this step.	_____	_____	__________
26. Decontaminated your hands.	_____	_____	__________
27. Reported and recorded your observations.	_____	_____	__________

Applying a Hot Pack

QUALITY OF LIFE

Name: ____________________

Date: ____________________

Remembered to:
- **Knock before entering the person's room**
- **Address the person by name**
- **Introduce yourself by name and title**

Pre-Procedure

	S	U	Comments
1. Followed Delegation Guidelines: Applying Heat and Cold. Viewed Safety Alert: Applying Heat and Cold.			
2. Explained the procedure to the person.			
3. Completed hand hygiene.			
4. Collected the following:			
• Commercial pack			
• Towel			
• Waterproof pad			
• Ties, tape, or rolled gauze if needed			
5. Heated the pack. Followed the manufacturer's instructions.			
6. Placed the pack in the cover.			
7. Identified the person. Checked the identification bracelet against the assignment sheet. Called the person by name.			
8. Provided for privacy.			

Procedure

	S	U	Comments
9. Placed the waterproof pad under the body part.			
10. Quickly applied the pack. Noted the time.			
11. Secured the pack in place with ties, tape, or rolled gauze. (Some packs secured with Velcro straps.)			
12. Placed the call bell within reach.			
13. Raised or lowered bed rails. Followed the care plan.			
14. Checked the area every 5 minutes. Checked for redness and complaints of pain, discomfort, or numbness. Removed the pack if any occurred. Told the nurse at once.			
15. Changed the pack if cooling occurred.			
16. Removed the pack after 20 minutes or as directed by the nurse. Patted the area dry. Lowered the bed rail for this step if it was up.			

Post-Procedure

	S	U	Comments
17. Provided for comfort.			
18. Unscreened the person.			
19. Raised or lowered bed rails. Followed the care plan.			
20. Placed the call bell within reach.			
21. Cleaned equipment. Discarded disposable items. Wore gloves for this step.			
22. Followed agency policy for soiled linen.			

Post-Procedure	S	U	Comments
23. Decontaminated your hands.	_____	_____	__________________
24. Reported and recorded your observations.	_____	_____	__________________
25. Cleaned a reusable pack. Followed agency policy and the manufacturer's instructions.	_____	_____	__________________

Applying an Aquathermia Pad

QUALITY OF LIFE

Name: ______________________

Date: ______________________

Remembered to:
- ◆ **Knock before entering the person's room**
- ◆ **Address the person by name**
- ◆ **Introduce yourself by name and title**

Pre-Procedure

	S	U	Comments
1. Followed Delegation Guidelines: Applying Heat and Cold. Viewed Safety Alerts: Applying Heat and Cold and The Aquathermia Pad.	____	____	__________
2. Explained the procedure to the person.	____	____	__________
3. Completed hand hygiene.	____	____	__________
4. Collected the following:			
• Aquathermia pad and heating unit	____	____	__________
• Distilled water	____	____	__________
• Flannel cover, pillowcase, or towel	____	____	__________
• Ties, tape, or roller gauze	____	____	__________
5. Identified the person. Checked the identification bracelet against the assignment sheet. Called the person by name.	____	____	__________
6. Provided for privacy.	____	____	__________

Procedure

	S	U	Comments
7. Filled the heating unit to the fill line with distilled water.	____	____	__________
8. Removed bubbles. Placed the pad and tubing below the heating unit. Tilted the heating unit from side to side.	____	____	__________
9. Set the temperature as the nurse directed, usually 105° F (40° C). Removed the key. Gave the key to the nurse after the procedure.	____	____	__________
10. Placed the pad in the cover.	____	____	__________
11. Plugged in the unit. Allowed the water to warm to the desired temperature.	____	____	__________
12. Set the heating unit on the bedside stand. Kept the pad and connecting hoses level with the unit. Made sure that the hoses did not have kinks.	____	____	__________
13. Applied the pad to the part. Noted the time.	____	____	__________
14. Secured the pad in place with ties, tape, or rolled gauze. Did not use pins.	____	____	__________
15. Unscreened the person. Placed the call bell within reach.	____	____	__________
16. Raised or lowered bed rails. Followed the care plan.	____	____	__________
17. Checked the person every 5 minutes. Checked the skin for redness, swelling, and blisters. Asked about pain, discomfort, or decreased sensation. Removed the pad if any occurred. Told the nurse at once.	____	____	__________
18. Removed the pad at the specified time. Lowered the nearest bed rail for this step if it was up.	____	____	__________

Post-Procedure	S	U	Comments
19. Provided for comfort.	_____	_____	__________
20. Unscreened the person.	_____	_____	__________
21. Raised or lowered bed rails. Followed the care plan.	_____	_____	__________
22. Placed the call bell within reach.	_____	_____	__________
23. Cleaned equipment. Discarded disposable items. Wore gloves for this step.	_____	_____	__________
24. Followed agency policy for soiled linen.	_____	_____	__________
25. Decontaminated your hands.	_____	_____	__________
26. Reported and recorded your observations.	_____	_____	__________

Applying an Ice Bag, Ice Collar, Ice Glove, or Dry Cold Pack

QUALITY OF LIFE

Name: ______________________

Date: ______________________

Remembered to:
- ◆ **Knock before entering the person's room**
- ◆ **Address the person by name**
- ◆ **Introduce yourself by name and title**

Pre-Procedure	S	U	Comments
1. Followed Delegation Guidelines: Applying Heat and Cold. Viewed Safety Alerts: Applying Heat and Cold and Commercial Cold Packs.	____	____	____________
2. Explained the procedure to the person.	____	____	____________
3. Completed hand hygiene.	____	____	____________
4. Collected a cold pack or the following:			
• Ice bag, collar, or glove	____	____	____________
• Crushed ice	____	____	____________
• Flannel cover, towel, or pillowcase	____	____	____________
• Paper towels	____	____	____________
5. Applied an ice bag, collar, or glove:			
a. Filled it with water. Put in the stopper. Turned the device upside down to check for leaks.	____	____	____________
b. Emptied the device.	____	____	____________
c. Filled the device one-half to two-thirds full with crushed ice or ice chips.	____	____	____________
d. Removed excess air. Bent, twisted, or squeezed the device, or pressed it against a firm surface.	____	____	____________
e. Securely placed the cap or stopper on.	____	____	____________
f. Dried the device with the paper towels.	____	____	____________
g. Placed the device in the cover.	____	____	____________
6. Applied a cold pack:			
a. Squeezed, kneaded, or struck the cold pack as directed by the manufacturer to release the cold.	____	____	____________
b. Placed the pack in the cover.	____	____	____________
7. Identified the person. Checked the identification bracelet against the assignment sheet. Called the person by name.	____	____	____________
8. Provided for privacy.	____	____	____________

Procedure

9. Applied the device. Secured it in place with ties, tape, or rolled gauze. Noted the time.	____	____	____________
10. Placed the call bell within reach. Raised or lowered bed rails. Followed the care plan.	____	____	____________
11. Checked the skin every 5 minutes. Checked for blisters; pale, white, or gray skin; cyanosis; and shivering. Asked about numbness, pain, or burning. Removed the device if any occurred. Told the nurse at once.	____	____	____________
12. Removed the device after 20 minutes or as directed by the nurse.	____	____	____________

Post-Procedure	S	U	Comments
13. Provided for comfort.	______	______	____________________
14. Unscreened the person.	______	______	____________________
15. Raised or lowered bed rails. Followed the care plan.	______	______	____________________
16. Placed the call bell within reach.	______	______	____________________
17. Cleaned equipment. Discarded disposable items. Wore gloves for this step.	______	______	____________________
18. Followed agency policy for soiled linen.	______	______	____________________
19. Decontaminated your hands.	______	______	____________________
20. Reported and recorded your observations.	______	______	____________________
21. Cleaned a reusable cold pack. Followed agency policy and the manufacturer's instructions.	______	______	____________________

Applying Cold Compresses

QUALITY OF LIFE

Name: ______________________

Date: ______________________

Remembered to:
- ◆ Knock before entering the person's room
- ◆ Address the person by name
- ◆ Introduce yourself by name and title

Pre-Procedure	**S**	**U**	**Comments**
1. Followed Delegation Guidelines: Applying Heat and Cold. Viewed Safety Alert: Applying Heat and Cold.	_____	_____	_____
2. Explained the procedure to the person.	_____	_____	_____
3. Completed hand hygiene.	_____	_____	_____
4. Collected the following:			
• Large basin with ice	_____	_____	_____
• Small basin with cold water	_____	_____	_____
• Gauze squares, washcloths, or small towels	_____	_____	_____
• Waterproof pad	_____	_____	_____
• Bath towel	_____	_____	_____
5. Identified the person. Checked the identification bracelet against the assignment sheet. Called the person by name.	_____	_____	_____
6. Provided for privacy.	_____	_____	_____
Procedure			
7. Placed the waterproof pad under the affected body part. Exposed the area.	_____	_____	_____
8. Placed the small basin with cold water into the large basin with ice.	_____	_____	_____
9. Placed the compresses into the cold water.	_____	_____	_____
10. Wrung out a compress.	_____	_____	_____
11. Applied the compress to the part. Noted the time.	_____	_____	_____
12. Checked the area every 5 minutes. Checked for blisters; pale, white, or gray skin; cyanosis; or shivering. Asked about numbness, pain, or burning. Removed the compress if any occurred. Told the nurse at once.	_____	_____	_____
13. Changed the compress when it warmed, usually every 5 minutes.	_____	_____	_____
14. Removed the compress after 20 minutes or as directed by the nurse.	_____	_____	_____
15. Patted area dry.	_____	_____	_____
Post-Procedure			
16. Provided for comfort.	_____	_____	_____
17. Unscreened the person.	_____	_____	_____
18. Raised or lowered bed rails. Followed the care plan.	_____	_____	_____
19. Placed the call bell within reach.	_____	_____	_____

Post-Procedure—cont'd	S	U	Comments
20. Cleaned equipment. Discarded disposable items. Wore gloves for this step.	______	______	______________
21. Followed agency policy for soiled linen.	______	______	______________
22. Decontaminated your hands.	______	______	______________
23. Reported and recorded your observations.	______	______	______________

Using a Pulse Oximeter

QUALITY OF LIFE

Name: ______________________

Date: ______________________

Remembered to:
- ◆ **Knock before entering the person's room**
- ◆ **Address the person by name**
- ◆ **Introduce yourself by name and title**

Pre-Procedure

	S	U	Comments
1. Followed Delegation Guidelines: Pulse Oximetry. Viewed Safety Alert: Pulse Oximetry.	____	____	____________
2. Explained the procedure to the person.	____	____	____________
3. Completed hand hygiene.	____	____	____________
4. Collected the following:			
• Oximeter and sensor	____	____	____________
• Nail polish remover	____	____	____________
• Cotton balls	____	____	____________
• SpO_2 flow sheet	____	____	____________
• Tape	____	____	____________
• Towel	____	____	____________
5. Identified the person. Checked the identification bracelet against the assignment sheet. Called the person by name.	____	____	____________
6. Provided for privacy.	____	____	____________

Procedure

	S	U	Comments
7. Removed nail polish from the finger or toenail. Used nail polish remover and a cotton ball.	____	____	____________
8. Dried the site with a towel.	____	____	____________
9. Clipped or taped the sensor to the site.	____	____	____________
10. Turned on the oximeter.	____	____	____________
11. Set the high and low alarm limits for SpO_2 and pulse rate. Turned on audio and visual alarms.	____	____	____________
12. Checked the person's pulse (apical or radial) with the pulse on the display. The pulses should be equal. Told the nurse if the pulses were not equal.	____	____	____________
13. Read the SpO_2 on the display. Noted the value on the flow sheet and your assignment sheet.	____	____	____________
14. Left the sensor in place for continuous monitoring. Otherwise, turned off the device and removed the sensor.	____	____	____________

Post-Procedure

	S	U	Comments
15. Provided for comfort.	____	____	____________
16. Placed the call bell within reach.	____	____	____________
17. Raised or lowered bed rails. Followed the care plan.	____	____	____________
18. Unscreened the person.	____	____	____________

Post-Procedure—cont'd	S	U	Comments
20. Returned the device to its proper place unless monitoring was continuous.	______	______	______
21. Decontaminated your hands.	______	______	______
22. Reported and recorded the SpO_2 and pulse rate, as well as your other observations.	______	______	______

Assisting With Coughing and Deep Breathing Exercises

QUALITY OF LIFE

Name: ______________________

Date: ______________________

Remembered to:
- ◆ Knock before entering the person's room
- ◆ Address the person by name
- ◆ Introduce yourself by name and title

Pre-Procedure

	S	U	Comments
1. Followed Delegation Guidelines: Coughing and Deep Breathing.	_____	_____	__________
2. Explained the procedure to the person.	_____	_____	__________
3. Completed hand hygiene.	_____	_____	__________
4. Identified the person. Checked the identification bracelet against the assignment sheet. Called the person by name.	_____	_____	__________
5. Provided for privacy.	_____	_____	__________

Procedure

	S	U	Comments
6. Helped the person into a comfortable sitting position: dangling, semi-Fowler's, or Fowler's.	_____	_____	__________
7. Asked the person to take deep breaths:			
a. Asked the person to place his or her hands over the rib cage.	_____	_____	__________
b. Asked the person to exhale. Explained that the ribs should move as far down as possible.	_____	_____	__________
c. Asked the person to take another deep breath. Made sure it was as deep as possible. Reminded the person to inhale through the nose.	_____	_____	__________
d. Asked the person to hold the breath for 3 seconds.	_____	_____	__________
e. Asked the person to exhale slowly through pursed lips. Made sure the person exhaled until the ribs moved down as far as possible.	_____	_____	__________
f. Asked the person to repeat inhaling and exhaling four more times.	_____	_____	__________
8. Asked the person to cough:			
a. Asked the person to interlace his or her fingers over the incision. Gave the person the option of holding a pillow or folded towel over the incision.	_____	_____	__________
b. Asked the person to take in a deep breath:			
• Asked the person to exhale. Explained that the ribs should move down as far as possible.	_____	_____	__________
• Asked the person to take another deep breath. Made sure it was as deep as possible. Reminded the person to inhale through the nose.	_____	_____	__________
c. Asked the person to cough strongly twice with the mouth open.	_____	_____	__________

Post-Procedure	S	U	Comments
9. Provided for comfort.	_____	_____	__________
10. Raised or lowered bed rails. Followed the care plan.	_____	_____	__________
11. Placed the call bell within reach	_____	_____	__________
12. Unscreened the person.	_____	_____	__________
13. Decontaminated your hands.	_____	_____	__________
14. Reported and recorded your observations.	_____	_____	__________

Setting Up for Oxygen Administration

Quality of Life

Name: ______________________

Date: ______________________

Remembered to:
- Knock before entering the person's room
- Address the person by name
- Introduce yourself by name and title

Pre-Procedure

	S	U	Comments
1. Followed Delegation Guidelines: Oxygen Administration Set-Up. Viewed Safety Alert: Oxygen Administration Set-Up.			
2. Completed hand hygiene.			
3. Collected the following:			
• Oxygen device with connecting tubing			
• Flowmeter			
• Humidifier if ordered			
• Distilled water if using a humidifier			
4. Identified the person. Checked the identification bracelet against the assignment sheet. Called the person by name.			
5. Explained the procedure to the person.			

Procedure

	S	U	Comments
6. Made sure the flowmeter was in the OFF position.			
7. Attached the flowmeter to the wall outlet or to the tank.			
8. Filled the humidifier with distilled water.			
9. Attached the humidifier to the bottom of the flowmeter.			
10. Attached the oxygen device and connecting tubing to the humidifier. Did not set the flowmeter, and did not apply the oxygen device on the person.			

Post-Procedure

	S	U	Comments
11. Discarded packaging.			
12. Made sure the cap was securely on the distilled water. Stored it according to agency policy.			
13. Provided for comfort.			
14. Placed the call bell within reach.			
15. Decontaminated your hands.			
16. Told the nurse when you were done. The nurse:			
• Turned on the oxygen and set the flow rate			
• Applied the oxygen device on the person			

Caring for Eyeglasses

QUALITY OF LIFE

Name: ______________________

Date: ______________________

Remembered to:
- ◆ Knock before entering the person's room
- ◆ Address the person by name
- ◆ Introduce yourself by name and title

Pre-Procedure	S	U	Comments
1. Followed Delegation Guidelines: Eyeglasses. Viewed Safety Alert: Eyeglasses.	____	____	____________
2. Explained the procedure to the person.	____	____	____________
3. Completed hand hygiene.	____	____	____________
4. Collected the following:			
• Eyeglass case	____	____	____________
• Cleaning solution or warm water	____	____	____________
• Tissues or cloth	____	____	____________

Procedure	S	U	Comments
5. Removed the glasses:			
a. Held the frames in front of the ear on both sides.	____	____	____________
b. Lifted the frames from the ears. Brought the glasses down away from the face.	____	____	____________
6. Cleaned the eyeglasses with the cleaning solution or warm water. Dried the lenses with tissues.	____	____	____________
7. Opened the eyeglass case.	____	____	____________
8. Folded the glasses. Put them in the case. Did not touch the clean lenses.	____	____	____________
9. Placed the glass case in the top drawer of the bedside stand or in the drawer of the overbed table, or put the glasses back on the person as follows:	____	____	____________
a. Unfolded the glasses.	____	____	____________
b. Held the frame at each side. Placed them over the ears.	____	____	____________
c. Adjusted the glasses so the nosepiece rested on the nose.	____	____	____________
d. Returned the eyeglass case to the drawer in the bedside stand or overbed table.	____	____	____________
10. Decontaminated your hands.	____	____	____________

Cleaning Baby Bottles

Name: ______________________

Date: ______________________

Pre-Procedure

	S	U	Comments
1. Completed hand hygiene.	____	____	____________
2. Collected the following:			
• Bottles, nipples, and caps	____	____	____________
• Funnel	____	____	____________
• Can opener	____	____	____________
• Bottle brush	____	____	____________
• Dishwashing soap	____	____	____________
• Other items used to prepare formula	____	____	____________
• Towel	____	____	____________

Procedure

	S	U	Comments
3. Washed the bottles, nipples, caps, funnel, and can opener in hot, soapy water. Washed other items used to prepare formula.	____	____	____________
4. Cleaned inside baby bottles with bottle brush.	____	____	____________
5. Squeezed hot, soapy water through the nipples to remove formula.	____	____	____________
6. Thoroughly rinsed all items in hot water. Squeezed hot water through the nipples to remove soap.	____	____	____________
7. Placed a clean towel on the counter.	____	____	____________
8. Stood bottles upside down to drain. Placed nipples, caps, and other items on the towel. Allowed the items to dry.	____	____	____________

Diapering a Baby

QUALITY OF LIFE

Name: ______________________

Date: ______________________

Remembered to:
- ◆ **Knock before entering the person's room**
- ◆ **Address any adult who is present by name**
- ◆ **Introduce yourself by name and title**

Pre-Procedure	**S**	**U**	**Comments**
1. Completed hand hygiene.	____	____	____________
2. Collected the following:			
• Gloves	____	____	____________
• Clean diaper	____	____	____________
• Waterproof changing pad	____	____	____________
• Washcloth	____	____	____________
• Disposable wipes or cotton balls	____	____	____________
• Basin of warm water	____	____	____________
• Baby soap	____	____	____________
• Baby lotion or cream	____	____	____________
3. Placed the changing pad under the baby.	____	____	____________

Procedure			
4. Put on the gloves.	____	____	____________
5. Unfastened the dirty diaper. Placed diaper pins out of the baby's reach.	____	____	____________
6. Wiped the genital area with the front of the diaper. Wiped from the front to the back.	____	____	____________
7. Folded the diaper to keep urine and feces inside. Set the diaper aside.	____	____	____________
8. Cleaned the genital area from front to back. Used a wet washcloth, disposable wipes, or cotton balls. Washed with mild soap and water for a large amount of feces or if the baby had a rash. Rinsed thoroughly and patted dry the area.	____	____	____________
9. Gave cord care and cleaned the circumcision.	____	____	____________
10. Applied cream or lotion to the genital area and buttocks. Made sure not to use too much and that caking did not occur.	____	____	____________
11. Raised the baby's legs. Slid a clean diaper under the buttocks.	____	____	____________
12. Folded a cloth diaper so extra thickness was in the front for a boy. For girls, folded the diaper so the extra thickness was at the back.	____	____	____________
13. Brought the diaper between the baby's legs.	____	____	____________
14. Made sure the diaper was snug around the hips and abdomen. Made sure that the diaper was loose near the penis if the circumcision had not healed and below the umbilicus if the cord stump had not healed.	____	____	____________
15. Secured the diaper in place. Used the tape strips or Velcro on disposable diapers. Made sure the tabs stuck in place. Used baby pins or Velcro for cloth diapers. Made sure that pins pointed away from the abdomen.	____	____	____________

Procedure—cont'd	S	U	Comments
16. Applied plastic pants if cloth diapers were worn. Did not use plastic pants with disposable diapers because they are water protected.	_____	_____	________________
17. Placed the baby in the crib, infant seat, or other safe location.	_____	_____	________________

Post-Procedure

	S	U	Comments
18. Rinsed feces from the cloth diaper in the toilet.	_____	_____	________________
19. Stored used cloth diapers in a covered pail. Put a disposable diaper in the trash.	_____	_____	________________
20. Removed the gloves. Completed hand hygiene.	_____	_____	________________
21. Reported and recorded your observations.	_____	_____	________________

Giving a Baby a Sponge Bath

QUALITY OF LIFE

Name: ______________________

Date: ______________________

Remembered to:
- ◆ Knock before entering the person's room
- ◆ Address any adult who is present by name
- ◆ Introduce yourself by name and title

Pre-Procedure	S	U	Comments
1. Completed hand hygiene.	____	____	____________
2. Placed the following in your work area:			
• Bath basin	____	____	____________
• Bath thermometer	____	____	____________
• Bath towel	____	____	____________
• Two hand towels	____	____	____________
• Receiving blanket	____	____	____________
• Washcloth	____	____	____________
• Clean diaper	____	____	____________
• Clean clothing for the baby	____	____	____________
• Cotton balls	____	____	____________
• Baby soap	____	____	____________
• Baby shampoo	____	____	____________
• Baby lotion	____	____	____________
• Gloves	____	____	____________

Procedure	S	U	Comments
3. Filled the bath basin with warm water. Made sure water temperature was 100° F to 105° F (38° C to 40.5° C). Measured water temperature with the bath thermometer, or used the inside of your wrist. Made sure the water felt warm and comfortable on your wrist.	____	____	____________
4. Provided for privacy.	____	____	____________
5. Identified the baby according to agency policy.	____	____	____________
6. Undressed the baby. Left the diaper on.	____	____	____________
7. Washed the baby's eyelids:			
a. Dipped a cotton ball into the water.	____	____	____________
b. Squeezed out excess water.	____	____	____________
c. Washed one eyelid from the inner part to the outer part.	____	____	____________
d. With new cotton ball, washed the other eyelid from the inner part to the outer part.	____	____	____________
8. Moistened the washcloth and made a mitt. Cleaned the outside of the ear and then behind the ear. Did the same for the other ear. Made sure all movements were gentle.	____	____	____________
9. Rinsed and squeezed out the washcloth. Made a mitt with the washcloth.	____	____	____________
10. Washed the baby's face. Cleaned inside the nostrils with the washcloth. Did not use cotton swabs to clean inside the nose. Patted the face dry.	____	____	____________

Procedure—cont'd	S	U	Comments
11. Picked up the baby. Held the baby over the bath basin, using the football hold. Supported the baby's head and neck with your wrist and hand.	____	____	________
12. Washed the baby's head:			
a. Squeezed a small amount of water from the washcloth onto the baby's head.	____	____	________
b. Applied a small amount of baby shampoo to the head.	____	____	________
c. Washed the head with circular motions.	____	____	________
d. Thoroughly rinsed the head by squeezing water from a washcloth over the baby's head. Made sure that you did not get soap in the baby's eyes.	____	____	________
13. Placed the baby on the table.	____	____	________
14. Put on the gloves.	____	____	________
15. Removed the diaper.	____	____	________
16. Washed the front of the body. Used a soapy washcloth, or applied soap to your hands, and washed the baby with your hands. Made sure that you did not get the cord wet. Rinsed thoroughly. Patted dry. Was sure to wash and dry all creases and folds.	____	____	________
17. Turned the baby to the prone position. Washed the back of the body. Used a soapy washcloth, or applied soap to your hands, and washed the baby with your hands. Rinsed thoroughly. Patted dry. Made sure to wash and dry all creases and folds.	____	____	________
18. Gave cord care. Cleaned the circumcision.	____	____	________
19. Applied baby lotion to the baby's body as directed by the nurse.	____	____	________
20. Put a clean diaper and clean clothes on the baby.	____	____	________
21. Wrapped the baby in the receiving blanket. Placed the baby in the crib or other safe area.	____	____	________

Post-Procedure

	S	U	Comments
22. Cleaned and returned equipment and supplies to the proper place. Completed this step when the baby was settled.	____	____	________
23. Removed the gloves. Completed hand hygiene.	____	____	________
24. Reported and recorded your observations.	____	____	________

Giving a Baby a Tub Bath

QUALITY OF LIFE

Name: ______________________

Date: ______________________

Remembered to:
- ◆ **Knock before entering the person's room**
- ◆ **Address any adult who is present by name**
- ◆ **Introduce yourself by name and title**

Pre-Procedure	**S**	**U**	**Comments**
1. Completed hand hygiene.	____	____	____________
2. Placed the following in your work area:			
• Bath basin	____	____	____________
• Bath thermometer	____	____	____________
• Bath towel	____	____	____________
• Two hand towels	____	____	____________
• Receiving blanket	____	____	____________
• Washcloth	____	____	____________
• Clean diaper	____	____	____________
• Clean clothing for the baby	____	____	____________
• Cotton balls	____	____	____________
• Baby soap	____	____	____________
• Baby shampoo	____	____	____________
• Baby lotion	____	____	____________
• Gloves	____	____	____________

Procedure			
3. Filled the bath basin with warm water. Made sure water temperature was 100° F to 105° F (38° C to 40.5° C). Measured water temperature with the bath thermometer or used the inside of your wrist. Made sure the water felt warm and comfortable on your wrist.	____	____	____________
4. Provided for privacy.	____	____	____________
5. Identified the baby according to agency policy.	____	____	____________
6. Undressed the baby. Left the diaper on.	____	____	____________
7. Washed the baby's eyelids:			
a. Dipped a cotton ball into the water.	____	____	____________
b. Squeezed out excess water.	____	____	____________
c. Washed one eyelid from the inner part to the outer part.	____	____	____________
d. Washed the other eyelid from the inner part to the outer part with a new cotton ball.	____	____	____________
8. Moistened the washcloth and made a mitt. Cleaned the outside of the ear and then behind the ear. Did the same for the other ear. Made sure all motions were gentle.	____	____	____________
9. Rinsed and squeezed out the washcloth. Made a mitt with the washcloth.	____	____	____________
10. Washed the baby's face. Cleaned inside the nostrils with the washcloth. Avoided using cotton swabs to clean inside the nose. Patted the face dry.	____	____	____________

Procedure—cont'd	S	U	Comments
11. Picked up the baby. Held the baby over the bath basin using the football hold. Supported the baby's head and neck with your wrist and hand.	_____	_____	____________
12. Washed the baby's head:			
a. Squeezed a small amount of water from the washcloth onto the baby's head.	_____	_____	____________
b. Applied a small amount of baby shampoo to the head.	_____	_____	____________
c. Washed the head with circular motions.	_____	_____	____________
d. Thoroughly rinsed the head by squeezing water from a washcloth over the baby's head. Made sure you did not get soap in the baby's eyes.	_____	_____	____________
13. Placed the baby on the table.	_____	_____	____________
14. Put on the gloves.	_____	_____	____________
15. Removed the diaper.	_____	_____	____________
16. Held the baby as follows:			
a. Placed one hand under the baby's shoulders. Made sure your thumb was over the baby's shoulder and your fingers were under the baby's arm.	_____	_____	____________
b. Supported the buttocks with your other hand. Slid your hand under the thighs. Held the far thigh with your other hand.	_____	_____	____________
17. Lowered the baby into the water feet first.	_____	_____	____________
18. Washed the front of the baby's body. Washed all folds and creases. Rinsed thoroughly.	_____	_____	____________
19. Reversed your hold. Used your other hand to hold the baby.	_____	_____	____________
20. Washed the baby's back. Rinsed thoroughly.	_____	_____	____________
21. Reversed your hold again. Held the baby with your other hand.	_____	_____	____________
22. Washed the genital area.	_____	_____	____________
23. Lifted the baby out of the water and onto a towel.	_____	_____	____________
24. Wrapped the baby in the towel, and covered the baby's head.	_____	_____	____________
25. Patted the baby dry. Dried all folds and creases.	_____	_____	____________
26. Applied baby lotion to the baby's body as directed by the nurse.	_____	_____	____________
27. Put a clean diaper and clean clothes on the baby.	_____	_____	____________
28. Wrapped the baby in the receiving blanket. Placed the baby in the crib or other safe area.	_____	_____	____________

Post-Procedure

	S	U	Comments
29. Cleaned and returned equipment and supplies to the proper place. Completed this step when the baby was settled.	_____	_____	____________
30. Removed the gloves. Completed hand hygiene.	_____	_____	____________
31. Reported and recorded your observations	_____	_____	____________

Weighing an Infant

Name: ______________________

Date: ______________________

Pre-Procedure	S	U	Comments
1. Completed hand hygiene.	_____	_____	__________
2. Collected the following:			
• Baby scale	_____	_____	__________
• Paper for the scale	_____	_____	__________
• Items for diaper changing	_____	_____	__________
• Gloves	_____	_____	__________
Procedure			
3. Identified the baby following agency policy.	_____	_____	__________
4. Placed the paper on the scale. Adjusted the scale to zero (0).	_____	_____	__________
5. Put on the gloves.	_____	_____	__________
6. Undressed the baby and removed the diaper. Cleaned the genital area.	_____	_____	__________
7. Placed the baby on the scale. Kept one hand over the baby to prevent falling.	_____	_____	__________
8. Read the digital display, or moved the pointer until the scale was balanced.	_____	_____	__________
9. Noted the measurement.	_____	_____	__________
10. Diapered and dressed the baby. Placed the baby in the crib.	_____	_____	__________
11. Removed and discarded the gloves. Completed hand hygiene.	_____	_____	__________
Post-Procedure			
12. Returned the scale to its proper place.	_____	_____	__________
13. Decontaminated your hands.	_____	_____	__________
14. Reported and recorded your observations.	_____	_____	__________

Adult CPR–One Rescuer

QUALITY OF LIFE

Name: ______________________

Date: ______________________

Remembered to:
- **Knock before entering the person's room**
- **Address the person by name**
- **Introduce yourself by name and title**

Procedure	S	U	Comments
1. Checked if the person was responding. Tapped or gently shook the person, called the person by name and shouted, "Are you OK?"	_____	_____	_____
2. Called for help. Activated the emergency medical service (EMS) or the agency's emergency response system.	_____	_____	_____
3. Turned the person to the supine position. Logrolled the person to avoid twisting the spine. Made sure the person was on a hard, flat surface. Placed the person's arms alongside the body.	_____	_____	_____
4. Opened the airway. Used the head-tilt/chin-lift maneuver.	_____	_____	_____
5. Checked for breathing. Observed whether the chest rose and fell. Listened for the escape of air. Felt for the flow of air on your check.	_____	_____	_____
6. Gave two slow breaths if the person was not breathing or was not adequately breathing. Made sure each breath took 2 seconds. Allowed the person's chest to deflate between breaths.	_____	_____	_____
7. Checked for a carotid pulse and for breathing, coughing, and moving. (This took 5 to 10 seconds.) Used your other hand to keep the airway open with the head-tilt/chin-lift method.	_____	_____	_____
8. Gave chest compressions at a rate of 100 per minute. Gave 15 compressions and then 2 slow breaths.	_____	_____	_____
a. Established a rhythm and counted out loud, "1 and 2 and 3 and 4 and 5 and 6 and 7 and 8 and 9 and 10 and 11 and 12 and 13 and 14 and 15."	_____	_____	_____
b. Opened the airway, and gave two slow breaths.	_____	_____	_____
c. Established a rhythm and counted out loud, "1 and 2 and 3 and 4 and 5 and 6 and 7 and 8 and 9 and 10 and 11 and 12 and 13 and 14 and 15."	_____	_____	_____
d. Opened the airway, and gave two slow breaths.	_____	_____	_____
e. Established a rhythm and counted out loud, "1 and 2 and 3 and 4 and 5 and 6 and 7 and 8 and 9 and 10 and 11 and 12 and 13 and 14 and 15."	_____	_____	_____
f. Opened the airway, and gave two slow breaths.	_____	_____	_____
g. Established a rhythm and counted out loud, "1 and 2 and 3 and 4 and 5 and 6 and 7 and 8 and 9 and 10 and 11 and 12 and 13 and 14 and 15."	_____	_____	_____
h. Opened the airway, and gave two slow breaths.	_____	_____	_____
9. Checked for a carotid pulse, and checked for breathing, coughing, and moving.	_____	_____	_____

Procedure—cont'd	S	U	Comments
10. Continued cardiopulmonary resuscitation (CPR) if the person showed no signs of circulation. Began with chest compressions. Continued the cycle of 15 compressions and 2 breaths. Checked for circulation every few minutes.	_____	_____	__________
11. Performed the following if the person showed signs of circulation:			
a. Checked for breathing.	_____	_____	__________
b. Positioned the person in the recovery position, if the person was breathing.	_____	_____	__________
c. Monitored breathing and circulation.	_____	_____	__________
12. Performed the following if the person had signs of circulation but breathing was absent:			
a. Gave one rescue breath every 5 seconds. (This was at a rate of 10 to 12 breaths per minute.)	_____	_____	__________
b. Monitored circulation.	_____	_____	__________

Adult CPR—Two Rescuers

QUALITY OF LIFE

Name: ______________________

Date: ______________________

Remembered to:
- Knock before entering the person's room
- Address the person by name
- Introduce yourself by name and title

Procedure	S	U	Comments
1. Checked if the person was responding. Tapped or gently shook the person, called the person by name, and shouted, "Are you OK?" One rescuer activated the EMS or the agency's emergency response system.	____	____	____________
2. Opened the airway and checked for breathing. Used the head-tilt/chin-lift method.	____	____	____________
3. Gave two slow rescue breaths if the person was not breathing or was not adequately breathing. Allowed the person's chest to deflate between breaths.	____	____	____________
4. Checked for a carotid pulse, and checked for breathing, coughing, and moving.	____	____	____________
5. Performed two-person CPR if the person showed no signs of circulation:			
a. The first rescuer gave chest compressions at a rate of 100 per minute. Counted out loud in a rhythm, "1 and 2 and 3 and 4 and 5 and 6 and 7 and 8 and 9 and 10 and 11 and 12 and 13 and 14 and 15."	____	____	____________
b. The second rescuer gave 2 slow breaths after 15 compressions. Paused for the breaths. Continued chest compressions after the breaths.	____	____	____________
6. One rescuer does the following after 4 cycles of 15 compressions and 2 breaths:			
a. Gave two slow breaths.	____	____	____________
b. Checked for circulation—carotid pulse, breathing, coughing, and moving.	____	____	____________
7. Continued with 15 compressions and 2 slow breaths if the person showed no signs of circulation. Started with chest compressions.	____	____	____________

Infant CPR–One Rescuer

QUALITY OF LIFE

Name: ______________________

Date: ______________________

Remembered to:
- ◆ Knock before entering the person's room
- ◆ Address any adult who is present by name
- ◆ Introduce yourself by name and title

Procedure	S	U	Comments
1. Checked whether the infant was responding. Shouted at the infant. Gently tapped an arm or leg.	____	____	____________
2. Activated the EMS or the agency's emergency response system if help was available.	____	____	____________
3. Knelt at the infant's side near the head.	____	____	____________
4. Logrolled the infant onto his or her back. Kept the head, neck, and spine straight. Turned the infant in the supine position on a hard, flat surface.	____	____	____________
5. Opened the airway. Used the head-tilt/chin-lift method if injury was not suspected. Used the jaw-thrust method if injury was suspected.	____	____	____________
6. Checked for breathing. Observed whether the chest rose and fell. Listened for the escape of air. Felt for the flow of air on your cheek.	____	____	____________
7. Covered the infant's nose and mouth with your mouth for rescue breathing.	____	____	____________
8. Gave two slow rescue breaths. Used enough force to make the chest rise. Took 1 to 1 1/2 seconds for each breath. Allowed the chest to deflate between breaths.	____	____	____________
9. Checked for circulation using the brachial pulse, and checked for breathing, coughing, and moving.	____	____	____________
10. Located hand position for chest compressions. Kept the airway open with one hand.			
a. Drew an imaginary line between the nipples. Found the sternum (breastbone).	____	____	____________
b. Placed two fingers on the sternum about one finger-width below the imaginary line.	____	____	____________
11. Gave 5 chest compressions followed by 1 slow breath. Gave 100 chest compressions per minute and 20 rescue breaths per minute.			
a. Used the two fingers on the sternum for chest compressions. Pressed the sternum down about 1/3 to 1/2 the depth of the chest (about 1/2 to 1 inch).	____	____	____________
b. Released pressure after each compression. Kept your fingers on the chest.	____	____	____________
c. Counted out loud in a rhythm, "1, 2, 3, 4, 5."	____	____	____________
d. Gave one breath after every five chest compressions.	____	____	____________
12. Checked for circulation after 1 minute.	____	____	____________

Procedure—cont'd	S	U	Comments
13. Performed the following if no signs of circulation were observed:			
a. Activated the EMS or emergency response system.	______	______	______________________
b. Continued CPR.	______	______	______________________
14. Gave one rescue breath every 3 seconds if there were signs of circulation but breathing was absent or inadequate. Gave 20 rescue breaths per minute.	______	______	______________________

Child CPR–One Rescuer

QUALITY OF LIFE

Name: ______________________

Date: ______________________

Remembered to:
- **Knock before entering the person's room**
- **Address the child or any adult by name**
- **Introduce yourself by name and title**

Procedure	S	U	Comments
1. Checked whether the child was responding. Shouted at the child. Gently tapped an arm or leg.	____	____	____________
2. Activated the EMS or the agency's emergency response system if help was available.	____	____	____________
3. Knelt at the child's side near the head.	____	____	____________
4. Logrolled the child onto his or her back. Kept the head, neck, and spine straight. Turned the child in the supine position on a hard, flat surface.	____	____	____________
5. Opened the airway. Used the head-tilt/chin-lift method if injury was not suspected. Used the jaw-thrust method if injury was suspected.	____	____	____________
6. Checked for breathing. Observed whether the chest rose and fell. Listened for the escape of air. Felt for the flow of air on your cheek.	____	____	____________
7. Covered the child's mouth with your mouth. Pinched the nostrils shut.	____	____	____________
8. Gave two slow rescue breaths. Used enough force to make the chest rise. Took 1 to 1½ seconds for each breath. Let the chest deflate between breaths.	____	____	____________
9. Checked for circulation. Used the carotid pulse. Checked for breathing, coughing, or moving.	____	____	____________
10. Located hand position for chest compressions. Kept the airway open with one hand.			
a. Found the middle of the sternum (breastbone).	____	____	____________
b. Placed the heel of one hand over the lower half of the sternum. Kept your fingers off the chest.	____	____	____________
11. Gave 5 chest compressions followed by 1 slow breath. Gave 100 chest compressions per minute and 20 rescue breaths per minute.			
a. Used the heel of your hand on the sternum for chest compressions. Pressed the sternum down about ⅓ to ½ the depth of the chest (about 1 to 1½ inches).	____	____	____________
b. Released pressure after each compression. Kept the heel of your hand on the chest.	____	____	____________
c. Counted out loud in a rhythm ("1, 2, 3, 4, 5").	____	____	____________
d. Gave one breath after every five chest compressions.	____	____	____________
12. Checked for circulation after 1 minute.	____	____	____________

Procedure—cont'd	S	U	Comments
13. Performed the following if no signs of circulation were observed:			
a. Activated the EMS or emergency response system.	______	______	____________________
b. Continued CPR.	______	______	____________________
14. Gave 1 rescue breath every 3 seconds if there were signs of circulation, but breathing was absent or inadequate. You gave 20 rescue breaths per minute.	______	______	____________________

FBAO—The Responsive Adult

QUALITY OF LIFE

Name: ______________________

Date: ______________________

Remembered to:
- ◆ **Knock before entering the person's room**
- ◆ **Address the person by name**
- ◆ **Introduce yourself by name and title**

Procedure	S	U	Comments
1. Asked the person if he or she is choking.	____	____	____________
2. Asked the person if he or she could cough or speak.	____	____	____________
3. Gave abdominal thrusts:			
a. Stood behind the person.	____	____	____________
b. Wrapped your arms around the person's waist.	____	____	____________
c. Made a fist with one hand.	____	____	____________
d. Placed the thumb side of the fist against the abdomen. Made sure the fist was in the middle above the navel and below the end of the sternum (breastbone).	____	____	____________
e. Grasped your fist with your other hand.	____	____	____________
f. Pressed your fist and hand into the person's abdomen with a quick, upward thrust.	____	____	____________
g. Repeated thrusts until the object was expelled or the person lost consciousness.	____	____	____________
4. Lowered the unresponsive person to the floor or ground. Positioned the person supine.	____	____	____________
5. Activated the EMS or the agency's emergency response system.	____	____	____________
6. Performed a finger sweep to check for a foreign object:			
a. Opened the person's mouth. Used the tongue-jaw lift method.	____	____	____________
• Grasped the tongue and lower jaw with your thumb and fingers.	____	____	____________
• Lifted the lower jaw upward.	____	____	____________
b. Inserted your other index finger into the mouth along the side of the cheek and deep into the throat. Make sure your finger is positioned at the base of the tongue.	____	____	____________
c. Formed a hook with your index finger.	____	____	____________
d. Tried to dislodge and remove the object. Tried not to push it deeper into the throat.	____	____	____________
e. Grasped and removed the object if it was within reach.	____	____	____________
7. Opened the airway with the head-tilt/chin-lift method.	____	____	____________
8. Gave one or two rescue breaths.	____	____	____________
9. Repositioned the person's head if the chest did not rise. Gave one or two rescue breaths.	____	____	____________
10. Gave up to five abdominal thrusts.	____	____	____________

Procedure—cont'd	S	U	Comments
11. Repeated finger sweeps to recheck for a foreign object until rescue breathing was effective. Started CPR if necessary.	____	____	____
a. Opened the person's mouth. Used the tongue-jaw lift method.	____	____	____
• Grasped the tongue and lower jaw with your thumb and fingers.	____	____	____
• Lifted the lower jaw upward.	____	____	____
b. Inserted your other index finger into the mouth along the side of the cheek and deep into the throat. Made sure your finger was positioned at the base of the tongue.	____	____	____
c. Formed a hook with your index finger.	____	____	____
d. Tried to dislodge and remove the object. Tried not to push it deeper into the throat.	____	____	____
e. Grasped and removed the object if within reach.	____	____	____

FBAO—The Unresponsive Adult

QUALITY OF LIFE

Name: ______________________

Date: ______________________

Remembered to:
- ◆ **Knock before entering the person's room**
- ◆ **Address the person by name**
- ◆ **Introduce yourself by name and title**

Procedure	S	U	Comments
1. Checked if the person was responding.	____	____	____________
2. Called for help. Activated the EMS or the agency's emergency response system.	____	____	____________
3. Logrolled the person to the supine position with his or her face up. Positioned the arms at the sides.	____	____	____________
4. Opened the airway. Used the head-tilt/chin-lift method.	____	____	____________
5. Checked for breathing.	____	____	____________
6. Gave one or two slow rescue breaths. Repositioned the person's head and opened the airway if the chest did not rise. Gave one or two rescue breaths.	____	____	____________
7. Gave five abdominal thrusts if you could not ventilate the person:			
a. Straddled the person's thighs.	____	____	____________
b. Placed the heel of one hand against the abdomen. Made sure your heel was positioned in the middle above the navel and below the end of the sternum (breastbone).	____	____	____________
c. Placed your second hand on top of your first hand.	____	____	____________
d. Pressed both hands into the abdomen with a quick, upward thrust. Gave five thrusts.	____	____	____________
8. Performed a finger sweep to check for a foreign object.			
a. Opened the person's mouth. Used the tongue-jaw lift method.	____	____	____________
• Grasped the tongue and lower jaw with your thumb and fingers.	____	____	____________
• Lifted the lower jaw upward.	____	____	____________
b. Inserted your other index finger into the mouth along the side of the cheek and deep into the throat. Made sure your finger is positioned at the base of the tongue.	____	____	____________
c. Formed a hook with your index finger.	____	____	____________
d. Tried to dislodge and remove the object. Tried not to push it deeper into the throat.	____	____	____________
e. Grasped and removed the object if within reach.	____	____	____________

Procedure—cont'd	S	U	Comments
9. Repeated rescue breaths, abdominal thrusts, and finger sweeps until rescue breathing was effective. Started CPR if necessary.	_____	_____	_____
a. Gave one or two slow rescue breaths. Repositioned the person's head and opened the airway if the chest did not rise. Gave one or two rescue breaths.	_____	_____	_____
b. Gave five abdominal thrusts if you could not ventilate the person:	_____	_____	_____
i. Straddled the person's thighs.	_____	_____	_____
ii. Placed the heel of one hand against the abdomen. Made sure the heel was in the middle above the navel and below the end of the sternum (breastbone).	_____	_____	_____
iii. Placed your second hand on top of your first hand.	_____	_____	_____
iv. Pressed both hands into the abdomen with a quick, upward thrust. Gave five thrusts.	_____	_____	_____
c. Performed a finger sweep to check for a foreign object.	_____	_____	_____
i. Opened the person's mouth. Used the tongue-jaw lift method.	_____	_____	_____
• Grasped the tongue and lower jaw with your thumb and fingers.	_____	_____	_____
• Lifted the lower jaw upward.	_____	_____	_____
ii. Inserted your other index finger into the mouth along the side of the cheek and deep into the throat. Made sure your finger should be at the base of the tongue.	_____	_____	_____
iii. Formed a hook with your index finger.	_____	_____	_____
iv. Tried to dislodge and remove the object. Tried not to push it deeper into the throat.	_____	_____	_____
v. Grasped and removed the object if it was within reach.	_____	_____	_____

FBAO—The Responsive Infant

QUALITY OF LIFE

Name: ______________________

Date: ______________________

Remembered to:
- **Knock before entering the person's room**
- **Address any adult who is present by name**
- **Introduce yourself by name and title**

Procedure	**S**	**U**	**Comments**
1. Held the infant face down over your forearm. Knelt or sat to support your arm on your thigh. The infant's head is lower than the trunk. Held the infant's jaw to support the head.	_____	_____	__________
2. Gave up to five back blows using the heel of your hand. Gave the back blows between the shoulder blades. Stopped the back blows if the object was expelled.	_____	_____	__________
3. Turned the infant as a unit.			
a. Supported his or her head, neck, jaw, and chest with one hand.	_____	_____	__________
b. Supported the back with your other hand.	_____	_____	__________
c. Turned the infant as a unit. Turn the infant in the back-lying position on your forearm.	_____	_____	__________
4. Gave up to five chest thrusts:			
a. Located hand positions for chest compressions.	_____	_____	__________
b. Compressed the chest upward toward the head. Used two or three fingers.	_____	_____	__________
c. Stopped chest thrusts if the object was expelled.	_____	_____	__________
5. Gave five back blows followed by five chest thrusts until the object was expelled or the child became unresponsive.	_____	_____	__________
6. Perform the following if the infant became unresponsive:			
a. Activated the EMS or the agency's emergency response system if you had help.	_____	_____	__________
b. Opened the airway with the tongue-jaw lift method. Gave a rescue breath.	_____	_____	__________
7. Looked in the throat for an object. If an object was observed, removed it with a finger-sweep.	_____	_____	__________
8. Repeated rescue breathing, back blows, chest thrust, and tongue-jaw lift maneuver, and performed the finger sweep for a visible object until one of the following occurred:	_____	_____	__________
a. The object was expelled.	_____	_____	__________
b. The infant started breathing.	_____	_____	__________
c. You had to start CPR.	_____	_____	__________
9. Activated the EMS or the agency's emergency response system after following the procedure for 1 minute.	_____	_____	__________
10. Continued the FBAO procedure or CPR until emergency personnel arrived.	_____	_____	__________

FBAO–The Responsive Child

QUALITY OF LIFE

Name: ______________________

Date: ______________________

Remembered to:
- Knock before entering the person's room
- Address the child or any present adult by name
- Introduce yourself by name and title

Procedure	S	U	Comments
1. Determined whether the child was choking and if he or she could speak. Told the child that you would help.	____	____	____________
2. Stood behind the child.	____	____	____________
3. Wrapped your arms under the child's underarms and around the chest.	____	____	____________
4. Made a fist with one hand. Placed the thumb side of the fist on the child's abdomen. Positioned your fist in the middle above the navel and below the sternum (breastbone).	____	____	____________
5. Grabbed the fist with the other hand.	____	____	____________
6. Gave a quick inward and upward thrust.	____	____	____________
7. Repeated abdominal thrust until the object was expelled or until the child became unresponsive.	____	____	____________
8. Performed the following if the child became unresponsive:			
a. Activated the EMS or the agency's emergency response system if you had help.	____	____	____________
b. Opened the airway with the tongue-jaw lift method. Gave a rescue breath.	____	____	____________
9. Searched the throat for an object. If an object was found, removed it with a finger sweep.	____	____	____________
10. Repeated rescue breathing, abdominal thrusts, and tongue-jaw lift maneuver, and performed the finger sweep for a visible object until one of the following occurred:	____	____	____________
a. The object was expelled.	____	____	____________
b. The child started breathing.	____	____	____________
c. You needed to start CPR.	____	____	____________
11. Activated the EMS or the agency's emergency response system after following the procedure for 1 minute.	____	____	____________
12. Continued the FBAO procedure or CPR until emergency personnel arrived.	____	____	____________

FBAO—The Unresponsive Infant or Child

QUALITY OF LIFE

Name: ______________________

Date: ______________________

Remembered to:
- ◆ Knock before entering the person's room
- ◆ Address any adult who is present by name
- ◆ Introduce yourself by name and title

Procedure	S	U	Comments
1. Checked whether the infant or child is responding.	____	____	____________
2. Activated the EMS or the agency's emergency response system if you had help.	____	____	____________
3. Opened the airway.	____	____	____________
4. Checked for breathing. Observed whether the chest rose and fell. Listened for the escape of air. Felt for the flow of air on your cheek.	____	____	____________
5. Gave a rescue breath. Repositioned the head if the chest did not rise. Opened the airway, and gave a rescue breath.	____	____	____________
6. Performed one of the following:			
a. For an infant—gave up to five back blows and five chest thrusts.	____	____	____________
b. For a child—gave up to five abdominal thrusts.	____	____	____________
7. Opened the airway with the tongue-jaw maneuver. Gave a rescue breath.	____	____	____________
8. Searched the throat for an object. If an object is found, removed it with a finger-sweep.	____	____	____________
9. Repeated rescue breathing, abdominal thrusts (back blows and chest thrusts for an infant), and tongue-jaw lift maneuver, and performed the finger sweep for a visible object until one of the following occurred:	____	____	____________
a. The object was expelled.	____	____	____________
b. The infant or child started breathing.	____	____	____________
c. You needed to start CPR.	____	____	____________
10. Activated the EMS or the agency's emergency response system after following the procedure for 1 minute.	____	____	____________
11. Continued the FBAO procedure or CPR until emergency personnel arrived.	____	____	____________

Assisting With Postmortem Care

Name: ______________________

Date: ______________________

Pre-Procedure	S	U	Comments
1. Completed hand hygiene.	____	____	____________
2. Collected the following:			
• Postmortem kit (shroud or body bag, gown, identification tags, gauze squares, safety pins)	____	____	____________
• Bed protectors	____	____	____________
• Washbasin	____	____	____________
• Bath towels and washcloths	____	____	____________
• Tape	____	____	____________
• Dressings	____	____	____________
• Gloves	____	____	____________
• Cotton balls	____	____	____________
• Gown	____	____	____________
• Valuables envelope	____	____	____________
3. Provided for privacy.	____	____	____________
4. Raised the bed for body mechanics.	____	____	____________
5. Made sure the bed was flat.	____	____	____________

Procedure

6. Put on the gloves.	____	____	____________
7. Turned the body to the supine position. Positioned the arms and legs straight. Placed a pillow under the head and shoulders.	____	____	____________
8. Closed the eyes. Gently pulled the eyelids over the eyes. Applied moist cotton balls gently over the eyelids if the eyes would not stay closed.	____	____	____________
9. Inserted dentures if it is the agency policy. If not, placed the dentures in a labeled denture container.	____	____	____________
10. Closed the mouth. If necessary, placed a rolled towel under the chin to keep the mouth closed.	____	____	____________
11. Followed agency policy about jewelry. Removed all jewelry, except for wedding rings if this was agency policy. Listed the jewelry that you removed. Placed the jewelry and a list of valuables in an envelope.	____	____	____________
12. Placed a cotton ball over the rings. Taped them in place.	____	____	____________
13. Removed drainage containers. Left tubes and catheters in place if an autopsy is to be performed. Asked the nurse about removing tubes.	____	____	____________
14. Bathed soiled areas with plain water. Dried thoroughly.	____	____	____________
15. Placed a bed protector under the buttocks.	____	____	____________

Procedure—cont'd	S	U	Comments
16. Removed soiled dressings. Replaced them with clean ones.	____	____	____
17. Put a clean gown on the body. Turned the body to the supine position as before with arms and legs straight. Placed a pillow under the head and shoulders.	____	____	____
18. Brushed and combed the hair if necessary.	____	____	____
19. Covered the body to the shoulders with a sheet if the family is to view the body.	____	____	____
20. Gathered the person's belongings. Placed them in a bag labeled with the person's name.	____	____	____
21. Removed supplies, equipment, and linens. Straightened the room. Provided soft lighting.	____	____	____
22. Removed the gloves. Decontaminated your hands.	____	____	____
23. Allowed the family to view the body. Provided for privacy. Returned to the room after the family left.	____	____	____
24. Decontaminated your hands. Put on gloves.	____	____	____
25. Filled out the identification tags. Tied one to the ankle or to the right big toe.	____	____	____
26. Placed the body in the body bag or covered it with a sheet, or applied the shroud:			
a. Brought the top down over the head.	____	____	____
b. Folded the bottom up over the feet.	____	____	____
c. Folded the sides over the body.	____	____	____
d. Pinned or taped the shroud in place.	____	____	____
27. Attached the second identification tag to the shroud, sheet, or body bag.	____	____	____
28. Left the denture cup with the body.	____	____	____
29. Pulled the privacy curtain around the bed, or closed the door.	____	____	____

Post-Procedure

30. Removed the gloves. Decontaminated your hands.	____	____	____
31. Stripped the unit after the body had been removed. Wore gloves for this step.	____	____	____
32. Removed the gloves. Decontaminated your hands.	____	____	____
33. Reported the following to the nurse:			
• Time the body was taken by the funeral director.	____	____	____
• What was done with jewelry and personal items.	____	____	____
• What was done with dentures.	____	____	____